Ketogenic Diet and Intermittent Fasting Weight Loss Guide

(5 Manuscripts In 1 Book)

The Keto Diet For Beginners

Intermittent Fasting with Keto Diet

Intermittent Fasting For Women

Fast Keto Diet

The Complete Guide To Intermittent Fasting

Will Ramos & Gin Fung

Jason Legg

Suzanne Summers

Table Of Contents

Keto Diet

For Beginners

How To Go On The Ketogenic Diet

Will Ramos

Keto Diet For Beginners
How To Go On The Ketogenic Diet

Chapter 1:
Starting Your Keto Journey

The Ketogenic Diet – or Keto Diet for short – is powerful. It's life changing in every sense of the word. While weight loss is probably one of the reasons you picked up this book, it's just one of the unexpected and beautiful side effects of eating in a way that benefits your entire physical well being

What else can you expect when eating the Keto Diet way?

You'll regain your health. We'll go into this in much more detail throughout the following chapters, but suffice it to say, the way you're eating today – and the way you've largely been taught to eat in this American culture – is not healthy. You probably already have this belief yourself, as you're surrounded by fast food restaurants, fried food eateries, convenience stores that sell every non-healthy item, and even your own grocery store is to blame, stuffed with nutritionally deficient food products.

Yuck!

But after being on the Ketogenic Diet for one month – that's right, just four weeks – you'll see a remarkable difference in your health. You'll regain it and feel better overall – more energy, sleeping better, waking up refreshed, and weight loss, too.

What You'll Find Here

Inside this Ketogenic Diet book, you'll find all of the following and more:

- Dietary information backed up by real science, not bogus claims peddled by 'get rich quick' diet gurus
- A breakdown of why your body functions best in ketosis
- The exact Keto Diet success formula you'll follow
- Learning all about the ingredients you'll buy to stock your kitchen
- Not just one 4 week meal plan, but two – a basic plan and a 30-minute meal plan
- A complete and detailed step-by-step plan to get your body into ketosis
- Help and troubleshooting to mitigate potential side effects (none of which are harmful!)
- Dozens of helpful tips and tricks to fully integrate the Keto diet into not your neighbor's life – but yours!

Think of this book as the Ketogenic Diet all-in-one handy manual you've been looking for! We're not going to give you some vague advice, three recipes, and send you out into the confusing food landscape to fend for yourself. Nope, not at all! This book is here to guide you, help you, and encourage you every step of the way. There are big dietary changes in store for you, so come with us and enjoy the journey!

Trying Diet After Diet

The diet merry-go-round is confusing, dizzying, and doesn't get you anywhere. You just keep going in circles. Even if you do make a little bit of progress for a few weeks or months, it's not enough progress and doesn't motivate you.

That doesn't mean you are destined to fail at diets or will never be able to succeed on one.

It just means the diet is flawed!

It's hard to try another diet, because behind you in your past is a bunch of dieting mistakes that haven't worked. Diets are disappointing. You see the "before and after" pictures of people in magazines, on TV, and online, and you want that to be you.

A diet is just a meal plan. Right now, you're already on a diet. But it's not working. It's not bringing you the results that you want, it's not bringing you the body you want, and it's not bringing you any closer towards the future that you want.

So, let's try a new diet, one which will work. It will bring you closer to the results you want.

A Diet Based on Your Actual Body

What is this new diet? It's called the Ketogenic Diet, or Keto Diet for short. It's called the ketogenic diet because we'll be changing your body's natural metabolic processes from using unhelpful fuel to using helpful fuel (as well as stored fuel, too!)

Your body is amazing and needs lots of fuel every day to keep you mentally alert, keep your body systems functioning properly, to physically move you, and to do all the things you need to do throughout your life. Everything you eat becomes this fuel.

But some fuel is better than others. Some fuel (carbohydrates, sugars) is going to give you a quick burst of energy, and then the rest get stored. Other fuel (good fats, proteins) is going to not only give you better, more sustained and long-lasting energy, but will also start up a whole new metabolic process in your cells that burns the stored fuel. Pretty cool, huh?

We're not bashing carbs and sugars here, but they're just not sufficient enough for the complex and wonderful physical body you have. They're largely insufficient as a fuel source. It would be like trying to run a campfire on twigs. Sure, you get a little heat and light. But, wouldn't you want more substantial fuel, like thick logs? That's basically why the Ketogenic Diet switches up your fuel source from carbohydrates and sugars to fats and proteins. You can't run your body on twigs!

The Ketogenic Diet is designed to put your body into a metabolic state called *ketosis*. Ketosis is not a singular bodily function, but rather a series of processes that activate certain cells to stop doing things they were before and start doing new things. When your body goes into ketosis, it's kind of like having a change in an upper level position. New management comes in to switch policies around.

Your body is going to be using different energy sources than it was before.

Your Metabolism Process

So, ketosis is a metabolic state. But, what exactly does that mean?

When we're talking about your metabolism, we're actually talking about specifically how your body takes in energy from the foods you eat, processes it, and either stores it or uses it for fuel. Your metabolism takes this entire energy life cycle into account. When we say, "Oh, she has a high metabolism," we mean that the entire process of assimilating foods and using them for energy is functioning at its peak potential.

You can see the process listed out here:

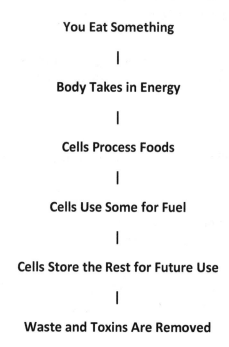

You Eat Something

|

Body Takes in Energy

|

Cells Process Foods

|

Cells Use Some for Fuel

|

Cells Store the Rest for Future Use

|

Waste and Toxins Are Removed

This cycle is continuously operating every day of your life. Every time you eat something, the nutrients in those foods enter the metabolic cycle and go through the whole process. Your body is like a metabolism factory, continuously processing incoming shipments. Those 'shipments' are the different chemical components of the foods that you eat: fats, proteins, carbohydrates, sugars, starches, fiber, vitamins, and minerals.

A Storage Solution That Works Against You

Many storage solutions are very helpful. But, unfortunately, the body's natural ability to store extra energy is working against you in the fight to lose weight.

If our bodies didn't have a built-in storage function, then none of us would ever need to lose weight! It wouldn't be stored in our cells in the first place. But, this was a survival mechanism from thousands of years ago, when obtaining foods year round was much more difficult than it is today. Your body developed 'storage spaces' for cells to deposit that unused energy to use it for a future time. Without out, Homo sapiens would surely have died out during the long, cold European winters. We absolutely needed that stored energy.

The problem today is, of course, our lifestyles have become so convenient, every single type of food is so plentiful, and we don't have enough natural exercise integrated into that lifestyle. We don't have a starvation winter period in our lives anymore. We just keep eating what we want every day. But, our body's metabolic process hasn't changed. It doesn't know that it's the 21st century. Your body still thinks it's 30,000 years ago and keeps storing and storing. That storage gets larger and larger, resulting in weight gain.

This is why it's so easy to gain weight in the 21st century. You have an ancient survival mechanism to fight against.

How do we change this process?

There is a way – and that's by changing your metabolic state to go into ketosis.

Ketosis utilizes that stored energy *in addition to* the energy that you're eating that day. It's burning the fat your body stored two weeks ago, two months ago, or even two years ago. Ketosis changes the metabolism cycle – and changes how your body uses that stored energy.

What is This Stored Energy?

The stored energy in your cells doesn't come from every single food you eat. It only comes from foods containing glucose, which is primarily found in carbohydrates. Glucose is a small sugar molecule.

That's right – carbohydrates become glucose, which becomes extra stored energy, isn't burned off by your normal daily body functions, and makes you gain weight.

The Carbohydrate Life Cycle

Let's look at the metabolic life cycle of a carbohydrate in your body.

Step 1:

You're at a birthday party and decide to eat a slice of cake. Hey, it's super yummy! Cake is made with white flour and sugar, both of which are carbohydrates. It also has eggs.

Step 2:

As soon as the cake enters your stomach, those nutrients are broken down. The protein and fat in the eggs is used as energy. The carbohydrates from the flour and sugar are turned into glucose.

Step 3:

You need more energy to have fun at the party, so a small amount of glucose is used as energy that day. But not all of it is needed. Plus, your body is specifically designed to store extra glucose. You might need that energy later.

Step 4:

The extra glucose is deposited into your cells for storage, causing you to gain weight from eating the cake.

Step 5:

The weight that you are trying to lose is still there. Your body didn't use it as energy at the party. Also, now you've added to the weight by eating more carbohydrates. There's also a huge chance you won't go through a 'starvation period' in the near future. You'll go back to step 1, eating more carbohydrates and only using the glucose as energy that day, never touching the stored fat you want to lose.

Yes, it's frustrating to be stuck in this type of carbohydrate metabolic cycle. It's happening every day when you eat bread, pasta, white flour goods, rice, and other whole grains. These carbohydrates have nowhere to go but right into the storage areas. They're not utilized by your cells. Also, your body isn't using the existing energy storage, either. It's just piling more and more glucose molecules into your cells. The number on the scale goes up, and not even a weekly exercise routine helps it go back down again.

That's why you need to switch your body from a carbohydrate metabolic state to a ketosis metabolic state.

So, What Exactly is Ketosis?

When your body is in ketosis, your liver is the organ that helps you out the most. It starts producing ketones that work in tandem with your energy storage cells to take that energy out of the cells and use it.

Ketones are a byproduct that's created when your body breaks down 'good fats' for energy while at the same time your carbohydrate intake (glucose intake) is low. We'll talk more about 'good fats' to eat later in this chapter.

When you stop eating carbohydrate heavy foods, you drastically reduce the amount of glucose entering your system. Your body is naturally wired to use glucose for fuel, right? So, when there isn't a lot of it coming in, your body has to look elsewhere for fuel.

In this case, it's fat – the stored energy in your cells.

So, your body goes to those fat storage cells and starts using those for energy. This process is called beta-oxidation because it uses oxygen atoms. After beta-oxidation is finished, what you get is a ketone. That ketone is then used as fuel for your daily energy. This whole new metabolic cycle is called ketosis.

Let's take a look at all the steps in this process:

You Eat Good Fats

|

Fats Enter the Stomach

|

Liver Breaks Down Fats For Energy (Beta-Oxidation)

|

Liver Produces Ketones

|

Ketones Used As Fuel

|

Liver Also Uses Stored Fat to Make Ketones

|

Ketones Used As Fuel

The Ketogenic Diet reduces carbohydrates to such a tiny amount in your diet and raises your 'good fat' intake to such a high percentage of your diet, that it kicks your body into ketosis.

Ketosis is the metabolic state that helps you burn stored energy – and gain all those wonderful benefits.

My Ketogenic Story

There are so many hidden carbohydrates (including all kinds of sugars) lurking in the foods you eat, that even someone who appears healthy on the outside can suffer from unexpected and severe health problems on the inside.

That's exactly what happened to me. I was a hale and healthy male athlete in my teens! I was playing sports, getting outside a lot, didn't carry any extra weight, and my BMI was totally normal. If you saw me, you'd have no idea that I was secretly unhealthy. I sure didn't know.

So, imagine my total surprise when I was suddenly diagnosed with diabetes.

Wait, what?

Yeah, whatever stereotypes you think about the average diabetes sufferer, that surely wasn't me. But suddenly, it was. I now had a disease that radically changed my relationship with food. I'd always exercised frequently, that I just didn't think it was necessary or important to care about what was on the plate. I just burned all those calories, anyway.

But diabetes has nothing to do with calories, being thin, exercising, or sports. That was eye-opening. I was thrown for a loop and struggled with my life into my early adulthood, trying everything I could think of to lessen my symptoms and get my diabetes under control. It took longer than I want to admit (especially to you!) to finally realize there was this incredible link between diet and health. Hey, I was a teenager okay?

Yet, once I recognized this link, my whole outlook changed immediately. I started with the Atkins Diet, which was popular at the time, then shortly thereafter started exploring the Keto Diet. This was around the early 2000s. The Ketogenic Diet sounded weird and extreme to me, with its ridiculously high fat contents and ridiculously low carb contents, but hey – I was already experimenting, so why not?

Well, needless to say, that Keto Diet experiment turned into a full tilt obsession as soon as my diabetes numbers started looking healthier. The more I ate this diet, the better my numbers got. Each doctor visit I was improving. I read everything I could get my hands on, including all about the nutrition, the science, the practical application, the recipes, and the meal plans. I absorbed this knowledge even better than a sponge, because my own health was at stake!

My experiments and personal field tested knowledge paid off. You might not believe me, but it's the truth:

The diabetes is gone. A long gone memory by this point.

And, I've been on the Ketogenic Diet for fourteen years.

I changed the metabolic process in my own body, I'm in ketosis 100% of the time, and I've never been healthier. On the inside and the outside this time.

Your Future Story

Ten years from now, you're going to be telling a story about your health to someone. "Back ten years ago, I'd never been on the Ketogenic Diet, but I was struggling with my weight and health. As soon as I got on it, I felt better and have never looked back."

Let's make that your real story. Let's eat for your real body and what it needs every day of your life. Let's go Keto – and never look back!

Chapter 2:
Why You Want Get Into The Keto Lifestyle

Besides weight loss, there are many other benefits to being in a ketosis metabolic state on the Ketogenic Diet. They can be basically grouped into two categories:

- Health
- Lifestyle

We'll go into each one of these in detail, so that you get a complete understanding of how this diet can help you.

7 Benefits of Keto for Your Health

1. Keto for Diabetes

The sugar in your blood sugar is insulin, which also comes from carbohydrates. When you eat too many carbohydrates, then you also increase the amount of insulin in your blood stream. This creates a spike of energy, which you might think of as a 'sugar high.' But after every high comes a crash. Then you reach for more carbohydrates and sugars to spike again. This spike-crash-spike-crash cycle is bad for your health. Staying in ketosis stabilizes your blood sugar.

When you think 'blood sugar,' you've got to also think about your body's energy that's processed as part of your overall metabolism. Your blood moves along the interior highway of your artery and vein system, carrying nutrients from the food you eat to every part of your body.

However, just like a polluted river, blood can also become clogged with too much glucose. That glucose wasn't processed by your liver, so it ends up in your blood stream, elevating your blood sugar levels. The sugars and carbs you eat end up in your blood stream, spiking your energy levels.

You spike your blood sugar, you receive a spike of energy. That doesn't seem so bad. A quick burst of energy is good from time to time. But with every spike comes an opposite reaction of the crash. That crash is not healthy and represents too much of a change in your blood sugar. It also makes you feel sluggish, mentally foggy, drained, and it also interferes with your natural sleep cycle. As a result, in order to feel that burst of energy again, you're naturally going to – you guessed it – reach for something else to spike your blood sugar.

If you repeat this spike-crash-spike-crash cycle too often, you're sending your blood sugar on an unnecessary and unhealthy roller coaster that can have long-term negative consequences. However, if you go into the ketosis metabolic state, your blood sugar won't get stuck in this cycle, thus preventing and helping diabetes.

2. Keto for Metabolic Syndrome

The Ketogenic Diet helps those who struggle with metabolic syndrome and its problems: an expanded waistline, low HDL levels, and high blood pressure, triglyceride levels, and blood sugar. This diet will lower your insulin levels, stabilize your blood sugar, and reduces your blood pressure. It's ideal for metabolic syndrome.

3. Keto for Brain Health

It goes without saying that your brain is unbelievably important – and when your diet doesn't support brain health, you can feel it. You have problems with memory, nerve function, your vision, alertness, and struggle with brain fog. On the Keto Diet, your brain is fueled both by protein and ketones. Also, since your brain requires so much energy, your liver will start producing making new glucose in a process called gluconeogenesis. Your liver takes the glycerol from the fatty acids present in triglycerides, which are the fats your body stores, turns them into glucose, and sends them to the brain as fuel. In fact, the Keto Diet was first developed for those suffering with epilepsy – because it helps the brain so much.

4. Keto for Cancer

How can this new eating plan help cancer? Some initial research has linked the Keto Diet with slowing down the growth of tumors. Cell biologist Otto Warburg discovered cancer cells flourish due to their ability to ferment glucose. In other words, one of a cancer cell's primary food sources is – you guessed it – sugar. Eliminate the sugars and carbs from the diet, and the cancer cells become weakened and starved. More research in this area is required, but suffice it to say, it only makes sense that Keto helps reduce cancer.

5. Keto for Reduced Inflammation

When the body has difficulty healing itself and struggles to protect itself from illnesses, that's when you get inflammation. Inflammation has also proven to be the first symptom for many chronic conditions, including rheumatoid arthritis, atherosclerosis, periodontitis, hay fever, and even some cancers. But being on the Keto Diet reduces sugars derived from carbohydrates, which are a huge source of inflammation. Less sugar equals less inflammation.

6. Keto to Manage Cholesterol and Blood Pressure

Stabilizing your blood sugar helps give you a much better circulatory system, which in turn both manages and lowers cholesterol and helps your blood pressure. It's common knowledge to assume that heart problems come from eating too much fat, but that's not true. It's too many carbohydrates that cause problems. When you reduce carbs and eat good fats and proteins, you're giving your heart what it needs.

A lot of people also think more fat equals higher cholesterol, but your body knows how to maintain cholesterol homeostasis. Those sugars stay in your bloodstream, while the cholesterol you eat (in the good fats mentioned in the next chapter) attaches to lipoproteins and is transported to your cells and organs. HDL is this high density lipoprotein. In essence, you want to eat these good fats, which we'll explain more in the chapter on your Macros! That helps balance your cholesterol and increase the overall health of your entire circulatory system.

7. Keto for Fatty Liver Disease

As you've read in this book, your liver is the main organ switching you from a carbohydrate metabolic state to a ketosis state. It produces ketones. Your liver acts as a filter, helping to separate good nutrients from bad and send the bad nutrients to your kidneys to be flushed out. Fatty liver disease comes when you're consuming so many sugars and carbs (usually through alcohol), that your body isn't burning any stored fat and instead is depositing it on your liver. Once you stop consuming such high quantities of carbohydrates, your body will then start burning the fat deposits on your liver – and any other organ as well.

7 Benefits of Keto for Your Lifestyle

1. Natural Weight Loss

This is definitely the most obvious benefit, and not just because you're cutting out nearly an entire food group! When your body is in ketosis, it's designed to burn the extra fat stores in your cells. That contributes to a natural and healthy weight loss. Your weight loss amounts will vary depending on how much weight you have to lose and the percentage of fat in your body. But you will see a difference!

2. Hunger Management

When you eat carbs and sugars, you enter the blood sugar spike-crash-spike cycle mentioned above. That quick energy doesn't sustain your appetite at all, which you've probably noticed. Those simple carbohydrates and sugars are burned so quickly that you get hungry again in a short period of time. But when you replace those ingredients with the good fats and proteins, your hunger pangs will be greatly reduced. Instead of reaching for toast or pancakes in the morning, try an egg omelet with bacon and cheese. You'll feel full for hours! We give plenty of breakfast options here to stave off hunger at any time of the day!

3. Better Appetite Control

You've probably tried diets in the past that left you constantly hungry. Low fat meals and simple carbohydrates like bread, biscuits, fruit, or cookies not only don't satisfy your hunger, they actually make you more hungry in the long run! That's why humans are more apt to develop sugar cravings rather than meat cravings. Calm your cravings down and help bring your appetite under control by following the Keto Diet. It's an unexpected and amazing benefit!

4. More Energy

Your body was not just built to store fat, but to use the 'good fats' effectively as fuel. This helps to give you much more energy. It won't be the spike-crash style of sugary laden energy, either. You will have plentiful, sustained energy that keeps you going all day and won't make you feel exhausted in the afternoon. The Keto Diet is built for a high performance lifestyle. This is also shown in nature, too; carnivores have to expend more energy than herbivores just to catch their prey, so they rely on a high fat, high protein diet. Humans are omnivores, but our brain and muscles require incredible amounts of calories for daily use. Switch those calories to the perfect Macro percentage, and you'll get more energy than you ever dreamed of.

You'll also avoid what's commonly nicknamed the 'carb coma,' which happens when you feel sleepy after consuming too many carbohydrates!

5. Mental Clarity

Your brain requires hundreds of calories per day to process all of its intricate functions. Not to mention when you decide to learn something new, take a class, speak a foreign language, or just need that gray matter to get through a stressful day at the office. When you eat 'good fats' and proteins, those nutrients give your mind the power it needs.

Thus, you not only feel more mentally alert, but everything associated with your brain is increased. You'll remember things better, you'll have an easier time coming up with new ideas, you'll retain more information, and overall, you'll learn better. This is especially important if you work in a field that requires heavy brainpower, like marketing, the arts, and other creative professions.

6. Burn Fat for Fuel

This benefit is the heart of what makes being in a ketosis metabolic state so incredible. Your cells aren't using just the fuel you're eating now; they're also using the stored fuel. When your body uses stored fat from your cells for fuel, that fat disappears off your body, thus decreasing your weight. That fat is gone – because it was used! Think of the Ketogenic Diet as a fat decluttering nutrition plan. You're cleaning out your cells of fat that's been stored there for a long time, perhaps even years. The longer you're in ketosis, the more frequently this process occurs. It's a win-win situation.

7. Better Mood and Emotions

If you've struggled with mood swings and emotions that frequently vacillate, then you'll find the Ketogenic Diet to be a breath of fresh air. You'll get out of the blood sugar spike-crash-spike cycle and you'll stabilize your emotions as well. Your brain will use protein and the ketones from your liver as fuel, which is excellent for the neurotransmitters in your brain to produce the 'good' hormones like serotonin, dopamine, and endorphins. That alone will do wonders for your mood and is a great, unexpected, and useful benefit

Is the Keto Diet for Everyone?

While being in ketosis is a metabolic state any human body can achieve, not everyone should be on the Keto Diet. As a disclaimer, we want to advise you to consult a doctor or certified nutritionist before beginning this diet. There are rare conditions like Muscular Dystrophy and conditions that affect certain organs like your kidneys, liver, or pancreas. Also, if you have a digestive disorder affecting your blood sugar, such as hypoglycemia or Type 1 diabetes. Yes, ketosis helped my diabetes, but I also want to caution you. As for Type 2 diabetes, I also advise you to consult a physician.

The Keto Diet is not recommended if you're pregnant, have gestational diabetes, or are nursing. Everything you eat affects your baby, so please don't change your diet until after your baby's been weaned. Suffering from an eating disorder wreaks havoc with both your mind and body, so don't attempt this diet at that time.

Once you've been cleared, then you're good to proceed!

Confusion Leads to Bad Press About Ketosis

You might have heard or read some bad press about the Keto Diet. It's jumped in popularity and has attracted its fair share of naysayers. They say that the diet is unhealthy, gives you weight gain rather than weight loss, messes with your blood sugar, leads to long term liver problems, and other negative claims.

Ketosis is NOT Ketoacidosis – Here's the Difference!

Most of this confusion comes from differentiating between two similar sounding conditions: ketosis and ketoacidosis. Ketosis is the metabolic state whereby your liver is producing ketones. By itself, it isn't harmful to your body at all. It just means you have a higher amount of ketones present in your blood and urine. But it isn't high enough to tip over into acidosis.

In fact, ketosis developed in our bodies thousands of years ago in human evolution as a way to use stored body energy during the winter, when fresh grains, sugars, and carbohydrates weren't plentiful. So, ketosis kept many of our ancestors alive in cold winters.

Ketoacidosis is completely different and yes, it is harmful. It's known as Diabetic Ketoacidosis (DKA). When your ketones are in dangerously high levels and your blood sugar is also too high, that makes your blood too acidic. When that happens, you have to seek medical attention immediately. But this condition usually only happens to those who not just have Type 1 or Type 2 diabetes, but whose bodies didn't produce any insulin or very poor amounts. If you produce insulin, then you're not in danger of your body developing DKA.

Symptoms of DKA include dehydration with extreme thirst and needing to urinate frequently, nausea, vomiting, stomach pain, low energy, and being short of breath. You'll be measuring your ketones using a breath meter or strips, so you'll know on a regular basis that you're in the good range.

So, ketosis is one of your body's natural functions (as a way to keep you alive during times of less food) and diabetic ketoacidosis is very harmful. They're very different!

What's the Keto Flu?

You'll find more in depth information about what's nicknamed the "Keto Flu" in Chapter 6, but briefly, this is the combination of flu-like symptoms you'll experience within the first 1-3 weeks of starting the Ketogenic Diet. Your body is adjusting to a completely new way of functioning, and it's a transition period.

These symptoms include:

- Low energy and fatigue
- Being brain foggy
- Headaches
- Being irritable and unmotivated
- Muscle cramps
- Nausea
- Sugar cravings (please don't give in!)

Luckily, these don't last too long and can be helped by drinking water with lemon to restore your electrolytes.

Now that you've read all about the benefits to being on the Keto Diet and how it's not harmful for your body, we're going to go into the practical advice. Read on to the next chapter to see what foods you can – and cannot eat!

Chapter 3:
Keto Foods: The Good And Bad

This chapter is when the rubber meets the road, and you'll find out exactly what you can – and can't – eat. We'll go food group by food group, navigating the confusing modern American landscape of food options from grocery stores to restaurants.

The Ketogenic Diet begins at the grocery store, and that's where you'll find the vast majority of ingredients to make recipes and meal plans.

But, before we send you off to stock up your cart, you need to be educated about what you're reading on food packages to find the best options.

Decoding Nutritional Labels

Food package nutritional labels give you all the information you need to say yes to Keto foods. Don't be blissfully unaware of the chemicals, additives, preservatives, and other food product 'bad guys' manufacturers shove into that brightly colored package. Yes, it looks enticing. But those aren't Keto Diet friendly food items. Study nutritional labels to really become familiar with what's exactly in the package. If you see carbs or sugars, put it back on the shelf.

Here are some red flag words to avoid:

- High Fructose Corn Syrup - It's nothing but sugar. Stay away!
- Enriched Flour / Wheat Flour / Corn Flour / Oat Flour - Carbs, carbs, and more carbs. Avoid anything with the word 'flour' in it.
- Partially Hydrogenated Oil – Stick to olive oil or coconut oil instead.
- Dextrose / Sucralose / Fructose / Lactose / Maltose – Anything with the suffix "ose" means sugar.
- Wheat Starch / Cornstarch – Starches are carbs.
- Aspartame / Saccharin / Acesulfame Potassium – Just fancy words for chemical sugars. Buy Stevia or anything with zero sugar.
- Lactitol / Sorbitol / Mannitol / Xylitol / Ethanol – More fancy words for sugar. These are sugar alcohols.
- Syrup – Liquid sugar. Yuck!

Food companies are pretty sneaky with the above ingredients. They'll stick them in supposedly harmless things like ketchup, barbecue sauce, ranch dressing, yogurt, and cheese. Get to know the red flag words, and you'll have a better chance on the Keto Diet.

Foods to Avoid

We thought we'd get the 'naughty list' out of the way first, so that you're aware of what you can't put in your grocery cart any longer. While this list is comprehensive, the foods you can eat is even more so!

Grains and Flours

Yes, this is the big "no no" category. Grain foods contain the highest amount of carbohydrates out of all the nutrition categories. Even if the product is gluten free, it's still not allowed on the Keto Diet.

Avoid:

- Bread
- Buns and rolls
- Bagels
- Biscuits
- Pasta and noodles
- Crackers of any flavor or shape
- Flour baked goods, like cakes, cookies, brownies, and pastries
- Pie crusts
- Pizza dough
- Donuts
- White flour and corn tortillas
- Cereals
- Rice
- Oats and oatmeal
- Other grains – barley, couscous, pilaf, pita, quinoa, etc.

Dairy

You get plenty of dairy options on the Ketogenic Diet, including an entire cheese selection. But there are a few dairy items you shouldn't have.

Avoid:

- Margarine in any form
- Cow's milk
- Sweetened milks
- Soymilk
- Evaporated milk
- Non-homemade whipped cream
- Ice cream
- Low-fat dairy items

Vegetables

We debunk the myth in this Ketogenic Diet book that all vegetables help you lose weight. But it is a pervasive myth, which is why we included our special veggie selection. Stick to those recommendations only. Otherwise, you'll be eating vegetables that are too high in carbs. Like these ones.

Avoid:

- Potatoes
- Sweet potatoes / yams
- Corn

- Carrots
- Leeks
- Peas
- Soybeans
- Beans – kidney beans, cannellini beans, black beans, etc.
- Any foods based on these vegetables, like refried beans, mashed potatoes, and French fries
- Any oils based on these vegetables, like corn oil and soybean oil

Fruits

Fruits are the second highest carbohydrate heavy foods. They just have way too much sugar. Think of fruits as colorful, sweet-smelling enemies that will subtly sabotage your diet!

Avoid:

- Apples
- Bananas
- Citrus – oranges, grapefruit, tangerines
- Melons – watermelon, honeydew, cantaloupe
- Grapes
- Pineapple
- Peaches
- All other fresh fruits – kiwi, papaya, mangoes, plums, etc.
- Fruit products – dried fruit, fruit juice, fruit popsicles, fruit candy, etc.

Packaged Meals

Packaged meals are some of the sneakiest items in the grocery store. They are often splashed with giant headlines like "all natural," "nutritious," and "complete meal." They're usually packed with carbs, sugars, and ridiculously high amounts of sodium.

Avoid:

- Canned soups
- Canned meals (Chef Boyardee, etc.)
- Boxed meal kits
- Frozen boxed meals
- Frozen breakfast sandwiches or wraps
- Frozen pizza
- Kids' lunch packaged meals
- Grocery store packaged foods or complete meals
- Pre-packaged sauce mixes
- Dried soup mixes

Snacks

Food manufacturers are incredibly good at getting you to buy their products by making them colorful, crunchy, and completely addicting. Some of these snacks say they're organic, all natural, healthy, or other bogus claims. Bypass them all. They'll not only stop your weight loss, they'll reverse it.

Avoid:

- Potato chips of any flavor
- Cheesy crunchy snacks (Cheetos, Cheese puffs, etc.)
- Pretzels
- Popcorn
- Tortilla chips
- Doritos of any flavor
- Rice cakes
- Cheese crackers, like Cheez-its and Goldfish
- Air popped crunchy snacks
- Any other packaged salty or cheesy snack food

Sweets

Sweet foods contain massive amounts of sugar, which will knock your body out of ketosis. Yeah, you don't want to do that. Although it seems counter-intuitive since many sweets are fat free, they are actually fattening to you. Please don't put these sugary sweets in your grocery cart.

Avoid:

- Candy
- Ice cream
- Frozen ice cream treats
- Popsicles
- Gum
- Canned cake frosting
- Plain white sugar
- Brown sugar
- Milk chocolate with a high sugar content
- Honey
- Any sweetener besides Stevia

Beverages

Americans love drinking our calories! Whether it's a grande latte in Starbucks, a soda at the movie theater, or an energy drink to help you through class, beverages are packed with sugars. Most of them are definitely on the avoid list.

Avoid:

- Soda, even if it says zero calories
- Energy drinks
- Sports drinks
- Coffee drinks

- Fruit juices
- Bottled or canned iced tea
- Alcohol, unless it's the occasional glass of approved wine

Foods You Can Eat!

So, we got the bad news out of the way with the foods you can't eat, but you have plenty of other options! We'll go through each of the major food groups and tell you exactly which foods you can have. If you were thinking that many Keto Diet ingredients are expensive and hard to find, then think again. You'll be purchasing produce, meats, dairy, herbs / spices, and some condiments. Find most of these are in your neighborhood grocery store. Some specialty ingredients might be found in a health food store or ordered online.

Beverages

Almond Milk - Regular cow's milk is not recommended on the Keto Diet, but you can definitely have almond milk. It comes in different flavors, like plain and vanilla. Be sure to get it unsweetened!

Coffee - Sheesh, a diet without coffee? Not the Keto Diet! Coffee by itself has an extremely low carb count, so you're safe to have your morning cup. Add a pinch of Stevia to sweeten it and pour on the heavy cream.

Tea - You might want to stock up your tea selection with a nice variety – black teas, green teas, herbal teas, and chai teas. A cup of English tea in the afternoon with a slice of lemon or a splash of heavy cream is a great pick-me-up.

Water – Make sure you're getting plenty of water on your Keto Diet. It helps flush out toxins, and your whole body needs it. You can have it with lemon or lime slices for some flavor and electrolytes.

Wine - Yes, you can have a little bit of wine on the Keto Diet. On average, wines have between 3 and 4 grams of carbohydrates per serving. White wines have less than red wines. Stick with Pinot Noir as a dry red and Pinot Blanc as a dry white. A small glass once or twice a week, as long as you factor in the carbs as part of your diet, can help you not feel deprived. You can use wine in cooking, too.

Meat, Fish & Eggs

Chicken – Chicken is such a huge source of both protein and fat that it must be included on here. Chicken also, well, tastes like chicken, so it takes to marinades and slow roasts really well.

Bacon – I know what you're thinking. A diet that helps me lose weight has *bacon* in it? Yes! In fact, bacon (look for nitrate-free and high quality bacon) is encouraged. Bacon has a magical mixture of both high fats and protein to give you the energy you need in the morning.

Beef – Yes, you can make Keto Diet burgers! Don't forget chili, too. Get some ground beef, roast beef, pot roast, sirloin tips, and steaks to cook and serve on the Keto Diet.

Eggs – One whole egg has 6 grams of protein and plenty of the good fats, so have fun eating eggs. They're a lot lower in protein than beef, pork, or chicken.

Fish – There are plenty of fish options on the Keto Diet, including cod, haddock, halibut, salmon, sea bass, trout, ahi tuna, and tilapia. Whatever kind of fish you purchase, make sure it is certified wild caught and hasn't been coated in carb heavy breading or fried.

Ham – You can get some ham to dice up for omelets and soups. Ham also makes a wonderful pairing with different cheeses. Make sure you're not getting ham with any sugar or honey curing.

Hot Dogs – Yep, good old fashioned beef franks are allowed on the Ketogenic Diet! Splurge on an all natural brand with the fewest fillers and the most fat.

Lamb – Ground lamb can be used as an alternative to ground pork or ground beef or ground turkey in a regular recipe to switch up your flavors! You can also purchase lamb chops and lamb tenderloin.

Meat Broth/Bouillon – Vegetable broth has too many carbs, so for making Keto soups, buy chicken broth and beef broth. Check the nutritional labels on chicken, beef, or fish bouillon cubes for their carb count. Some of them are made with wheat or whey powder.

Pork – Pork is delicious and carb free. There are many ways you can purchase it, including ground pork, pork shoulder, and pork tenderloin. You can also have pork rinds.

Prosciutto – Two slices of this popular Italian ham have 3 grams of fat.

Sausage – Store bought sausage often is stuffed with not just meat, but carb fillers. There's a recipe here in this book to make your own, which is a lot easier than you think!

Shrimp – Shrimp is a staple protein on the Ketogenic Diet, so stock up on either fresh or frozen. Homemade, unsweetened cocktail sauce goes very well with shrimp as a low carb appetizer.

Seafood – Besides fresh or frozen plain shrimp, you can also purchase many other types of seafood: scallops, crabs, mussels, clams, and even lobster. None of them have any carbs and make yummy dinner entrees.

Turkey – Turkey is not as high in fat as other forms of protein, so eat the dark meat only. One serving of roast dark meat has 5 grams of fat. You can also buy ground turkey.

Dairy

Brie – If you've never had this luscious, creamy cheese before, you're in for a tummy-pleasing treat. Definitely add it to your grocery cart.

Butter - For all of you butter lovers out there, this is the diet to be on! The Keto Diet encourages you to eat 70% of your calories from fat, and there is no fat tastier than butter. Buy unsalted, good quality butter in sticks or fresh from a farm.

Cheddar Cheese – One of the most popular cheeses in the world, you can purchase any style you like, except for a low fat version of course!

Colby Jack Cheese – A mild orange and white cheese that can be used in hundreds of recipes or eaten plain as a snack.

Cottage Cheese – Skip the low-fat version and go for the full fat instead, plain and with no fruit or flavorings added.

Cream Cheese – You want the full fat cream cheese, either in tubs or in blocks. None of that low-fat diet stuff from Philadelphia!

Feta Cheese – A creamy, yummy Mediterranean cheese for salads or to cook with.

Ghee – Ghee is Indian clarified butter, concentrating both the flavor and the fat. Each tablespoon has a whopping 12.7 grams of fat.

Goat Cheese – A unique tangy flavor makes goat cheese a great addition to Keto salads or as a snack. A 1 ounce serving has 8 grams of fat.

Greek Yogurt – Unsweetened and plain Greek yogurt is a yummy addition to the Keto Diet. It also provides probiotics to help balance good bacteria in your digestive tract.

Gruyere – Originally from Switzerland, this European cheese has 9 grams of fat per slice.

Heavy Cream – Say goodbye to low fat diets and hello to heavy cream. It has 12 grams of fat and no carbs, so add it to your tea, coffee, baked egg dishes, and soups.

Monterey Jack Cheese – This semi-hard cheese changes up regular flavors and is great with Mexican cuisine. It's filled with good fat, too.

Mozzarella Cheese – Even without pasta or garlic bread, you can still enjoy Italian food by having mozzarella cheese. Stringy and gooey, it's delicious.

Parmesan Cheese – A sprinkle of Parmesan brings wonderful Mediterranean flavor. Buy the full fat kind.

Sour Cream – With its light tang and creamy texture, sour cream is delicious in sauces, as a soup topping, and mixed with herbs for a dip.

Swiss Cheese – Holey Swiss cheese, Batman. You get 8 grams of fat per slice in this popular, tart cheese.

Vegetables

Arugula – This peppery tasting lettuce has 2.05 grams of carbohydrates and is a great base for Keto Diet friendly salads.

Asparagus – Only 1.78 grams of carbohydrates are in these fresh, crunchy vegetables. They're delicious when grilled, roasted, or wrapped in bacon.

Bell Pepper (Green) – The green bell peppers have less carbs than red, orange, or yellow, so buy that color only. They have 2.9 grams of carbs.

Bok Choy – This excellent Chinese vegetable is delicious in Asian soups or stir fries. Its carbohydrate count is only 1.18 grams. You can find it at Asian stores.

Broccoli – With 4 grams of carbs per cup, these little tree shaped veggies are a staple in the Keto kitchen. Buy them fresh or frozen.

Cabbage – With only 3 grams of carbohydrates, you can have cabbage on the Keto Diet. Only buy the green, since the red is much higher.

Cauliflower – You can chop up cauliflower, add cheese to it, or put it in stir fries. It has 2.9 carb grams per cup.

Chili Peppers – There are quite a few that are Keto diet friendly, including the small Thai red chilis, ghost peppers, and jalapenos. One cup of sliced jalapenos has 6 grams of carbs.

Celery – With 1.37 grams of carbs per stalk, this is one of the best Keto Diet friendly vegetables. That's great news, since it's such a delicious snack food.

Cucumber – Made of 96 percent water and 1.9 grams of carbohydrates, cucumbers are one of the healthiest and most refreshing veggies.

Dark Greens – Dark leafy greens like Swiss chard, mustard greens, and turnip greens each have less than 5 grams of carbohydrates per serving, making them both healthy and ideal for the Keto Diet.

Eggplant – Eggplant is a delicious Mediterranean vegetable and has a low carb count, at only 2.88 grams.

Green Beans – There are 7 grams of carbohydrates per 1 cup of 1/2" cut pieces of this sweet, popular legume. Get them frozen, since they still have plenty of nutritional value.

Iceberg Lettuce – There isn't much nutritional value to iceberg lettuce, but at only 0.2 carbs per serving, you can't go wrong adding chopped leaves to salads or as burger toppings.

Kohlrabi – This funny looking vegetable is super Keto friendly and has 2.6 grams of carbs. Chop it up with cabbage and iceberg lettuce to make a slaw.

Mushrooms – Regular white button mushrooms have only 2.26 grams of carbs, so you're welcome to eat them! They are great marinated in olive oil, stuffed with cheeses, or as a Keto pizza topping.

Onions – Although onions have 7.64 grams of carbohydrates, making them a bit high, they're an essential ingredient in cooking. Green onions have 1.1 grams and shallots have 1.7 grams, so use those whenever you can.

Romaine Lettuce – Pick up some Romaine for Keto salads, topping on burgers, and to make lettuce wraps. Romaine has 2.8 grams of carbs per serving.

Spinach – Fresh or frozen, delicious spinach is Ketogenic Diet approved, with only 1.43 grams of carbohydrates. Mix it with other dark greens and arugula for a base to salads.

Tomatoes – Yes, tomatoes are great on this diet. They have 2.69 grams of carbohydrates per serving. They're actually a fruit, but are way lower in carbs than most fruits.

Turnips – While a bit high at 4.63 grams of carbohydrates, turnips are still low enough to be enjoyed as an autumn treat. They're delicious roasted or mashed.

Zucchini – Yummy zucchini has 2.11 grams of carbs and can be mixed with herbs and spices for a quick roast or made into 'noodles' (zoodles) for veggie pasta.

Fruits

Avocado – Although it's green and looks like a vegetable, avocados are technically a fruit. They only have 1.84 grams of carbohydrates and are very high in good fats. You can slice them over salads or make your own guacamole.

Blackberries – The fruit with the lowest net carbs, at 4.3 grams per ¾ cup. Please be diligent when consuming these berries, since those carbs add up quickly.

Lemon – Lemons have a bit higher carb count since they are fruits, but a squeeze of fresh lemon juice here or there only adds a few grams.

Lime – One lime has 7 grams of carbs, so you can have a small occasional splash of lime juice to flavor Mexican dishes.

Raspberries – No fruit is no-carb, but raspberries are a delicious treat. One cup contains 15 grams of carbs, so factor those into your Macros.

Strawberries – A world without strawberries would be a sad one, indeed. Each cup contains 11 grams of carbohydrates, but the flavor is worth it!

Herbs & Spices

Basil – One tablespoon of fresh basil has 0.1 grams of carbs. The dried version has more carbs, but it is still worth purchasing to create Italian flavored dishes.

Bay Leaves – No carbs in bay leaves! Keto soups taste so good with these flavored herbs. Don't forget to take them out of the soup before serving.

Black Pepper – Black pepper has no carbohydrates. Pair it with the sea salt below to spice up foods.

Cajun Spices – Pick up a canister of no carb Cajun spices to dress up salmon, shrimp, beef, or chicken.

Chili Powder – Make chili, Mexican dishes, and other meat marinades with low carb chili powder, at 1.6 grams per teaspoon.

Cilantro – This peppery tangy herb has less than 1 gram of carbs per Tablespoon of fresh leaves. Make your own salsa with cilantro, tomatoes, and onions.

Cinnamon – Warm and comforting, cinnamon is also low carb and great for the Keto diet.

Cumin – There are no carbs in ground cumin! This incredible spice is essential in many Southwestern, Mexican, and Indian dishes.

Curry Powder – Curry powder has a wonderful yellow color and exotic flavor. Each teaspoon has 1.16 grams of carbs.

Garlic – Each fresh garlic clove has 1 gram of carbs, which is much less than garlic powder or salt. Garlic is an essential cooking ingredient, so stock your kitchen with fresh heads of garlic.

Lemon Pepper – There are no carbs in this popular spice blend. It's delicious on chicken.

Oregano – Together with basil, oregano is a popular and low carb Italian herb, at less than 1 gram per teaspoon.

Parsley – Dried parsley has no carbs! It's great to sprinkle over meats and add to soups.

Rosemary – A delicious herb when paired with beef, rosemary has no carbs!

Sage – Sage doesn't have any carbohydrates, either, so use as much as you want in your cooking.

Sea Salt – Don't buy the regular table salt, since that's not no-carb like sea salt. You can purchase different sea salt flake sizes and varieties like Himalayan pink sea salt.

Tarragon – Ground tarragon is usually found in a popular herb blend called Herbs de Provence, which also has marjoram, thyme, and parsley. It has less than 1 gram of carbohydrates per teaspoon.

Thyme – Both fresh and ground thyme are also low carb, with less than 1 gram per teaspoon.

Nuts and Seeds

Almonds - Almonds have a fairly low carb count and are one of the most versatile nuts. They're also delicious for snacking, too.

Chia Seeds – Chia seeds are slightly high in carbohydrates, featuring 12 grams per ounce, but they also have 9 grams of fat. You'll find recipes for them in this book.

Hemp Seeds – Two tablespoons adds 6 grams of good fats to your smoothies and other recipes.

Macadamia Nuts - Have you ever tried these nuts before? They are now going to be one of your staple snacks, since they're not only very low in carbs, they're also really high in Omega 3 essential fatty acids.

Nut Butters - Peanut butter is a bit high in carbs, but it is also high in fat, so that makes it less likely to spike your blood sugar glucose levels. Try other nut butters like almond butter and macadamia nut butter. If you've plateaued on your weight loss or are stalling, then keep nut butters to a bare minimum or cut them out completely. They do contain higher carbs than other snacks.

Pecans - Pecans are very good in a nutty snack mix, in baking, or by themselves by the handful. A 1 ounce serving contains 20.4 grams of fat.

Pumpkin Seeds – Full of good fats, pumpkin seeds are salty and crunchy. A 1 ounce serving has 5 grams of fat.

Sesame Seeds – You get 4.5 grams of fat in each Tablespoon of these tiny, crunchy seeds. They make an excellent salad topping and are perfect in Asian cooking.

Sunflower Seeds – Packed with 14 grams of fat per ounce, you'll want to snack on toasted or roasted sunflower seeds. Mix them with other nuts and seeds for a delicious Keto friendly trail mix.

Tahini - Tahini, or sesame seed butter, is a great snack with celery sticks. It provides plenty of the daily fats you need on the Keto Diet, while also being extremely low carb.

Walnuts - Whether sprinkled over a salad, folded into batter for baking, added to other nuts and seeds for a mix, or eaten alone, walnuts are delicious. Just 1 ounce has 28 grams of fat.

Oils, Vinegars, and Condiments

Apple Cider Vinegar - Since apple cider vinegar is high in acetic acid, that helps reduce the glycemic response of carbohydrates. It contains enzymes that enhance your metabolizing of proteins and fats. It's an excellent vinegar.

Barbecue Sauce – Made from either a ketchup or mustard base and loaded with spices, many barbecue sauces are Keto Diet friendly. Buy ones that have no sugar or carbs added.

Coconut Milk – Each 13.5 ounce can of full fat coconut milk has 2 grams of carbohydrates, so stock up your pantry. Canned coconut milk is dairy free and very creamy, making it perfect for Thai or Indian curries, soups, and sauces.

Coconut Oil - You want some cold-pressed coconut oil. Coconut oil is one of the most useful things you can have in the house. It also is an essential ingredient in Keto Fat Bombs.

Curry Paste – You can find jars of pre-made Thai curry pastes (yellow, red, green) in the Asian section of your grocery store or at an Asian food market. These pastes are made up of distinctly strong herbs and spices that form a base for making amazing curries. They have between 1 and 3 grams of carbs per Tablespoon, depending on the brand.

Dill Pickles - Pickles are part of the fermented food group, along with sauerkraut. Pickles have natural acids that stabilize your blood sugar. Go for dill pickles that aren't as sweet as other kinds.

Fish Sauce – Thai and Vietnamese dishes use fish sauce, which is extremely low carb, at less than 1 gram per Tablespoon. It's so strongly flavored, which you can smell as soon as you open the bottle, that you don't need much. Use fish sauce in Asian soups and curries.

Flavored Oils – Flavored oils can become marinades for meat or fish, cooking oils, or homemade salad dressings. You can add many flavors to your pantry, including garlic oil, chili oil, rosemary oil, oregano oil, thyme oil, and basil oil. Choose the ones with the highest fat contents. They have no carbs!

Horseradish Sauce – Its distinct flavor and very low carb count make horseradish sauce a great condiment. There are 1.7 grams of carbohydrates per Tablespoon.

Ketchup – If you can find a natural ketchup made without sugar or high fructose corn syrup, then add it to your Ketogenic Diet pantry. Ketchup is a bit higher in carbs than mustard or mayo, because it's made with tomatoes. Use sparingly as a treat.

Lemon Juice / Lime Juice – Bottled lemon and lime juice can also be stocked in your pantry. A little goes a long way with these citrusy, tangy juices. They have higher carb counts than other condiments, so use sparingly.

Mayonnaise – Did you know that regular full fat (not diet) mayo has 0.5 grams of carbohydrates? It's a very Keto Diet friendly condiment. You can make both egg and chicken salads with mayo.

Mustard – Both classic yellow mustard and high quality Dijon mustard are excellent condiments for a low carb pantry. They hardly have any carbohydrates and no sugar, either. Use on chicken, beef, or pork dishes.

Olive Oil – Regular full fat olive oil is going to be one of your best sources of the good fats in the Keto Diet. You can pan fry chicken, drizzle it over salads, or even make homemade beauty products with it. Check nutritional labels to purchase the olive oils with the highest fat content in grams.

Pesto – Pesto is made with basil, garlic, pine nuts, and sometimes a splash of lemon juice. It's a delicious combination that gives you Italian flavor for chicken or beef dishes.

Ranch Dressing – Its creamy texture comes from dairy products and not carbs, so ranch dressing is okay to have on the Keto Diet. Choose a brand with the lowest sugar content you can find.

Red Wine Vinegar – Balsamic vinegar has too many carbs for the Keto diet, so substitute red wine vinegar instead. You can mix it with flavored oils to create your own salad dressings.

Soy Sauce – Asian cuisine wouldn't be the same without salty, delicious soy sauce. It's a low carb condiment that you can use as a flavoring in soups or as a marinade for beef, chicken, pork, or shrimp. There's about 1 gram of carbohydrates per Tablespoon.

Sriracha – This popular red Asian hot sauce is also low carb, at 1 gram per teaspoon. Find a brand that is completely sugar free. Drizzle it over salads, eggs, meats, or fish.

Tabasco – Another popular hot sauce, Tabasco has no carbs!

Tamari – This is another kind of soy sauce and is both gluten free and carbohydrate free. Get the reduced sodium kind to cut out more salt.

Tartar Sauce – You can make your own tartar sauce with mayonnaise and diced dill pickles, or you can purchase it premade. If you do get it bottled, read the labels and buy the brand with no sugar or carbs. It's delicious on fish!

Tomato Sauce – Buy plain, unsweetened tomato sauce and diced tomatoes in cans or jars. You'll also want some tomato paste, too. Although tomato is a fruit, it's very low in carbohydrates.

White Vinegar – You can not only cook with white vinegar, you can clean with it, too! It has no carbs and is an essential ingredient if you want to pickle onions or cucumbers.

White Wine Vinegar – Not to be confused with white vinegar, you can definitely have white wine vinegar on the Keto Diet. Its carb count is less than 1 gram per Tablespoon. Mix with horseradish and cream to make a horseradish cream sauce for roast beef.

Worcestershire Sauce – Your Keto beef stews and soups will taste wonderful with a splash of Worcestershire sauce. One Tablespoon has 3.3 grams of carbohydrates.

Baking Ingredients

Almond Extract – There are no carbs in almond extract! It gives a nice nutty flavor to Keto Fat Bombs and baking.

Almond Flour – Every type of white or wheat based flour is off limits on the Keto Diet. But you can have almond flour! It's made up of ground almonds and gives a slight nutty taste to baking. For every ¼ cup, you get 6 grams of carbohydrates and 14 grams of the good fats. It is a bit high in carbs, so factor those into your daily Macro percentages.

Baking Powder – Your Keto bread doughs and pizza recipes won't rise without baking powder, so this is an ingredient to have in your kitchen. Baking powder has 1.3 grams of carbohydrates per teaspoon.

Cocoa Powder – High quality unsweetened cocoa powder will make your Keto Fat Bombs and baked goods taste delicious! Just one Tablespoon has 3 grams of carbs.

Coconut Flour – Coconut flour, made from coconuts, is another ingredient to substitute in baking for white flour. That way, you can make Keto breads and doughs. It has 16 grams of carbohydrates and 4 grams of fat per ¼ cup. That's a pretty high carb count, so use it sparingly.

Dark Chocolate – Yes, you can have chocolate on the Ketogenic Diet. Add it to baked goods, Keto hot chocolate, or have a small nibble as a snack when cravings strike. Look for high quality dark chocolate bars that have at least 80% cacao in them and the lowest amount of sugar you can find. Some companies make Keto friendly dark chocolate morsels and chips, too.

Flaxseed Meal – Flax seeds are very low carb and a crunchy topping for Keto salads. Flaxseed meal is an essential baking ingredient for several recipes, so you'll want to have some in your pantry. Two Tablespoons have 4 grams of carbohydrates.

Lemon Extract – Make Keto lemon cookies with carb free lemon extract. That hint of tartness really elevates your baking.

Psyllium Husk Powder – Psyllium husk is a form of fiber made from the husks of the Platago ovata plant's seeds. Psyllium husk powder can be mixed with other flours and baking ingredients to make Keto pizza dough. You probably won't find it in your local grocery store, but it can be in health food stores or purchased online.

Stevia – No white sugar or brown sugar allowed on the Ketogenic Diet. However, you can have a natural substitute. Stevia has 1 gram per 2 teaspoons, so it's okay to add a dash to your morning coffee, afternoon tea, or slip into Keto Fat Bombs. Go easy on the Stevia, but it can help you with sugar cravings.

Vanilla Extract – At less than 1 gram of carbs per teaspoon, you can add delicious vanilla flavor to your Keto Fat Bombs, bullet proof coffee, cookies, and cakes.

Other

Lard – Yep, the old-fashioned pig fat lard. It's full of healthy saturated fats. There are 13 grams of fat per Tablespoon.

MCT oil - This ingredient, called Medium-chain triglyceride oil, might not be found at your grocery store, although some specialty health food stores could carry it. It's easier to digest than other oils, a great source of energy, and supports the hormones in your body.

Olives – Green olives have 2.8 grams of carbohydrates and are packed with amazing good fats, so buy plenty! Black olives are higher in carbs, so stick with green ones only.

Getting Your Pantry Ready for the Keto Lifestyle

Time to give your kitchen a makeover! Ridding your cupboards, fridge, and freezer of carbs, fruits, and sugars is the best beginner tip for starting the Ketogenic Diet. You're able to give yourself a clean slate and start fresh with new foods that actually work with your body.

In this chapter, you've read all about ingredients that are Keto Diet friendly, so those are the only ones to keep. All the rest must go. If you feel guilty about throwing out perfectly good food, then call up a friend or family member and bring it over to them. You can donate canned beans and boxed pastas or grains to your local food bank.

Eating Out on the Keto Diet

Restaurants know that we crave their meals, and they pile on the sugar and carbs. You'd be amazed at how quickly a simple appetizer can derail your best laid plans for weight loss and health. How do you know which restaurants to pick that are Keto Diet friendly?

Take a walk around your neighborhood (or use a smartphone app or local website) to really look at your restaurant options. You'll see fast food places, soup and sandwich shops, pizza joints, international food restaurants, dinner restaurants, and sweets places like bakeries, cafes, and ice cream stands. Look up restaurant menus online to see which options they have that you can use on the Keto Diet.

Here are some general tips to ordering in a restaurant:

- Ask them to remove the bread.
- Crispy means fried and fried means the wrong types of oils and plenty of trans fats. Order grilled instead.
- Portions are way too big. Either share with a friend or ask the restaurant to box up half the meal to take home for lunch the next day.
- Put together several Keto friendly appetizers and sides instead of an entrée. You can choose from soups, salads, grilled meats, spice rubbed fish, and vegetables like broccoli or zucchini.
- "Breaded" is a code word for "coated in bread crumbs." Stay away from carbs.
- Many restaurants have gluten-free options to help you remove carbs. Ask your server.

Basically, when you order in a restaurant, think of the types of Keto friendly meals you make at home. Then, try as closely as possible to replicate those meals.

80% Keto Friendly Restaurants:

Choose these to find great menus filled with plenty of things to eat:

- Breakfast places – Eggs, bacon, sausage, ham, steak, and cheese galore.
- Steak house restaurants – Any protein grilled and served alongside broccoli or cauliflower is a good bet. No baked potatoes.

- Barbecue restaurants – Lots of protein options here: chicken, beef, pork, ham, or even fish. Skip the cornbread and mashed potatoes, and go for the collard greens instead.
- Seafood restaurants – Dip that lobster in butter! You can have any type of fish or shrimp with a Keto veggie side. Make sure it's not breaded.
- Asian restaurants – Thai, Vietnamese, Chinese, Japanese, and other Asian restaurants offer plenty of entrees with no carbs. Hold the rice and noodles.
- French restaurants – All that Brie, butter, heavy cream, shallots, and mushrooms are excellent on a Keto diet.
- Indian restaurants – You won't find any beef dishes, but there are delicious chicken, lamb, and vegetarian options. No rice or naan.

50% Keto Friendly Restaurants:

The following menus have limited Keto options, so you'll have to do a bit of navigating:

- Diners – Skip the dinner rolls and order either steak or chicken dishes with Keto veggie sides.
- Mexican restaurants – Navigate past the corn, beans, rice, and tortillas. Go for the grilled shrimp, salsa, and queso.
- Soup, Salad, and Sandwich places – Try ordering a cup of Keto friendly soup and a side salad. If they have lettuce wraps, go for it.
- Italian restaurants – Difficult, but you can order chicken parmesan with no pasta. Get creative!
- Mediterranean restaurants – Stay away from hidden carbs like pita, barley, quinoa, and couscous.
- Bars and pubs – You'll find lots of potatoes and bread, but you can order chicken wings in a pinch.
- Fast Food Burger Joints – Not easy, but we have faith you can order burgers with no buns!

No – No Restaurants:

Please avoid these on the Keto Diet!

- Pizza restaurants – Everything is served either on top of or alongside bread. Lots of bread.
- Coffee Shops – Turning plain coffee into dessert drinks. Step away from the breakfast pastries!
- Bakeries – Pretty self explanatory. Nothing but sugar and carbs.
- Ice Cream / Dessert places – Sugar, sugar, and more sugar.
- Carnivals – You won't find anything remotely healthy or Keto friendly in fair food. It's all carbs that are battered and fried.
- Movie Theaters – You get three terrible choices: soda, candy, or popcorn. No thanks!
- Sports stadium food – You might be able to get away with ballpark franks without the bun, but that's about it.
- Convenience Stores – Nothing but soda, candy, potato chips, and sugary packaged treats.
- Vending Machines – Just seeing if you're paying attention!

Just because you can't have pizza, baked goods, or pasta, doesn't mean there aren't amazing other options on the Ketogenic Diet! In your first month of eating on this plan, you might want to avoid most of these restaurants, so that you're not tempted to eat something you shouldn't.

Now that you've got your ingredients, your Keto friendly stocked kitchen and have successfully navigated the world of restaurants, how exactly will you be eating each day? In the next chapter, we'll get into the nitty gritty of getting into ketosis: Macros!

Chapter 4:
Come Here And Learn All About It!

Getting started on the Keto Diet is just the first step in an exciting journey! As you saw in the previous chapter, there are foods you can't eat. But you'll feel so good you won't be tempted to order a carb-heavy meal and kick yourself out of ketosis! You'll want to stay in this new metabolic state for life.

There are some basic tenets of the Keto lifestyle that can help you along the way. They're easy to memorize and can be repeated to yourself, similar to mantras.

"No Sugar Today – Feeling Sweet Tomorrow"

You'll get sugar cravings on the Keto diet. But, they do get better with time. If you can say no to a sugary item now, you'll feel sweet and look better tomorrow.

"It's Not About Can't – It's About Don't"

Forget saying, "I can't have carbs." Start saying: "I don't want carbs." It's a subtle, but necessary mindset shift. It'll really help you.

"I'm Just Not Hungry for That"

You can mentally trick your taste buds into finding a particular food distasteful. Some people love licorice; others hate it. Some people hate mushrooms; others love them. Try and mentally trick yourself into just not being hungry for some carb item that'll just sit in your stomach and make you feel sluggish.

You can come up with your own mantras, too. Been suffering from a health problem? Imagine feeling better once Keto has helped reduce your symptoms. Sick and tired of low energy? Create a mantra that focuses on what you want to use your new energy for. When you custom tailor a mantra, you're more likely to remember it.

To remember it even more, take a pen and write out your mantra on a piece of paper. Don't type it. Hand write it. That puts it into your memory.

Know Your Body

Each of us start out wanting to know exactly what state our body is in. When you assess where you are today, right now during the exact moment you're reading this, then that gives you a start point. It's like the first "Start" square on a gameboard. Today is when you'll begin. It also functions as a reference point for the progress you'll make throughout the next few weeks as you transition to this new eating plan.

Think of where you were just one year ago. You've progressed a long way since then. It might not be in the direction you want, but it is a different direction. Diets can be difficult, because they're measured on a longer time frame than many of us want them to be! We want to see results in days, whereas your body operates on a much more elongated calendar. Patience creates results.

So do metrics. Body metrics, specifically. In this beginning state, you're encouraged to get your full physical self assessed. This can be done through a simple physical at your doctor's. Please fill out the following:

Height:

Current Weight:

BMI:

You are also highly HIGHLY encouraged to keep a food diary. Just get a simple notebook from a store and write down everything you eat and drink. Beginning this simple habit is eye-opening.

After you have your numbers and metrics from your doctor visit, what's the next step?

The Keto Mindset

It's not just about numbers, as those of you who've dieted before well know. It also has so much to do with your mindset. While it may come across as mumbo-jumbo, uncovering your personal psychological reasons for why you want to get healthier and more slim and trim, plus your current emotional state, will help you so much later on, when you'll have to face the challenges of this diet (as any diet). Just like a Greek warrior gathering his magic sword and shield from the gods, so, too, will you gather the tools you need to fight against your old impulses, overcome them, and win!

Yes, fighting the carb battle is a battle. So, it is important that we discuss one powerful word:

WHY?

Why do you want to embark on this Ketogenic Diet? Although initially the reason might be that it looks cool, it's a neat fad, cutting out carbs is easier than ever, or whatever, you've got to come up with deeper reasons.

So, why?

Why do you want to succeed on the Keto Diet? Why do you want to start it in the first place? Why do you have strong feelings about this diet, as opposed to another one? Why do you want to be healthier?

It helps to raise your own stakes in this battle. Many people have a near-death experience before they make a radical change – and that's because they've realized there's high stakes involved. If they don't do X, it might harm or even kill them in the long run.

What are your high stakes? If you don't embark on this diet and make it a success, then what's your high stakes reason to keep going? It could be something personal, that you're doing this for you. It could be spiritual, that you feel you were given this physical body from a higher power and you want to treat it better. It could be relational, like you're doing this for your family member, friend, or other loved one. It could be physical, that you're simply sick and tired of being sick and tired. There's only so much you can take!

It would be helpful to write this down in a journal. That is an excellent place to more deeply explore your thoughts. Make it easy on yourself to remember your reason. How about tattooing it on your arm? Just kidding!

But seriously. Discipline comes from strong and compelling reasons. Find a reason stronger than the breadstick sitting on the table in front of you, strong enough to say no to a hundred breadsticks – and you'll find your own diet success.

Keto Diet Tools

You want to transition from a carbohydrate metabolic state to a ketosis metabolic state and stay there. Just because you're low carb doesn't mean your liver is producing ketones. To measure ketosis, there are several tools on the market that you can buy to help you:

- Blood Ketone Monitor
- Breath Ketone Monitor
- Ketone Urine Strips

These three tools can test your blood, breath, or urine. They're easy to test at home by yourself. Your ideal ketone level varies depending on your age, gender, height, weight, and other body factors.

The Blood Ketone Monitor is similar to diabetes insulin testing. Insert the strip into the monitor machine, prick your finger to put blood on the strip, and you'll get a reading pretty quickly. While this is the most expensive method, it's the most accurate method of determining you're in ketosis.

To use a Breath Ketone Monitor, you'll plug the device into a power source, blow on it until the light stops flashing, take a note of the color and how many times it blinks. This takes a bit longer and hasn't been researched as much as the other solutions.

For the Ketone Urine Strips, you'll just pee on a stick, wait about a minute, and then compare the color to the chart on the package. It's the least expensive of the three methods, but don't work after you enter ketosis.

It's up to you which one you prefer using. I recommend the Breath Ketone Monitor, since it isn't painful and it measures those ketones properly.

Ketogenic Diet Macros

I've got good news! No need to count calories on the Ketogenic Diet! You can if you want to. But it's not as important as tracking your Macros. So, we do need to learn how to calculate those.

This diet is made up of three Macronutrients, which are nicknamed Macros:

FATS – PROTEINS – CARBOHYDRATES

Yes, carbs are included. We're not going to eliminate them completely, just reduce them to a tiny percentage.

On a normal balanced diet, which is recommended by USDA nutritional guidelines, you'd be consuming 35% of your daily calories from carbohydrates, 35% of your daily calories from proteins, and about 5% of your daily calories from good fats.

But the Macros on a Ketogenic Diet are much different.

With fats, we're going to increase from 5% all the way up to 70% of your daily calories from good fats. We'll discuss what good fats are below.

With proteins, you'll reduce the 35% down to about 19% protein.

With the carbohydrates, you'll be reducing that 60% down to about 5% - 8% of your daily calories.

So, we're going from this:

5% FATS - 35% PROTEINS – 60% CARBOHYDRATES

To this:

70% FATS – 19% PROTEINS – 5% CARBOHYDRATES

That's your new diet, one that will keep your body in a ketosis state.

How does this break down into counts in grams?

It varies depending on your body factors (gender, age, height, weight, etc.), but in general, you should aim for:

MEN:

208g FATS – 125g PROTEINS – 31g CARBOHYDRATES

WOMEN:

167g FATS – 100g PROTEINS – 25g CARBOHYDRATES

You can find Keto Macro calculators online that give you the exact numbers. My main point is just to have you keep your Macro numbers in mind, especially during your first four weeks of transition. For some, these carb grams might be a bit high for ketosis. That's why you should be using the Ketone monitors mentioned above to make absolutely sure.

Now, let's talk about each Macro and what it's for in your body!

Let's Start with Protein

Protein is one of your body's most essential nutrients. It's also delicious, too – roasted, baked, and grilled meats get your mouth watering for a reason. There are two types of protein: animal and plant. On the Ketogenic Diet, your plant intake is reduced because many vegetables and fruits have too many carbs. So, you're primarily going to get your protein from animal sources: meat, fish, seafood, eggs, and high protein dairy foods.

What does protein do in your body? It is a general repairman and handyman. It repairs and builds tissue, makes enzymes, makes hormones, and builds bones, muscle, cartilage, skin, and blood. It also gives you energy. Your brain needs a lot of protein for basic mental functions, too.

While protein is essential, it's not the amazing nutrient that's frequently advertised by food manufacturers. Most Americans consume too much protein, trying to get to that nationally recommended 35% amount. To get into and stay in ketosis, protein is important, but not as important as fat. Excess protein can also be stored as excess weight in your cells, so too much of a good thing is, well, not a good thing.

On the Ketogenic Diet, we'll reduce your protein amount to between 19% and 22% of your diet. It's easy to go overboard with the protein. Meats do have high percentages of good fats, though.

Keep your protein calorie counts a bit lower than you're used to. The Keto Diet is not a high protein diet.

The Truth Behind Carbohydrates

Carbohydrates are made up of the same three atoms as fatty acids: carbon, hydrogen, and oxygen. By themselves, these don't seem like bad chemical components, and they're not. When we think carbs, we think bread or pasta or cereal, right? That's because you see the high carbohydrate count on these foods.

Carbohydrates are a group of sugars, starches, and cellulose called saccharides. Starch and sugar are basically the two most important carbohydrates in nutrition.

There are four chemical groups of saccharides: the monosaccharides, disaccharides, oligosaccharides, and polysaccharides. Those are pretty big chemical names, but we're primarily going to focus on how they function in your body.

Sugars and Starches

Polysaccharides store energy in your cells, in the form of starch and glycogen. It's the starch present in foods like potatoes, rice, and wheat that eventually becomes too much stored energy in your body, resulting in weight gain. Sugars have the "ose" suffix, and you'll see them as sucrose (table sugar), fructose (fruit sugar), and glucose (blood sugar). Some people are lactose intolerant, so they can't have milk sugar. There's also cellulose, which is plant sugar, and we'll talk more about that below.

Glycogen is the other type of energy stored in your cells, and it's also a carbohydrate. It's primarily found in both your liver and your muscles.

Carbs Are Actually Sugars

So, when you're walking by the bakery section in the grocery store or the goodies in the snack aisle, just remember that all of those carbohydrates are actually sugars that will add weight. They don't burn off the weight you're trying to lose, either.

It's so tempting, because we live in such a carb loving and carb heavy culture. You bypass them in the grocery store all the time. You drive by fast food restaurants advertising sandwiches and fries, you can barely order an entrée without carbs, every convenience store sells potato chips, and entire cuisines like Italian and Mexican are built on carbohydrate foundations of pasta, bread dough, and rice.

But they all just become glucose sugar molecules in your body and contribute to weight gain.

Leave the carbohydrates on the shelf!

Fat Doesn't Necessarily Make You Fat

Now, let's talk about your number one Macro: fat.

Fat can mean so many different things. It's not just about making you fat. It's also about what fatty acids inside the fats are good for you. And many of them are! These are the fats your liver needs to break down and make ketones.

Yes, it's weird to think eating a high fat diet helps you burn fat. But it's absolutely true.

At the chemical level, a fat is composed of two different kinds of smaller molecules. One of them is glycerol, and the other is fatty acids. Glycerol is a simple compound that's colorless, odorless, has a sweet taste and is non-toxic to humans. The fatty acids are long acids made up of chains of atoms that include different combinations of carbon, oxygen, and hydrogen atoms.

Did you know that fatty acids aren't actually found in humans naturally? We get them from our diet, and they're one of the primary sources of fuel for most of our cells.

The good fats also break down more slowly than carbohydrates in your digestive tract. That means you'll feel full longer.

Good Fats and Bad Fats

The food industry is confusing enough without having to explain the difference between good fats and bad fats. While you're on the Ketogenic Diet, you want to stick to the 'good' fats, which we'll talk about in this chapter. We'll also discuss the 'bad' fats and why they're bad.

As a general guideline, you'll want to stick to eating fats that are naturally occurring in plants, animals, and seafoods. Processed fats are created in food product factories to add taste and flavor to many foods, including margarine, fried foods, and processed cheese. Eating all natural fats is basically the way to go.

It's important to know the difference between good and bad fats, because the good ones will have a positive effect on your body and keep you in ketosis. The bad fats will have a negative effect on your body and contribute towards not just weight gain, but circulatory problems like blocked arteries and even heart disease. Bad fats aren't processed by the body and used as fuel the same way the good fats are.

So, let's discuss the differences and examine them at a chemical level.

Good Fats

The two good fats are saturated fats and monounsaturated fats. Natural polyunsaturated fats can also be added to this category. They are better for your body because of the amount of chains of fatty acids found in them. What are they and how do they help your body?

Saturated Fat

This type of fat is one that contains a high proportion of fatty acid molecules without double bonds. These double bonds link individual carbon atoms to hydrogen atoms, which changes the chemical properties. The reason they're called saturated is because the molecules are saturated with hydrogen atoms. They are solid at room temperature and have higher melting points. The fats from animals are mostly saturated, which is why you'll find saturated fats in animal products like meats and dairy. Saturated fats get a bad rap because they can also be found in processed foods. We'll advise you on which saturated fats to consume in the next chapter.

Monounsaturated Fat

The second type of good fat for the Keto Diet is monounsaturated fat. It also contains a high proportion of fatty acid molecules, but these come with just one double bond (where the prefix 'mono' comes in) that link carbon atoms to hydrogen ones. At room temperature, they are liquids and either semi-solid or solid when refrigerated. When your cells start to use monounsaturated fats for fuel, there's not as many calories as the saturated fats. These are good fats because they protect against cardiovascular disease and are better fuel for your cells.

Bad Fats

The fats to avoid are the processed polyunsaturated fats and the trans fats. You've probably heard of these two bad guys. They have become not just diet enemies, but health enemies as well.

Processed Polyunsaturated Fats

Polyunsaturated fats are similar to the monounsaturated fats above, in that they contain a high proportion of fatty acid molecules. But these ones have more than one double bond between carbon and hydrogen atoms. While carbon and hydrogen don't sound like a bad pairing, in this case, too much of a good thing becomes a bad thing. We listed the processed version of these fats as the real culprit, but naturally occurring polyunsaturated fats are okay to eat. The processed version is often found in certain oils, like corn oil, soybean oil, and other fatty foods like margarine. Naturally occurring polyunsaturated fats are encouraged for you to eat. You might know them better as Omega-3 and Omega-6 fatty acids.

Trans Fats

Trans fat is the nickname for trans-fatty acids, which are the worst kind of fats. They're so bad they're banned in restaurants around the world. They've been around since the 1950s, with the rise of quick frying and the food product industry. Trans fats come from better unsaturated fats, but they have even more double bonds. They directly contribute towards raising your LDL lipoprotein levels, which is called bad cholesterol, lowering your good cholesterol, and directly contributing towards diseases. Trans fats are used to make foods taste better and have a longer shelf life. Plenty of bad foods on any diet are full of trans fats, including microwaved butter popcorn, carnival fried foods, and frozen breakfast sandwiches.

As long as you stay away from these bad fats, you should do just fine!

What About Vegetables?

It's a myth that eating certain vegetables help you lose weight. Their carbohydrate contents are simply too high. To eat some of these vegetables would be the equivalent of having a slice of toast, which is also forbidden.

Yes, it's bizarre that high carbohydrate foods like potatoes and carrots are unhealthier for you than full fat butter! But when it comes down to the cellular differences in how your body actually processes carbohydrates vs. the good fats, it becomes obvious.

Cellulose is present in the cell walls of all plant materials, and it is also known as fiber to help maintain your healthy digestive system. But cellulose is also a carbohydrate, just like starch and sugar. Some vegetables, like potatoes and corn, have too much starch in relation to their cellulose levels. That's why they're not considered as part of the Ketogenic Diet. Those carbohydrate molecules will be too much stored energy in your body and will also kick you out of ketosis.

Forget Conventional Nutritional Information

In order to have success on the Ketogenic Diet, you're going to have to forget a lot of the conventional nutritional information that you've learned over the years. The Food Pyramid has too many carbohydrates and doesn't work, the USDA Food Nutrition Guidelines don't take into account how your body actually processes nutrients, and fats aren't your number one diet enemy. Whole grains aren't as healthy for you as you think. A grain is still a grain, and grains are made up of carbohydrates.

The Ketogenic Diet has its own rules for how your body really works when in a ketosis metabolic state.

The reason we went into so much detail about how your body processes fats, carbohydrates, starches, and sugars is because …

That's essentially what's going on at a cellular level when you eat foods on the Ketogenic Diet.

Stick to these three Macros and their percentages:

70% FATS – 19% PROTEINS – 5% CARBOHYDRATES

These Macros switch your body from that carbohydrate metabolic state to the ketosis metabolic state.

Right now, whenever you eat something, your body is using the same old energy storing techniques. Think of your body as a warehouse. Shipments of new carbohydrates, fats, proteins, and other molecules are continually coming into the warehouse. Whenever new carbohydrates come in, a few of those sugars and starches are used for energy. That's the brief burst of craziness you get after eating a candy bar or the temporary 'sugar high.' But mostly, the rest of those carbohydrates are stored in the warehouse, not to be used again. You eat something else with carbohydrates in it, and the cycle repeats itself. A fraction is used for energy, and the rest is stored in your cells.

Too much stored energy results in the weight gain you're experiencing. For those of you who've tried exercising to take off the weight, you become frustrated because spending 30 minutes at the gym four times a week isn't going to stop the storage warehouse cycle. It isn't going to magically switch your body from storing energy to burning energy.

But, being in ketosis does do that!

The Keto Diet basically switches your body from an energy storage container to an energy burning machine.

That's what we're going for in this book.

Creating Ketones For Weight Loss

Once you've entered a state of ketosis and your liver is producing ketones, you'll notice the weight will start to come off. It's almost effortless, and doesn't require any additional exercise (although some is recommended).

The best thing you can do for your body and especially your liver, is to monitor your Macros on the Ketogenic Diet. Stick to your high fat percentage, moderate protein percentage, and very low carbohydrate percentage.

Chapter 5:
Your First 4 Weeks on The Keto Diet

When getting started on the Keto Diet, this chapter will be your nitty gritty guide to making it work! We're going to go through everything you should be eating, doing, and monitoring, making this transition as easy and enjoyable as possible.

I know you feel you've got plenty of information already, you've got the foods you can eat, there's a meal plan in two chapters, and you can just fly off on your own, right? You'll be just fine.

Hold up there! Please be patient with yourself and your body and follow these steps. Remember your body is changing its entire metabolic state. That's a big transition. Take it slow for the first four weeks, and you'll be assured of greater success in the long run.

Week One

Yay, you're starting the diet! Lots of support and encouragement from me here. You're armed with quite a few tools, including your list of foods you can eat, the foods you cannot have, the meal plans, the recipes, and at least one monitoring device for ketosis. You feel ready to set off on this new diet adventure. The beginning is filled with both drive and enthusiasm.

However, you could also be experiencing a bit of the trepidatious fear of the unknown. What's life without bread, pasta, rice, potatoes, and corn? Is this diet really all it's cracked up to be? Will my body respond just like all those others who've been on the Ketogenic Diet? What will be my results?

Yep, lots of questions. That's why it's helpful to keep a food journal or diary to track this transition period.

Dealing with Hunger

Up until now, when you've been in the mood for a snack, you've reached for something with carbs in it. Potato chips, pretzels, popcorn, maybe a piece of toast, or some crackers.

But when those items are off the menu, what do you substitute them with? Hopefully, you followed the 'cleaning the pantry' suggestions in the Foods to Eat chapter above. You do have plenty of snack options – cheese, nuts, hard boiled eggs, fresh veggies with tahini.

Hungry for something sweet? Try a cup of tea with a pinch of Stevia in it, or by making one of the Fat Bombs in the recipes chapter. Having a sweet tooth on the Ketogenic Diet does get better as the days go by. Make sure you're getting enough fat, and that will help.

Carb and Sugar Withdrawal

As part of dealing with hunger pangs, you might go through carbohydrate withdrawals. This is definitely natural and expected. Eating all of those sugars affected your brain in such a profound chemical way that it's like you've been on a stimulating drug! The symptoms of withdrawal include:

- Rampant sugar cravings
- Obsessing over sweet or carb foods

- Mood swings
- Dizziness
- Irritability
- Fatigue

Luckily, you'll only feel these symptoms for a few days. By the end of the first week, those cravings and these negative feelings will be much subsided. Then you'll emerge from it being better than ever, your blood sugar will stabilize and calm down, and your overall well being will be much improved. I went through it, too.

Pass the Salt

Keep that salt shaker handy during your first week on the Keto Diet. You were probably getting a great deal of your daily recommended allowance of sodium from carb foods, like potato chips and French fries.

By limiting your carbohydrates to around 30 grams per day, you're not eating large amounts of glucose. That means your body's not producing as much insulin. However, insulin not only is in conjunction with your blood sugar, but also your blood sodium levels by helping sodium get absorbed into the body. Without it, you'd just pee out the salt. It is a mineral, after all!

Having low insulin while in ketosis means that you're going to be urinating out much more sodium. This means you're also losing lots of electrolytes. So, you need to increase your salt intake. Aim for between 2000 mg and 4000 mg per day.

Fortunately, there's many yummy solutions: salty cheeses, salty nuts, salted meats, salted fish, salted butter, and sprinkling salt on salads. You can sip on salty chicken or beef broth between meals, too. This will also help to relieve lots of those carb withdrawal symptoms discussed above.

Keep your salt intake nice and high during not just your first week, but the entire time you're in ketosis on the Keto Diet. Don't forget to stay hydrated, too!

Week One Foods:

In addition to your salty foods, you'll want to slowly ease into the diet within your first week by choosing different foods and meals that are no carb.

MCT Oil

One of the foods discussed above was MCT Oil. It's worth it to pick up a bottle of this unusual supplement. MCT (medium-chain triglycerides) oil is found in coconut oil or it can be purchased separately at a health food store or online. MCT oil is a fat similar to olive oil that can be rapidly absorbed. It goes right to your liver, which is either immediately used for energy or converted right into ketones. Start with a lower dosage to see how it interacts with your body, and then gradually increase.

It supplies plenty of good nutrients your body needs for the transition. Right when you're fresh out of bed is when it can work the best. Keep up this practice for at least 14 days straight, and you'll achieve ketosis even faster.

More Butter ... and Then More

One of the many changes is wrapping your mind around the previous off limits foods you're now encouraged to eat. When cooking, reach for the butter. Put lots of butter (and salt!) on vegetables. Dip shellfish like crab, shrimp, or lobster into butter. Create a garlic butter sauce for fish or chicken. Butter is amazing and will help you get through the first week on the Keto Diet.

Drink Bullet Proof Coffee

What's bullet proof coffee? It's a simple cup of Joe that's been jolted with extra Keto friendly ingredients to turn it into a caffeinated and high performance drink. One serving has a whopping 28.5 fat grams, and only 1 gram of carbohydrates. You'll need 1 cup of black coffee, 1 Tablespoon of high quality grass fed unsalted butter, 1 Tablespoon coconut or MCT oil, ½ Tablespoon heavy cream, and ½ teaspoon vanilla extract. Mix everything in a blender or by hand and drink. It gives you so many good fats and is an excellent healthy start to your day. Pairing it with a high fat, low carb breakfast is one of the best ways to start on your Keto Diet. I also include a second recipe for Almond Bullet Proof Coffee in this book I think you'll love, too!

Nuts About Nuts

I've mentioned eating nuts several times to help you get through your first week. They provide a salty, meaty crunch as a snack food, plus they're packed with good fats and very low or no carbohydrates. Macadamia nuts, almonds, and walnuts can be mixed with low carb chocolate chips and seeds to create a yummy snack mix that will see you through your first week.

Cheesy and Delicious

Cheese really is delicious. You can snack on cheddar, goat cheese, cottage cheese, Colby Jack, mozzarella sticks, or any other creamy cheeses in the Foods to Eat chapter above. Having a few pieces of cheese boosts your fat intake. Don't forget melted cheese, too. Sprinkle shredded cheese on top of salads, chicken, or ground beef dishes. You can also create baked cheese dips for veggies.

Week One Tips

Hopefully, these tips and tricks will help you get through your first week on the Keto Diet. You might see a pound or two of initial weight loss, but you might not. This first week is more about slowly but steadily changing your mindsets around foods, increasing your fat intake, and trying new ways to get your ideal Macros through MCT oil and bullet proof coffee.

As another practical tip, read through the recipes in this book and make sure you've purchased the items you need to make all the meals. You'll need mini muffin tins or candy molds for the Fat Bombs, a blender for smoothies, and it helps to have a large crock pot for busy week nights. That way, by next week, you'll be able to make all the recipes.

It's not a race, so go slow. Your main objective is to reduce those carbohydrates and rid your home of them, and steadily increase your fat intake. Stock your cupboards with new foods and start experimenting with the recipes. It's helpful to start on a weekend day, so you have more time to go Keto for a full day.

Week Two

Good! You got through Week One! You knew that was going to be the hardest, and for some of you, the cravings and withdrawal symptoms were not easy to get through. But, you've made it – and this week is when your diet can start to change your body in new ways and better than you thought possible.

How does it do that?

Well, you're going to start seeing results. Physical results that come from changing to such a low carb lifestyle. The initial pounds that you lose this second week will first come from water weight loss. That is because glycogen from those carbohydrates you were previously eating was stored with H2O water cells throughout your body. You'll notice a drop in weight and a general feeling of lightness after the water weight is shed. Don't expect it to be too much, but it could be noticeable.

However, if this water weight loss doesn't happen, that's also normal. Not to worry! You might not have had that issue in your body. Each person will have a different range of experiences within the first two weeks of going Ketogenic.

Micromanage Your Macros

What truly is the most important thing you should do this second week is to watch your Macros very closely. By now, you should have calculated the exact grams using an online Macros calculator or by going off the guidelines in the previous chapter. This is when you've got to apply some of that discipline to track what you're eating and keep the Macros in your mind at all times.

Fortunately, I've made this super easy on you! Just follow the four-week meal plans in this book! You get two of them, either a regular meal plan or one for busy 30 minute meals. Week Two is an excellent time to start following that meal plan to the letter. The recipes for the meals are also in this book, as well as grocery lists. Please use these tools to your full advantage.

You'll also want to keep monitoring your ketone production using the blood, breath, or urine. Make sure you're not eating that many carbs. Those grams add up quickly.

It's also normal to not feel all that hungry as your body shifts. Just make sure you're getting enough calories and try not to skip meals or try drastic low calorie rations. It's okay to eat this much fat!

The good news is, once you stick to the Macros ratios and keep your grams consistent, it will happen eventually. Your body has this ability to go into ketosis, so keep at it.

The Keto 'Flu'

Since the Ketogenic Diet has become more popular, many dieters on it have talked about what's affectionately nicknamed the Keto Flu. It's not the real flu or influenza, in that there's no virus or bug you caught.

The Keto Flu is a collection of flu-like symptoms many experience after they start this new eating plan. This flu only lasts a few days and shouldn't be enough to call out sick from work or have to miss important appointments. It's simply your body's way of letting you know it's changing metabolic cycles.

When you have the Keto Flu, the first symptom you'll notice will be tiredness. That comes from the switch in metabolism. You also might get a headache and have other mental ailments like difficulty concentrating and brain fog. That's because your brain has been using glycogen for fuel and is now switching to ketones. Your brain requires a massive amount of protein and calories, so it's in essence pulling resources and trying to search for alternative fuel sources. The change in calorie source can also make you irritable, for the same reason being hungry can. You'll also have to urinate more, since your insulin levels are dropping.

While the Keto Flu isn't pleasant while you're experiencing it, count that as a good sign. Your body is effectively switching gears. Within a few days, your body will get the idea that there aren't more glucose or other sugar sources of fuel coming in, and it's time to switch to using the fat stores.

Most people do just fine with this Week Two transition. But, if you're having difficulty with the Keto Flu, read below.

Keto Flu Remedies

Replenishing Electrolytes and Salt

You're losing electrolytes because your insulin levels are dropping. So, slice up some lemons in water and drink that to rehydrate yourself and get those electrolyte levels up again. If the Keto Flu persists, that's a good indication that you're not hydrated enough. Get as much water as you can.

You'll also want to increase your salt intake. Warm up regular sodium (not low sodium) chicken broth or consommé and sip that throughout the day.

Replenishing both your electrolytes and salt will also help with another Keto Flu problem: muscle cramps. Your muscles are also attempting to switch from glycogen as fuel to fat as fuel, and that can cause them to shrink and contract. Muscle cramps might keep you awake at night. Drink as much water as you can and especially water with lemon to make sure you're getting the nutrients you need.

Due to this, you'll find you have to urinate much more frequently! Stay near a bathroom and try not to schedule any long trips or other situations where you can't have access to a restroom.

Bad Breath

Low carbohydrate diets can cause bad breath. It isn't an oral hygiene issue; your digestive system and liver are to blame. It's the ketones your liver emits that are causing the breath, which is why you can measure ketosis through the breath.

To combat this, brush and floss more frequently. Mint is an excellent remedy for bad breath, and chocolate works for some people as well. You can purchase a mint gel or use actual freshly washed mint leaves to rub around the gums and help freshen your breath. Mouth wash can also help. The breath problems do subside after you're fully in ketosis.

The Keto Rash

If your Keto Flu also comes with an overwhelming new sense of itchiness, then you also have the Keto Rash, too. It's a condition that's not dangerous and is called *prurigo pigmentosa*. You may experience some small itchy, raised skin lesions that vary in color between reddish pink to light brown. Yes, they itch. They're not life-threatening, dangerous, or should cause alarm. I just want you to be aware of them. It can increase in intensity from a few spots to a large rash spread over the skin. It does go away after a couple of weeks, and you can use talc-free baby powder to help stop the itch. The ketones are the main cause, so give your body time to adjust to this new diet.

Feast on Good Fats

Increase your fat consumption as well. Make yourself several batches of the Fat Bombs recipes in this book and make sure you're eating plenty of those. Snack on full fat cheeses, nuts, and hard boiled eggs. Track your fat gram Macros.

<u>No Going to the Gym</u>

In addition to eating better and staying hydrated, slow down on your physical activity. It puts a strain on your body to make this transition and exercise at the same time. This is only temporary and just until the Keto Flu symptoms pass away. Then you can return to your favorite high energy workout schedule.

<u>Catch More Zzzzs</u>

Just like when you went through puberty, your body is going through major changes in this early transition period towards ketosis. As a result, you may feel very tired. Some minor insomnia and night time sleeplessness is to be expected. Schedule in an extra nap or two into your day, if you can. Get in plenty of sleep, and that will not only help the Keto Flu symptoms go away, but you'll also feel more refreshed, too.

To help with sleeplessness, try taking a natural sleep aid supplement that has ingredients like Melatonin, valerian root, or chamomile. Eat some turkey just before bed time, which has the tryptophan in it to help lull you to sleep. You can also drink an herbal tea.

Week Two Tips

By week two, you should be fully on your Macros, watching those like a hawk, and keeping track of your grams and percentages. You might feel the Keto Flu symptoms, but stay on the diet.

If you've been sneaking a bit of carbs here and there during this Week Two and are in 'ketosis limbo,' where you're not exactly feeling well but you're not in full ketosis, then there's a good chance your Keto Flu symptoms will stick around longer. Unfortunately, there's no other remedy than to kick those carbs to the curb! This is not a 'cheat day' diet like some others. You really do have to slash your carb count.

Week Three

Congratulations for getting through the first two weeks of the Keto Diet! Those beginning 14 days were going to be some of the toughest, so getting over that is a reason to celebrate. If you did experience the Keto Flu, those symptoms should be starting to subside. If they're not, just read over the list of remedies above and drink as much water with lemon as you can.

This is also a good time to invest in a Keto Breath Monitor or Keto Blood Monitor, if you haven't already done so. The Ketosis Urine Strips only help during the transition. Once you're in ketosis, check your breath or blood every two or three days.

By Week Three, you should also be very familiar with how to count and calculate your Macros in each meal. If you've not started to follow the meal plans in the book, then please do so. Don't make this diet too hard on yourself! Just grocery shop for the ingredients, cook the dishes, and enjoy the new balance of flavors present in each meal.

Weight Loss

For most newbie Keto Dieters, it's really Week Three where they start to see the weight loss. You might even see several pounds come off within these first three weeks. Once your body has gotten the message that it should be in ketosis, that's when the magic happens.

Have fun tracking your weight loss! Set up a calendar with goal weights and rewards. When you've hit five pounds lost, treat yourself to something small. When you reach ten pounds lost, reward yourself again.

Keep up the positive reinforcement, so you have something to look forward to. Don't forget to take "before" and "after" pictures, too. Show off your progress. You deserve it!

Boosting Fat Intake

You've become very familiar with the foods you can and cannot eat! You've probably also gone out to restaurants by now and (hopefully) bypassed all that bread and pasta to go for the Keto approved meals.

Now, it's time to make sure that you're keeping your fat intake nice and high. If the day is passing by and you haven't eaten enough fat grams, then reach for another Fat Bomb, piece of cheese, extra slice of bacon, or a dosage of the MCT oil. It really is that important.

Week Three Tips

With the Keto Flu symptoms under control and ketosis finally achieved by watching your Macros and tracking using a monitor, you're well on your way towards being successful as a Keto Dieter.

The best tip this week is just to follow a meal plan to the letter. You can use the ones in this book, or you can make up your own if you feel confident enough! But make sure it's one that inspires you to stick with it. It's one thing to have a low carb meal plan; it's another to eat those meals each day.

Another excellent Week Three tip is to track your weight loss. That will help inspire you as well!

Week Four

If you weren't out of the Keto Flu last week, this is when those icky symptoms finally disappear. Your body has now successfully transitioned from a carbohydrate metabolic state to a ketosis metabolic state! You've got your Keto Monitor and are making sure you're staying in ketosis. You've also been cooking and eating Keto meals, ordering Keto items in restaurants, and even experienced some initial weight loss, too.

Now, you're going to start seeing all those benefits we've been talking about in this book! Your hard work will start to pay off, and you'll experience:

- Better Mental Clarity
- More Energy – some even call it 'lung bursting' energy!
- More Weight Loss
- Increased Sense of Well Being
- Stabilized Moods
- Stabilized Blood Sugar

The Ketogenic Diet has worked for thousands of people who've struggled through the first three weeks, only to get to Week Four and say, "Okay, now I get it! This is what everyone's been talking about!"

Intermittent Fasting

Once you've gotten the hang of the entire Keto diet lifestyle, you can try intermittent fasting. Intermittent fasting is a great way to jolt your body into ketosis. The meal plans in Chapter 7 provide you with plenty of daily food options. But, you're also encouraged to fast one day a week if you're able to, or skip a meal here and there. While fasting, remember to consume plenty of water and help yourself to a cup of bone broth if you're feeling hungry.

Keto in the Kitchen

While Week Four is full of rewards, it also has one potential pitfall: this diet can get repetitive for people who don't cook or aren't as comfortable cooking. That's perfectly understandable! Cooking can seem like just one more chore to add to your busy life.

But, with YouTube videos, television cooking shows, and a little time to devote to your new hobby, you'll grow to like cooking. Here are tips to have fun being Keto in your own kitchen:

- Watch YouTube videos on how to prepare vegetables, and just start practicing. Learn to slice and dice onions, tomatoes, and other veggies.
- With baking, you have to follow recipes and measure everything exactly.
- But with cooking, you can add a little more seasoning or substitute for an ingredient. There's a lot more leeway.
- Become familiar with your oven's temperature. Some ovens are colder than others, so a dish will take longer to cook.
- Clean as you go! While waiting for a pan to heat up, wipe down the counter. Cooking is much more enjoyable in a clean kitchen.
- Learn what flavors go together. Each cuisine (Italian, Mexican, French, Indian, Thai, etc.) has their own core ingredients.

With a little practice and following the recipes, you'll be making Keto recipes in no time. It gets easier and quicker!

I really like to cook! It makes my house smell good, I like the different sounds of meat sizzling or cheese bubbling, and it's quite a sensory experience. Plus, at the end, you get a delicious meal that makes you lose weight, live healthier, and feel better. What's not to love?

Week Four Tips

Week Four is all about getting past the Keto Flu and turning the corner towards a better future on the Keto Diet. You'll stop feeling deprived of carbs and start feeling great because you're seeing the results.

The best tip this week is to make the recipes, stick to the meal plans, and try new dishes. Treat the Keto Diet as an exploration of new flavors and ingredients that you might not have tried before. The average American diet is pretty bland. The ho-hum ingredients are boosted with sugar and carbs to make them taste better.

But when you choose better ingredients and then put them in improved recipes? That's when you'll start to fall in love with your new eating plan.

So, sit down, buckle in, and enjoy the Keto ride!

Chapter 6:
Proven Tips for Staying in Ketosis

In addition to following your first four weeks on the Ketogenic Diet in the previous chapter, this chapter is all about helping you on this diet. We're going to troubleshoot some frequently stated issues that dieters have had and offer solutions that have worked. So, no matter if you're just starting out and struggling or have been in Keto for six months and need a boost, let's get you back on track and make this a success!

Common Issues with the Ketogenic Diet

Not Getting Into Ketosis

Being stuck in 'ketosis limbo' is no fun, even when you're trying to eat as low carb as possible and following the meal plans in the next chapter. Make sure you're out of ketosis by checking with a Keto Monitor your blood, breath, or urine.

With this issue, it all comes down to numbers. Specifically, your Macros numbers. Track each of your Macros (fats – proteins – carbohydrates) and calculate your grams and percentages every day. Watch your food intake for these three, and write down absolutely everything you eat, including all beverages and serving portions, too.

With this, you'll also watch out for gluconeogenesis, a fancy term for your liver making new sugars and using amino acids for energy rather than ketones. This happens when you're eating too much protein. That's why it's important to track this Macro. Try reducing your protein intake by a couple of grams and measure your ketones again with a Keto Monitor.

Food manufacturers stuff hidden carbs and sugars into so many items. You'll have to keep a diligent eye on food labels and make sure you're not consuming anything you're not supposed to. Even a few extra grams makes a big difference. Try to stay within 30 grams of net carbs a day (give or take a gram or two).

Keep a detailed food diary, calculate your Macros, tweak and refine your diet as needed, and you'll get back into ketosis.

The Difference Between Net Carbs and Full Carbs

Curious about the difference between net carb count and gross carb count?

In order to easily calculate the net carbs in a recipe, subtract the insoluble fiber from the total carbohydrate and total fiber counts. We do this because fiber is technically not a carbohydrate. It's the portion of plant derived food that isn't completely broken down by the digestive enzymes in your stomach and intestines. Insoluble fiber doesn't dissolve in water. It's made of non-starch polysaccharides, which means it's not a starch or a carb.

Next, take a look at the sugar alcohol content. If the total sugar alcohol content exceeds 5 grams, subtract half of that number from the total carb count. That yields your net carbs.

Online nutritional calculators are free, easy to use resources that will help keep your carb count low. If you're not losing weight or staying in ketosis, try calculating your full gross carbs. You might be eating too many. Let your body adapt, and then you can slowly switch back to calculating your net carbs.

Insufficient Fat Intake

We talked previously in this book about how 'fat' doesn't make you fat. But this mindset is so deep in American culture, that it can be difficult to keep buying and eating products with good fats in them. You subconsciously avoid them because you don't want to get fat!

But on the Keto Diet, fat is your number one Macro, and you must consume a lot of it. If you have a concern that fats aren't healthy, refer back to Chapter 4 and re-read the section on good fats / bad fats. To ensure that you're eating the healthiest good fats, stick with the monounsaturated fats instead. This does mean you're cutting out the foods that have incredible flavor and taste, since it's the saturated fat that's the yummiest!

I encourage you to follow the meal plans in the next chapter, because each day gives you plenty of fat grams and satisfies the Keto Diet intake. Keep a food diary and track this Macro, since it's the most important one!

Eating Too Much or Too Often

Just because I heartily encourage you to eat lots of fat grams and a good amount of protein doesn't mean you should go crazy and consume lots of food at once!

I'm of the belief that restaurants have contributed to most Americans not really understanding proper portion and serving sizes. For example, a serving of chicken is 3-4 ounces, the size of a deck of cards. But order a chicken entrée in a restaurant, and they serve at least double that. Oh, and forget about burger sizes! Those are enormous. Portions are just way too big. Watch your serving sizes on the Keto Diet. Eating too much of any one thing, but especially carbs or protein, will keep you out of ketosis.

When you first start on the Keto Diet, you'll be eating the regular 3 meals a day, plus a drink, snack, or dessert. But being in ketosis helps reduce a ravenous appetite, so don't be surprised if you drop back down to just 2 or 2 ½ meals a day. It naturally suppresses your hunger.

Your Body's Carbohydrate Tolerance

The reason the Macros percentages are approximate, is because everybody has a slightly different carbohydrate tolerance. You might be doing the Keto Diet with a friend and notice he or she is able to eat 10 more grams of carbs than you and still lose weight. Consuming lots of carbohydrates also has resulted in metabolic damage to the body, but that exists in varying degrees. Your friend could have less damage and a better tolerance than you, or vice versa.

The good news is, the longer you're keeping your body in a ketosis state, the more it adapts to such a low carb diet. You might even find you can sneak in an extra gram or two of carbohydrates and still stay in ketosis. However, don't cheat for at least your first two months. Give your body time to fully adapt.

Why Aren't I Losing Weight?

Yes, it can be frustrating to pass up on all those carby, sugary treats you used to eat all the time, and the numbers on the scale aren't budging! It's a slippery slope towards feeling deprived, which then can cause you to throw up your hands and make a beeline for the nearest piece of bread. Stop!

Consider this for a moment. Your body could actually be in perfect balance. The energy you're consuming is on one side of the scale and the energy you're expending is on the other side. If those two numbers equal each other, that means no weight loss. You will gain the health benefits in this equalized state. To increase weight loss, try a little bit of exercise (but only after your Keto Flu symptoms have gone away). A few daily walks around the block could be all it takes to tip the scale in your favor.

You may not be fully in ketosis, either. Check with one of the Keto Monitors to be sure. If you're still experiencing the Keto Flu, that's the culprit. Return to diligently tracking your Macros.

Help! My Cholesterol is Out of Whack!

So, you've been to the doctor, they've done their tests, and now they've told you that both your HDL and LDL cholesterol levels have risen considerably. No cause for alarm! About one third of Keto Dieters experience this.

However, cholesterol is actually used by the body as a substance for repair and healing, similar to protein. It's a general handyman. So, when your LDL cholesterol levels rise, that could be a response to more repair going on in your body. That's a good thing! Your body is now working to repair the metabolic damage from eating too many carbohydrates.

So, not to worry about cholesterol levels. It doesn't mean plaque is building up in your arteries or your organs are at risk. It just indicates your LDL cholesterol 'handy men' are hard at work fixing you.

The Keto Lifestyle

If you fall out of ketosis, it isn't the end of the world. You can return to tracking your Macros, saying no to carbs and sugars, and reaching for more healthy fats at any time.

You've now been fully prepped and informed about what it takes to make the Keto Diet a success. It's more of a lifestyle, in that you'll be spending each day preparing and eating a whole new way. The Keto Diet favors those who stick with it over a long period of time. Your body will become more and more adapted, you'll lose weight, you'll feel better, and you'll be healthier, too.

Now, it's time to give you one of the most helpful tools in this book: a meal plan. In the next chapter, you'll get 8 weeks of meals, split into two different meal plans. That's 56 days of Keto Diet eating!

I want nothing but success for you on this health journey.

Chapter 7:
The 4 Week Meal Plans

Having these two excellent meal plans in this chapter ensures your success on the Ketogenic Diet. You get two plans, each for four weeks:

1. Basic Meal Plan – Four weeks of breakfast, lunch, snack, dinner, and dessert options.
2. 30-Minute Meal Plan – Four weeks of quick meals for busy families and households. Food on the table in 30 minutes or less!

You'll see some recipe overlap between the two meal plans. Both are entirely Ketogenic Diet friendly. Please see the Appendix for the grocery lists for both meal plans, split into two-week intervals to make it easier and cheaper for shopping.

The Basic Meal Plan will help you as you begin your journey into the Keto lifestyle! Each day includes three meals plus one snack, dessert, or drink. Each recipe lists the calories and Macros, plus totals them up. The meal plan is based on a daily intake of 1500 to 2,000 calories (give or take 100 calories) and an approximate Macro ratio of 70% to 80% fat, 10% to 20% protein, and 5% to 10% carbohydrates.

4-Week Basic Meal Plan

Week 1 Meal Plan				
Day	Breakfast	Lunch	Dinner	Snack/Dessert	Calories/Macros
1	Strawberry Cow Smoothie 301 cal 28.6 g fat 2.8 g protein 9 g carbs	Cilantro Lime Shrimp and Avocado Salad 529 cal 35.6 g fat 26 g protein 5 g carbs	Spinach Stuffed Cod 407 cal 13.7 g fat 65.6 g protein 1 g carbs	Seed Crackers & Guacamole 280 cal 24 g fat 8 g protein 3 g carbs	Calories: 1517 Fat: 101.9 g Protein: 82.4 g Net Carbs: 18 g

2	Coconut Macadamia Smoothie Bowl 362 cal 33.5 g fat 3.2 g protein 8 g carbs	Cream of Leek Soup with Seed Crackers 175 cal 14.5 g fat 4.3 g protein 3 g carbs	Roast Chicken (1 serving) with Butter Tossed Asparagus 280 cal 30 g fat 14 g protein 3 g carbs	Almond Butter Fat Bombs (2) 378 cal 38.2 g fat 6.4 g protein 2.8 g carbs	Calories: 1195 Fat: 116.2 g Protein: 31.1 g Net Carbs: 18.2 g
3	Almond Butter Smoothie 483 cal 34.6 g fat 5.5 g protein 4 g carbs	Chicken Salad 367 cal 25 g fat 34 g protein 2 g carbs	Beef Fajita Bowl 360 cal 12 g fat 48 g protein 11 g carbs	Nordic Seed Bread 369 cal 31.5 g fat 10 g protein 5 g carbs	Calories: 1579 Fat: 103.1 g Protein: 85.5 g Net Carbs: 22 g
4	Keto Eggs Benedict with Quick Hollandaise Sauce 757 cal 68 g fat 35 g protein 5 g carbs	Asian Salad with Asian Nut Dressing 579 cal 55.4 g fat 5 g protein 9 g carbs	Chicken Avocado Pesto Pasta 440 cal 40 g fat 36 g protein 3 g carbs	Almond Butter Fat Bomb 189 cal 19.1 g fat 3.2 g protein 1.4 g carbs	Calories: 1965 Fat: 182.5 g Protein: 79.2 g Net Carbs: 18.4 g
5	Beef Frittata (from leftover Beef Fajita Bowl) 584 cal 42 g fat 39 g protein 9.7 g carbs	Avocado and Chicken Salad 663 cal 55 g fat 28 g protein 6 g carbs	Pork Chops with Green Bean Fries 481 cal 37 g fat 39 g protein 2 g carbs	Celery and Almond Butter 230 cal 18 g fat 8 g protein 4 g carbs	Calories: 1958 Fat: 152 g Protein: 114 g Net Carbs: 21.7 g

6	Avocado Pesto Eggs 404 cal 37 g fat 4 g protein 4.6 g carbs	Pork Chopped Salad 681 cal 57.9 g fat 29 g protein 9 g carbs	Greek Lamb Burger 542 cal 40 g fat 36 g protein 5 g carbs	Chocolate Smoothie 575 cal 44 g fat 34 g protein 3 g carbs	Calories: 2202 Fat: 178.9 g Protein: 103 g Net Carbs: 21.6 g
7	Vanilla Smoothie 669 cal 70.8 g fat 5.5 g protein 4 g carbs	Lettuce Wrapped Lamb Burgers 513 cal 37 g fat 34 g protein 9 g carbs	Thai Chicken Coconut Red Curry 310 cal 26 g fat 14 g protein 7 g carbs	Raspberry Chia Pudding 642 cal 50 g fat 15.9 g protein 8 g carbs	Calories: 2134 Fat: 183.8 g Protein: 69.4 g Net Carbs: 28 g

		Week 2 Meal Plan			
Day	Breakfast	Lunch	Dinner	Snack/Dessert	Calories/Macros
8	2 Eggs (any style) and 2 strips of Bacon with Bulletproof Coffee 585 cal 56.5 g fat 21 g protein 3 g carbs	Cream of Mushroom Soup 222 cal 15.6 g fat 7.8 g protein 11 g carbs	Lamb Chops with Buttery Mustard Sauce 429 cal 27 g fat 25 g protein 9 g carbs	Seed Crackers & Guacamole 280 cal 24 g fat 8 g protein 3 g carbs	Calories: 1516 Fat: 123.1 g Protein: 61.8 g Net Carbs: 26 g
9	Pink Power Smoothie 310 cal 29.9 g fat 3.8 g protein 9 g carbs	Lemon Thyme Salmon Salad with Lemon Thyme Vinaigrette 402 cal 21.1 g fat 41.7 g protein 9.1 g carbs	Indian Butter Chicken with Roasted Cauliflower 592 cal 52 g fat 24 g protein 6 g carbs	Nordic Seed Bread 369 cal 31.5 g fat 10 g protein 5 g carbs	Calories: 1673 Fat: 134.5 g Protein: 79.5 g Net Carbs: 29.1g
10	Breakfast Sausages 326 cal 28 g fat 19 g protein 0 g carbs	Creamy Tomato Soup 135 cal 10.1 g fat 2.5 g protein 6 g carbs	Goat Cheese Stuffed Chicken Breasts 646 cal 44.5 g fat 55.9 g protein 3 g carbs	Raspberry Chocolate Fudge 74 cal 8.1 g fat 0.6 g protein 0.9 g carbs	Calories: 1181 Fat: 90.7 g Protein: 78 g Net Carbs: 9.9 g

11	Mushroom and Bacon Skillet 591 cal 47.7 g fat 36 g protein 3 g carbs	Italian Chopped Salad 469 cal 44 g fat 14 g protein 4 g carbs	Beef Stuffed Tomatoes 350 cal 15.5 g fat 36 g protein 5 g carbs	Mediterranean Fat Bomb 155 cal 15 g fat 3 g protein 1.2 g carbs	Calories: 1565 Fat: 122.2 g Protein: 89 g Net Carbs: 13.2 g
12	Coconut Macadamia Smoothie Bowl 362 cal 33.5 g fat 3.2 g protein 8 g carbs	Baja Style Halibut Salad 740 cal 40 g fat 95 g protein 7 g carbs	Baked Eggs with Kale and Tomato 187 cal 15.3 g fat 9 g protein 3 g carbs	Vanilla Smoothie 669 cal 70.8 g fat 5.5 g protein 4 g carbs	Calories: 1958 Fat: 159.6 g Protein: 112.7 g Net Carbs: 22 g
13	Bell Pepper Eggs 298 cal 26.2 g fat 11.9 g protein 4 g carbs	Kale Salad 322 cal 30.9 g fat 2.9 g protein 9 g carbs	Fish Tacos 740 cal 40 g fat 95 g protein 7 g carbs	Salted Macadamias 224 cal 22 g fat 3 g protein 1 g carbs	Calories: 1584 Fat: 119.1 g Protein: 112.8 g Net Carbs: 21 g
14	Breakfast Beef Skillet 705 cal 58.7 g fat 36.4 g protein 4 g carbs	Nicoise Salad 273 cal 20 g fat 23 g protein 2 g carbs	Jerk Chicken 524 cal 33.9 g fat 44 g protein 5 g carbs	Cheesy Fondue 376 cal 32 g fat 19.5 g protein 4.4 g carbs	Calories: 1878 Fat: 144.6 g Protein: 122.9 g Net Carbs: 15.4 g

		Week 3 Meal Plan			
Day	Breakfast	Lunch	Dinner	Snack/Dessert	Calories/Macros
15	Caprese Omelet 393 cal 35.9 g fat 11.3 g protein 6 g carbs	Leftover Jerk Chicken 524 cal 33.9 g fat 44 g protein 5 g carbs	Beef Kababs 219 cal 15.7 g fat 16 g protein 2 g carbs	Strawberry Chia Pudding Popsicles 277 cal 24.9 g fat 5 g protein 3 g carbs	Calories: 1413 Fat: 110.4 g Protein: 76.3 g Net Carbs: 16 g
16	Cream Cheese and Herb Pancakes with Smoked Salmon and Dill 417 cal 35.8 g fat 20 g protein 3 g carbs	Steak and Avocado Salad with Cilantro Lime Dressing 663 cal 44 g fat 50 g protein 7 g carbs	Thai Chicken Coconut Red Curry 310 cal 26 g fat 14 g protein 7 g carbs	Golden Milk Smoothie 460 cal 25.3 g fat 1.7 g protein 1.4 g carbs	Calories: 1850 Fat: 131.1 g Protein: 85.7 g Net Carbs: 18.4 g
17	Cuban Frittata 282 cal 21.6 g fat 17.7 g protein 3 g carbs	Avocado and Chicken Salad 663 cal 55 g fat 28 g protein 6 g carbs	Beef Stew 450 cal 30.4 g fat 35 g protein 4.5 g carbs	Nordic Seed Bread 369 cal 31.5 g fat 10 g protein 5 g carbs	Calories: 1764 Fat: 138.5 g Protein: 90.7 g Net Carbs: 18.5 g

18	Nordic Seed Bread Breakfast Sandwich 434 cal 40 g fat 32 g protein 4 g carbs	Warm Zucchini and Goat Cheese Salad 395 cal 35.5 g fat 14.8 g protein 6 g carbs	Parmesan Crusted Halibut 266 cal 14.8 g fat 30 g protein 1.2 g carbs	Almond Butter Cookies 98 cal 10 g fat 4 g protein 1.4 g carbs	Calories: 1193 Fat: 115.5 g Protein: 80.8 g Net Carbs: 12.6 g
19	Scotch Eggs 442 cal 46 g fat 25 g protein 0 g carbs	Creamy Cauliflower and Seafood Chowder 540 cal 52 g fat 28 g protein 7 g carbs	Chicken Kababs 270 cal 17.2 g fat 25 g protein 2 g carbs	Tahini Sauce with Veggies 555 cal 58.5 g fat 4 g protein 8 g carbs	Calories: 1807 Fat: 173.7 g Protein: 82 g Net Carbs: 17 g
20	Strawberry Cow Smoothie 301 cal 28.6 g fat 2.8 g protein 9 g carbs	Scallop and Mushroom Salad with Goat Cheese Vinaigrette 498 cal 38.8 g fat 32.7 g protein 4.4 g carbs	Beef Vindaloo 436 cal 30.4 g fat 35 g protein 3.5 g carbs	Seed Crackers and Guacamole 280 cal 24 g fat 8 g protein 3 g carbs	Calories: 1515 Fat: 121.8 g Protein: 78.5 g Net Carbs: 19.9 g
21	Cream Cheese and Lox Omelet 731 cal 61.9 g fat 40.9 g protein 3.5 g carbs	Cream of Mushroom Soup 222 cal 15.6 g fat 7.8 g protein 11 g carbs	Chicken Avocado Pesto Pasta 440 cal 40 g fat 36 g protein 3 g carbs	Raspberry Chia Pudding 642 cal 50 g fat 15.9 g protein 8 g carbs	Calories: 2035 Fat: 167.5 g Protein: 100.6 g Net Carbs: 25.5 g

			Week 4 Meal Plan		
Day	Breakfast	Lunch	Dinner	Snack/Dessert	Calories/Macros
22	2 Eggs (any style), 2 Strips of Bacon, and Bulletproof Coffee 585 cal 56.5 g fat 21 g protein 3 g carbs	Chicken Kale Wrap 415 cal 32.1 g fat 26.3 g protein 5.3 g carbs	Thai Coconut Cod 482 cal 34 g fat 42.5 g protein 5 g carbs	Almond Butter Fat Bomb 189 cal 19.1 g fat 3.2 g protein 1.4 g carbs	Calories: 1671 Fat: 141.7 g Protein: 93 g Net Carbs: 14.7 g
23	Almond Butter Smoothie 300 cal 31 g fat 7 g protein 4 g carbs	Thai Coconut Cod Lettuce Wraps 592 cal 46 g fat 35 g protein 6 g carbs	Cheese Stuffed Burgers 681 cal 44.7 g fat 63.1 g protein 3.7 g carbs	Green Bean Fries 113 cal 6 g fat 9 g protein 2 g carbs	Calories: 1686 Fat: 127.7 g Protein: 114.1 g Net Carbs: 15.7 g
24	Mushroom and Goat Cheese Omelet 818 cal 74.1 g fat 35.8 g protein 3 g carbs	Kale Salad 322 cal 30.9 g fat 2.9 g protein 9 g carbs	Keto Chinese Beef and Broccoli 273 cal 17 g fat 24 g protein 3 g carbs	Chocolate Smoothie 575 cal 44 g fat 34 g protein 3 g carbs	Calories: 1988 Fat: 166 g Protein: 96.7 g Net Carbs: 18 g

25	Avocado Breakfast Sandwich 698 cal 61 g fat 24.1 g protein 5.5 g carbs	Creamy Tomato Soup 135 cal 10.1 g fat 2.5 g protein 6 g carbs	Sea Bass with Prosciutto and Herbs 586 cal 16.2 g fat 40 g protein 6 g carbs	Almond Butter Cookies 98 cal 10 g fat 4 g protein 1.4 g carbs	Calories: 1517 Fat: 97.3 g Protein: 70.6 g Net Carbs: 18.9 g
26	Pink Power Smoothie 310 cal 29.9 g fat 3.8 g protein 9 g carbs	Steak and Avocado Salad 663 cal 44 g fat 50 g protein 7 g carbs	Goat Cheese Stuffed Chicken Breasts 646 cal 44.5 g fat 55.9 g protein 3 g carbs	Celery and Almond Butter 230 cal 18 g fat 8 g protein 4 g carbs	Calories: 1849 Fat: 136.4 g Protein: 117.7 g Net Carbs: 23 g
27	Bell Pepper Eggs 298 cal 26.2 g fat 11.9 g protein 4 g carbs	Leftover Goat Cheese Chicken Breasts 646 cal 44.5 g fat 55.9 g protein 3 g carbs	Steak and Avocado Taco Cups 650 cal 53 g fat 40 g protein 6 g carbs	Veggies with Spicy Mayo 90 cal 10 g fat 0 g protein 0 g carbs	Calories: 1684 Fat: 133.7 g Protein: 107.8 g Net Carbs: 13 g
28	Chocolate Smoothie 575 cal 44 g fat 34 g protein 3 g carbs	Cream of Leek Soup 175 cal 14.5 g fat 4.3 g protein 3 g carbs	Chicken Avocado Pesto Pasta 440 cal 40 g fat 36 g protein 3 g carbs	Nordic Seed Bread 369 cal 31.5 g fat 10 g protein 5 g carbs	Calories: 1559 Fat: 130 g Protein: 84.3 g Net Carbs: 14 g

Busy households will definitely appreciate the 30 minute fast meal plan. This is excellent for Keto dieters with a family, a demanding job, or when it's summer and too hot to cook in the kitchen!

4-Week Fast Meal Plan With 30-Minute Meals

			Week 1 Meal Plan		
Day	Breakfast	Lunch	Dinner	Snack/Dessert	Calories/Macros
1	Strawberry Cow Smoothie 301 cal 28.6 g fat 2.8 g protein 9 g carbs	Cilantro Lime Shrimp and Avocado Salad 529 cal 35.6 g fat 26 g protein 5 g carbs	Beef Stuffed Tomatoes 350 cal 15.5 g fat 36 g protein 5 g carbs	Almond Butter Fat Bomb 189 cal 19.1 g fat 3.2 g protein 1.4 g carbs	Calories: 1369 Fat: 98.8 g Protein: 68 g Net Carbs: 20.4 g
2	Coconut Macadamia Smoothie Bowl 362 cal 33.5 g fat 3.2 g protein 8 g carbs	Cream of Mushroom Soup 222 cal 15.6 g fat 7.8 g protein 11 g carbs	Beef Fajita Bowl 360 cal 12 g fat 48 g protein 11 g carbs	Mediterranean Fat Bomb 155 cal 15 g fat 3 g protein 1.2 g carbs	Calories: 1099 Fat: 76.1 g Protein: 62 g Net Carbs: 29 g
3	Almond Butter Smoothie 300 cal 31 g fat 7 g protein 4 g carbs	Beef Fajita Lettuce Wraps 513 cal 37 g fat 34 g protein 9 g carbs	Chicken Avocado Pesto Pasta 440 cal 40 g fat 36 g protein 3 g carbs	Veggies and Green Tahini 43 cal 3.9 g fat 0.7 g protein 0.3 g carbs	Calories: 1296 Fat: 111.9 g Protein: 77.7 g Net Carbs: 16.3 g

4	Beef Frittata 584 cal 42 g fat 39 g protein 9.7 g carbs	Asian Salad with Asian Nut Dressing 579 cal 55.4 g fat 5 g protein 9 g carbs	Greek Lamb Burger 542 cal 40 g fat 36 g protein 5 g carbs	Chocolate Smoothie 575 cal 44 g fat 34 g protein 3 g carbs	Calories: 2280 Fat: 181.4 g Protein: 114 g Net Carbs: 26.7 g
5	Vanilla Smoothie 669 cal 70.8 g fat 5.5 g protein 4 g carbs	Avocado and Chicken Salad 663 cal 55 g fat 28 g protein 6 g carbs	Cod Bruschetta 341 cal 18.2 g fat 28.4 g protein 3.5 g carbs	Raspberry Chia Pudding 642 cal 50 g fat 15.9 g protein 8 g carbs	Calories: 2315 Fat: 194 g Protein: 77.8 g Net Carbs: 21.5 g
6	2 Eggs (any style) and 2 Strips of Bacon with Bulletproof Coffee 585 cal 56.5 g fat 21 g protein 3 g carbs	Lettuce Wrapped Lamb Burgers 513 cal 37 g fat 34 g protein 9 g carbs	Thai Chicken Coconut Red Curry 310 cal 26 g fat 14 g protein 7 g carbs	Chocolate Smoothie 575 cal 44 g fat 34 g protein 3 g carbs	Calories: 1983 Fat: 163.5 g Protein: 103 g Net Carbs: 22 g
7	Pink Power Smoothie 310 cal 29.9 g fat 3.8 g protein 9 g carbs	Lemon Thyme Salmon Salad with Lemon Thyme Vinaigrette 402 cal 21.1 g fat 41.7 g protein 9.1 g carbs	Mushroom and Bacon Skillet 591 cal 47.7 g fat 36 g protein 3 g carbs	Celery and Almond Butter 230 cal 18 g fat 8 g protein 4 g carbs	Calories: 1533 Fat: 116.7 g Protein: 89.5 g Net Carbs: 25.1 g

		Week 2 Meal Plan			
Day	Breakfast	Lunch	Dinner	Snack/Dessert	Calories/Macros
8	Caprese Omelet 393 cal 35.9 g fat 11.3 g protein 6 g carbs	Nicoise Salad 273 cal 20 g fat 23 g protein 2 g carbs	Beef Stuffed Tomatoes 350 cal 15.5 g fat 36 g protein 5 g carbs	Raspberry Chocolate Fudge 74 cal 8.1 g fat 0.6 g protein 0.9 g carbs	Calories: 1090 Fat: 79.5 g Protein: 70.9 g Net Carbs: 13.9 g
9	Breakfast Sausages 326 cal 28 g fat 19 g protein 0 g carbs	Baja Style Halibut Salad 740 cal 40 g fat 95 g protein 7 g carbs	Keto Chinese Beef and Broccoli 273 cal 17 g fat 24 g protein 3 g carbs	Golden Milk Smoothie 460 cal 25.3 g fat 1.7 g protein 1.4 g carbs	Calories: 1799 Fat: 110.3 g Protein: 109.7 g Net Carbs: 11.4 g
10	Cream Cheese and Herb Pancakes with Smoked Salmon and Dill 417 cal 35.8 g fat 20 g protein 3 g carbs	Egg Salad 242 cal 18.6 g fat 11.4 g protein 8 g carbs	Fish Tacos 740 cal 40 g fat 95 g protein 7 g carbs	Salted Macadamias 224 cal 22 g fat 3 g protein 1 g carbs	Calories: 1623 Fat: 116.4 g Protein: 99.4 g Net Carbs: 19 g

11	Bell Pepper Eggs 298 cal 26.2 g fat 11.9 g protein 4 g carbs	Kale Salad 322 cal 30.9 g fat 2.9 g protein 9 g carbs	Lamb Chops with Buttery Mustard Sauce 429 cal 27 g fat 25 g protein 9 g carbs	Vanilla Smoothie 669 cal 70.8 g fat 5.5 g protein 4 g carbs	Calories: 1718 Fat: 154.9 g Protein: 45.3 g Net Carbs: 26 g
12	Lemon Cream Pancakes 351 cal 30.3 g fat 6.7 g protein 4 g carbs	Leftover Lamb Chops 429 cal 27 g fat 25 g protein 9 g carbs	Steak and Avocado Salad 663 cal 44 g fat 50 g protein 7 g carbs	Raspberry Chia Pudding 642 cal 50 g fat 15.9 g protein 8 g carbs	Calories: 2085 Fat: 151.3 g Protein: 97.6 g Net Carbs: 28 g
13	Coconut Macadamia Smoothie Bowl 362 cal 33.5 g fat 3.2 g protein 8 g carbs	Cream of Mushroom Soup 222 cal 15.6 g fat 7.8 g protein 11 g carbs	Steak and Avocado Taco Cups 650 cal 53 g fat 40 g protein 6 g carbs	Chocolate Smoothie 575 cal 44 g fat 34 g protein 3 g carbs	Calories: 1809 Fat: 146.1 g Protein: 85 g Net Carbs: 28 g
14	Avocado Breakfast Sandwich 698 cal 61 g fat 24.1 g protein 5.5 g carbs	Italian Chopped Salad 469 cal 44 g fat 14 g protein 4 g carbs	Thai Coconut Cod 482 cal 34 g fat 42.5 g protein 5 g carbs	Almond Butter Fat Bomb 189 cal 19.1 g fat 3.2 g protein 1.4 g carbs	Calories: 1838 Fat: 158.1 g Protein: 83.8 g Net Carbs: 15.9 g

		Week 3 Meal Plan			
Day	Breakfast	Lunch	Dinner	Snack/Dessert	Calories/Macros
15	Keto Breakfast Bowl 489 cal 35 g fat 29 g protein 4 g carbs	Thai Coconut Cod Lettuce Wraps 592 cal 46 g fat 35 g protein 6 g carbs	Chicken Avocado Pesto Pasta 440 cal 40 g fat 36 g protein 3 g carbs	Almond Butter Smoothie 300 cal 31 g fat 7 g protein 4 g carbs	Calories: 1821 Fat: 152 g Protein: 107 g Net Carbs: 17 g
16	Avocado Pesto Eggs 404 cal 37 g fat 4 g protein 4.6 g carbs	Lemon Thyme Salmon Salad with Lemon Thyme Vinaigrette 402 cal 21.1 g fat 41.7 g protein 9.1 g carbs	Beef Fajita Bowl 360 cal 12 g fat 48 g protein 11 g carbs	Almond Butter Cookies 98 cal 10 g fat 4 g protein 1.4 g carbs	Calories: 1264 Fat: 97.7 g Protein: 80.1 g Net Carbs: 26.1 g
17	Scotch Eggs 442 cal 46 g fat 25 g protein 0 g carbs	Beef Fajita Lettuce Wraps 513 cal 37 g fat 34 g protein 9 g carbs	Thai Chicken Coconut Red Curry 310 cal 26 g fat 14 g protein 7 g carbs	Strawberry Cow Smoothie 301 cal 28.6 g fat 2.8 g protein 9 g carbs	Calories: 1566 Fat: 137.6 g Protein: 75.8 g Net Carbs: 25 g

18	Coconut Porridge 400 cal 39 g fat 13 g protein 5 g carbs	Kale Salad 322 cal 30.9 g fat 2.9 g protein 9 g carbs	Mushroom and Goat Cheese Omelet 818 cal 74.1 g fat 35.8 g protein 3 g carbs	Chocolate Smoothie 575 cal 44 g fat 34 g protein 3 g carbs	Calories: 2115 Fat: 188 g Protein: 85.7 g Net Carbs: 20 g
19	Baked Eggs with Kale and Tomato 187 cal 15.3 g fat 9 g protein 3 g carbs	Italian Chopped Salad 469 cal 44 g fat 14 g protein 4 g carbs	Crab Stuffed Avocado 319 cal 25.7 g fat 9.4 g protein 6 g carbs	Mediterranean Fat Bomb 155 cal 15 g fat 3 g protein 1.2 g carbs	Calories: 1130 Fat: 100 g Protein: 35.4 g Net Carbs: 14.2 g
20	Cuban Frittata 282 cal 21.6 g fat 17.7 g protein 3 g carbs	Nicoise Salad 273 cal 20 g fat 23 g protein 2 g carbs	Greek Lamb Burger 542 cal 40 g fat 36 g protein 5 g carbs	Veggies with Tahini Sauce 555 cal 58.5 g fat 4 g protein 8 g carbs	Calories: 1652 Fat: 140.1 g Protein: 80.7 g Net Carbs: 18 g
21	Vanilla Smoothie 669 cal 70.8 g fat 5.5 g protein 4 g carbs	Lettuce Wrapped Lamb Burger 513 cal 37 g fat 34 g protein 9 g carbs	Mushroom and Bacon Skillet 591 cal 47.7 g fat 36 g protein 3 g carbs	Green Bean Fries 113 cal 6 g fat 9 g protein 2 g carbs	Calories: 1886 Fat: 161.5 g Protein: 84.5 g Net Carbs: 18 g

Day	Breakfast	Lunch	Dinner	Snack/Dessert	Calories/Macros
			Week 4 Meal Plan		
22	2 Eggs (any style), 2 strips of Bacon, and Bulletproof Coffee 585 cal 56.5 g fat 21 g protein 3 g carbs	Green Salad with Green Goddess Dressing 316 cal 32 g fat 2 g protein 2 g carbs	Thai Coconut Cod 482 cal 34 g fat 42.5 g protein 5 g carbs	Golden Milk Smoothie 460 cal 25.3 g fat 1.7 g protein 1.4 g carbs	Calories: 1843 Fat: 147.8 g Protein: 67.2 g Net Carbs: 11.4 g
23	Caprese Omelet 393 cal 35.9 g fat 11.3 g protein 6 g carbs	Thai Coconut Cod Lettuce Wraps 482 cal 34 g fat 42.5 g protein 5 g carbs	Beef Stuffed Tomatoes 350 cal 15.5 g fat 36 g protein 5 g carbs	Raspberry Chocolate Fudge 74 cal 8.1 g fat 0.6 g protein 0.9 g carbs	Calories: 1299 Fat: 106.5 g Protein: 90.4 g Net Carbs: 16.9 g
24	Baked Eggs with Kale and Tomato 187 cal 15.3 g fat 9 g protein 3 g carbs	Cilantro Lime Shrimp and Avocado Salad 529 cal 35.6 g fat 26 g protein 5 g carbs	Thai Chicken Coconut Red Curry 310 cal 26 g fat 14 g protein 7 g carbs	Celery and Almond Butter 230 cal 18 g fat 8 g protein 4 g carbs	Calories: 1256 Fat: 94.9 g Protein: 57 g Net Carbs: 19 g

25	Coconut Porridge 400 cal 39 g fat 13 g protein 5 g carbs	Avocado and Chicken Salad 663 cal 55 g fat 28 g protein 6 g carbs	Cod Bruschetta 341 cal 18.2 g fat 28.4 g protein 3.5 g carbs	Chocolate Smoothie 575 cal 44 g fat 34 g protein 3 g carbs	Calories: 1979 Fat: 101.75 g Protein: 83.4 g Net Carbs: 17.5 g
26	Scotch Eggs 442 cal 46 g fat 25 g protein 0 g carbs	Italian Chopped Salad 469 cal 44 g fat 14 g protein 4 g carbs	Keto Chinese Beef and Broccoli 273 cal 17 g fat 24 g protein 3 g carbs	Almond Butter Fat Bomb 189 cal 19.1 g fat 3.2 g protein 1.4 g carbs	Calories: 1373 Fat: 126.1 g Protein: 66.2 g Net Carbs: 8.4 g
27	Almond Butter Smoothie 300 cal 31 g fat 7 g protein 4 g carbs	Crab Stuffed Cucumbers 179 cal 17.4 g fat 3.1 g protein 3 g carbs	Chicken Avocado Pesto Pasta 440 cal 40 g fat 36 g protein 3 g carbs	Salted Macadamias 224 cal 22 g fat 3 g protein 1 g carbs	Calories: 1143 Fat: 110.4 g Protein: 49.1 g Net Carbs: 11 g
28	Lemon Cream Pancakes 351 cal 30.3 g fat 6.7 g protein 4 g carbs	Kale Salad 322 cal 30.9 g fat 2.9 g protein 9 g carbs	Lamb Chops with Buttery Mustard Sauce 429 cal 27 g fat 25 g protein 9 g carbs	Strawberry Cow Smoothie 301 cal 28.6 g fat 2.8 g protein 9 g carbs	Calories: 1403 Fat: 116.8 g Protein: 37.4 g Net Carbs: 29 g

Chapter 8:
K For Keto Recipes

After looking at the meal plans in the previous chapter, I hope you're excited to get cooking! In this chapter, you'll see the following seven sections:

- Breakfast
- Soups and Salads
- Pork and Poultry
- Beef and Lamb
- Seafood
- Desserts and Drinks
- Snacks and Sides

There are over 100 recipes here to inspire you. Think of these as launch points for your brand new Ketogenic adventure. Have fun with them, experiment with them, and make them your own.

Bon Appetit!

Breakfast

Keto Breakfast Bowl

Protein and flavor packed, this breakfast bowl will keep you full and satisfied for hours! It's really good for you and really delicious, too.

Serving: 1

Serving Size: whole recipe

Prep Time: 5 minutes

Cook Time: 5 minutes

Ingredients

> 2 eggs
>
> 50 g smoked salmon
>
> 1/2 avocado
>
> 2 cups kale
>
> 1 teaspoon olive oil

1 teaspoon coconut oil

Instructions

Start by chopping and washing the kale. Heat up a pan on medium heat with a little bit of olive oil and add the kale for about 5 minutes. While the kale is sautéing prepare the eggs the way you like them (scrambled, sunny side up, fried, etc..). Lastly slice up half an avocado and measure out 50 grams of smoked salmon. Once everything is ready combine in a wide bowl and enjoy.

Nutrition: 489 calories, 35g fat, 29g protein, 4g net carbs

Coconut Porridge

This porridge has a great consistency, and comes together very easily.

Serving: 2

Serving Size: 1 cup

Prep Time: 5 minutes

Cook Time: 10 minutes

Ingredients

¼ cup coconut flour

¼ cup ground flax

1 egg, beaten

1 ½ cups water

1 Tablespoon butter

2 Tablespoons heavy cream

1 Tablespoon Stevia

Instructions

Mix together the water, coconut flour and flax in a medium sized saucepan. Turn the heat on to high, and bring to a boil. Reduce heat to low, and simmer until it begins to thicken, about 5 minutes. Beat in the egg until smooth. Add in the butter, cream and sweetener right away, and stir until smooth.

Nutrition: 400 calories, 39 g fat, 13 g protein, 5 g net carbs

Coconut Macadamia Smoothie Bowl

This satisfying smoothie is a great snack or breakfast option! The creamy, crunchy macadamia nuts go really well with the smooth coconut milk, giving this bowl lots of great texture and flavor!

Serving: 1

Serving Size: whole recipe

Prep Time: 10 minutes

Cook Time: 0 minutes

Ingredients

> ½ cup coconut milk
>
> 1 teaspoon Stevia
>
> ¼ cup macadamia nuts
>
> 1 Tablespoon coconut flakes
>
> ¼ teaspoon salt
>
> 1 teaspoon cinnamon

Instructions

Whisk together the coconut cream, coconut milk, Stevia, salt and cinnamon. Spoon the mixture into a bowl, and top with the macadamia nuts and coconut flakes. Serve immediately, or keep in the fridge for up to a day.

> Nutrition: 362 calories, 33.5 g fat, 3.2 g protein, 8g net carbs

Caprese Omelet

Try this yummy omelet with a side of hash browns or sausage! This is a basic omelet recipe you can dress up with all kinds of Keto friendly ingredients: spinach and feta, mushroom and sausage, bacon and onion, Mexican salsa, etc. Have fun in the kitchen.

Serving: 2

Serving Size: half recipe

Prep Time: 5 minutes

Cook Time: 10 minutes

Ingredients

> 3 eggs
>
> ¼ cup butter
>
> ¼ cup heavy cream
>
> ¼ cup mozzarella, shredded
>
> 2 Tablespoons parmesan
>
> 4 cherry tomatoes, sliced in half
>
> Handful basil, chopped roughly

Instructions

Whisk together the eggs and cream. Season with salt and pepper. Preheat a medium pan over medium high heat, and melt the butter. Pour in the egg mixture, and let cook 3-4 minutes. Gently flip, cooking the other side.

Top with the cheeses, tomato and basil, and gently fold. Cook another 3-4 minutes. Cut in half. Serve immediately.

Nutrition: 393 calories, 35.9 g fat, 11.3 g protein, 6 g net carbs

Mushroom and Goat Cheese Omelet

Such a yummy classic French recipe! You can add some sliced shallots and a sprinkle of light shredded cheddar if you have it, too.

Serving: 2

Serving Size: Half Omelet

Prep Time: 5 minutes

Cook Time:10 minutes

Ingredients

6 eggs

½ cup mushrooms, sliced

¼ lb goat cheese

2 Tablespoons butter

1 Tablespoon olive oil

1 cup heavy cream

Instructions

Beat together the eggs and cream. Preheat a medium pan over medium heat. Drizzle in the oil and melt in the butter. Sauté the mushrooms with a pinch of salt until soft, about 1 minute. Pour in the egg mixture and cook for 3-5 minutes, until the bottom has set. Flip, and cook the other side. Lay the goat cheese on top, and fold the omelet. Serve warm.

Nutrition: 818 calories, 74.1 g fat,35.8 g protein, 3 g net carbs

Cream Cheese and Lox Omelet

Lox- also known by its more official term Smoked Salmon- is a high fat, high flavor breakfast favorite! This omelet combines creamy cream cheese with smoked salmon and dill for a fun, fast breakfast option!

Serving: 2

Serving Size: ½ omelet

Prep Time: 5 minutes

Cook Time: 10 minutes

Ingredients

½ lb smoked salmon, cut into ribbons

2 Tablespoons butter

6 eggs

1 cup heavy cream

¼ cup cream cheese

Handful dill, chopped

Instructions

Preheat a medium sized pan over medium heat. Drizzle in the oil and melt the butter. Mix the eggs and cream with a bit of salt, and pour the mixture into the pan. Allow the bottom to set, about 3 minutes, then flip. Cook until the other side has set, about 3 minutes longer. Spoon the cream cheese over top, followed by the smoked salmon and dill. Fold the omelet in half. Cook until the cheese starts to melt and ooze, about 3 minutes. Serve warm.

Nutrition: 731 calories, 61.9 g fat, 40.9 g protein, 3.5 g net carbs

Breakfast Sausage

The problem with store bought sausage is that it's normally full of sugar, carb-laden fillers, and other Keto no nos! Luckily, making your own sausage is a snap! These sausages are delicious, full of great fat, and can be made in batches and kept in the fridge for up to a week, or the freezer for up to 4 months.

Serving: 4

Serving Size: 2 Patties

Prep Time: 5 minutes

Cook Time: 10 minutes

Ingredients

1 lb ground pork

1 Tablespoon Italian herbs

1/2 Tablespoon garlic powder

1/2 Tablespoon onion powder

2 teaspoons fennel

1/2 teaspoon salt

1/2 teaspoon pepper

Instructions

In a large bowl combine the ground pork with all of the seasonings. Mix the seasoning into the meat as well as possible and then form 8 patties. Heat a pan on medium heat and add the coconut oil. Once the coconut oil is melted add all of the patties or if you can only fit 4 save half of the oil for the second batch. Fry the patties for 3-5 minutes on each side or until cooked through and golden brown on the outside. Serve warm, or store in an airtight container in the fridge for up to a week.

Nutrition: 326 calories, 28g fat, 19g protein, 0g net carbs

Scotch Eggs

Scotch eggs are traditionally soft-boiled eggs that have been coated in sausage and breading, and deep fried! The perfect Scotch egg is gooey in the center, and crispy on the outside with a thick coating of perfectly seasoned sausage all around! Using the base recipe for Breakfast Sausages, these eggs come together quickly and easily, and are the perfect addition to a keto friendly brunch!

Serving: 4

Serving Size: 1 egg

Prep Time: 5 minutes

Cook Time: 10 minutes

Ingredients

> 1 serving Breakfast Sausage, uncooked
>
> 4 eggs
>
> 1 cup ground pork rinds
>
> 6 cups oil, for frying

Instructions

Soft boil the eggs- In a medium sized saucepan with 1 cup of water in the bottom, boil the eggs for 4 minutes. Transfer to an ice bath, and allow to cool. Peel carefully, making sure not to break the egg. Divide the sausage meat into four portions, as you would for patties, and gently pack each portion around each egg. Next, pour the oil into a large pot and bring to a temperature of 350f on the stove, using a candy thermometer. Roll the sausage-coated eggs in the pork rinds, and fry for 2-4 minutes, until the eggs begin to float. Remove from heat, drain on a paper towel, and serve immediately.

> Nutrition: 442 calories, 46g fat, 25g protein, 0g net carbs

Baked Eggs with Kale and Tomato

This hearty skillet is the perfect thing for a chilly morning! You can substitute spinach for the kale, but make sure it's fresh.

Serving: 2

Serving Size: ½ skillet

Prep Time: 5 minutes

Cook Time: 10 minutes

Ingredients

> ½ tomato, diced

¼ cup kale, chopped

1 teaspoon garlic powder

2 Tablespoons butter

4 eggs

1 cup cream

1 teaspoon salt

1 teaspoon pepper

1 cup parmesan, shredded

Instructions

Preheat oven to 350F. Preheat a medium pan over medium heat. Melt in the butter, and sauté the kale, tomato and garlic butter together with the salt and pepper. Cook until the kale has wilted down slightly, about 3 minutes. Pour in the cream, and cook for another 3-4 minutes. Pour the mixture evenly into four ramekins. Crack an egg into each ramekin, and top with the cheese. Place the ramekins on a baking sheet, and bake for 15 minutes until the eggs are cooked and the yolks are still runny, and the cheese is bubbling. Serve warm.

Nutrition: 187 calories, 15.3 g fat, 9 g protein, 3 g net carbs

Bell Pepper Eggs

These eggs are adorable, and so easy to make! They're a variation on Toad in a Hole, where an egg is cooked in a bread ring.

Serving: 2

Serving Size: 2 eggs

Prep Time: 5 minutes

Cook Time: 15 minutes

Ingredients

1 green bell pepper, cut into ¼" rings

4 eggs

3 Tablespoons butter

Instructions

Preheat a medium pan over medium high heat. Melt in the butter, and lay the peppers down. Crack an egg into each pepper ring, and allow to cook until the whites have set and the yolk is still runny. Season with salt and pepper, and serve warm.

Nutrition: 298 calories, 26.2 g fat, 11.9 g protein, 4 g net carbs

Breakfast Beef Skillet

This hearty skillet is the perfect thing for a chilly morning!

Serving: 2

Serving Size: ½ skillet

Prep Time: 5 minutes

Cook Time: 10 minutes

Ingredients

½ green pepper, diced

½ tomato, diced

¼ red onion, diced

¼ lb ground beef

2 Tablespoons butter

1 Tablespoon olive oil

1 teaspoon ground cumin

1 teaspoon salt

4 eggs

Instructions

Preheat a medium sized pan over medium heat. Drizzle in the oil and melt in the butter. Add in the veggies, and sauté for 2 minutes. Add the beef and cumin, along with the salt, and cook until the beef is done, about 3-4 minutes. Crack in the eggs, and cook until the whites have set and the yolks are still runny, about 3 minutes. Serve warm.

Nutrition:705 calories, 58.7 g fat,36.4 g protein, 4 g net carbs

Mushroom and Bacon Skillet

Sautéing mushrooms and yummy bacon in a skillet with an egg packs in the protein and gives you a fully tummy for the rest of your day. Also makes a super easy dinner.

Serving: 1

Serving Size: whole recipe

Prep Time: 10 minutes

Cook Time: 10 minutes

Ingredients

1 cup mushrooms, sliced

4 slices bacon, diced

1 teaspoon salt

1 egg

1 Tablespoon butter

Instructions

Melt the butter into a skillet over medium high heat. Add in the mushrooms and bacon, and sauté until done- about 5 minutes. Crack in the egg, mixing well. Season with salt and pepper.

Nutrition: 591 calories, 47.7 g fat, 36 g protein, 3 g net carbs

Nordic Seed Bread Breakfast Sandwich

When you have leftover Nordic Seed Bread, then combine it with the following ingredients to make your own breakfast sandwich, excellent for busy weekday mornings!

Serving: 1

Serving Size: whole recipe

Prep Time: 5 minutes

Cook Time: 5 minutes

Ingredients

1 egg, beaten

1 teaspoon mayonnaise

1 teaspoon mustard

1 small handful arugula

1 piece Nordic Seed Bread, cut in half

Instructions

Beat the egg in a small bowl, and cover. Microwave on high for 40 seconds, until fully cooked. Spread the mustard and mayo onto each slice of the seed bread. Sandwich together with the egg and arugula. Serve immediately.

Nutrition: 434 calories, 40 g fat, 32 g protein, 4g net carbs

Keto Eggs Benedict

Nordic seed bread is a great alternative to toast, making this classic recipe Keto friendly! Make the hollandaise in advance, and keep it in an airtight container in the fridge for up to four days for an easy weekday breakfast. To reheat the hollandaise, simply microwave on low for 10 second intervals until warm, or whisk in a bowl over simmering water for 10 minutes.

Serving: 1

Serving Size: whole recipe

Prep Time: 5 minutes

Cook Time: 5 minutes

Ingredients

1 serving Quick Hollandaise Sauce

1 egg

¼ cup water

1 serving Nordic Seed Bread (from Snacks section)

Instructions

If making the hollandaise from scratch, use the Quick Hollandaise Sauce recipe. If you already have this sauce made in the fridge, remove it from the fridge and place it in a heat-proof bowl. Bring a pot of water to a simmer, and place the bowl over top, whisking it gently for about 5 minutes until it is warm. For a quick and easy breakfast, poach the egg using the microwave technique- pour the ¼ cup of water into a microwave safe mug. Crack the egg in, and cover the mug with a plate. Microwave on high for 55 seconds. To serve, lay the seed bread onto a plate, and gently place the poached egg on top with a spoon. Spoon the hollandaise sauce over top. Serve immediately.

Nutrition: 757 calories, 68 g fat, 35 g protein, 5g net carbs

Quick Hollandaise Sauce

This sauce is the perfect topper for Keto Eggs Benedict, but can also be used at your discretion with smoked salmon and cream cheese pancakes, roasted veggies, or anything else!

Serving: 4

Serving Size: ¼ recipe

Prep Time: 5 minutes

Cook Time: 5 minutes

Ingredients

4 egg yolks

1 Tablespoon lemon juice

½ cup butter, melted

1 teaspoon cayenne

1 teaspoon salt

Instructions

In a heatproof bowl, whisk the egg yolks and lemon juice well until slightly light in color. Bring a pot of water to a simmer over medium low heat. Place the bowl with the egg yolk mixture over top of the pot of simmering water, making sure the bottom of the bowl does not touch the water. Continue to whisk quickly, and slowly whisk in the melted butter, a small bit at a time, whisking well between each addition. Whisk in the cayenne and the salt. Set aside.

Nutrition: 260 calories, 27.6 g fat, 3g protein, 1g net carb

Avocado Pesto Eggs

This fun, flavor packed recipe uses up leftover Chicken Avocado Pesto Pasta, for a fun, crispy baked egg breakfast!

Serving: 1

Serving Size:

Prep Time: 5 minutes

Cook Time: 15 minutes

Ingredients

> 1 serving Avocado Pesto Pasta
>
> 1 Tablespoon butter
>
> 1 egg

Instructions

Preheat oven to 350F. In a small pan over medium high heat, melt the butter, and toss the Avocado Pesto Pasta in, cooking for 3-4 minutes until crispy and fragrant. Transfer the crispy pasta to a small ramekin, and press in well. Crack the egg into the center of the pasta, and bake for 10 minutes. Serve immediately.

> Nutrition: 404 calories, 37 g fat, 4 g protein, 4.6 g net carbs

Cream Cheese and Herb Pancakes with Smoked Salmon and Dill

These savory pancakes are the perfect thing for brunch, breakfast or lunch. The smoked salmon, fresh dill and cream cheese compliment these pancakes beautifully!

Serving: 4

Serving Size: 2-4 pancakes (depending on size of pancake)

Prep Time: 5 minutes

Cook Time: 20 minutes

Ingredients

> 1 cup almond flour
>
> ½ Tablespoon dried tarragon
>
> ½ Tablespoon dried thyme
>
> 1 egg, beaten
>
> 1 cup heavy cream
>
> 1 teaspoon baking powder
>
> ¼ teaspoon salt
>
> ¼ cup butter, melted

For the sauce:

> ¼ cup cream cheese

> 1 teaspoon dried tarragon

> ½ teaspoon garlic powder

To top:

> 4 oz smoked salmon

> Handful fresh dill, thyme, basil or chopped chives

Instructions

Start by making the pancakes. Whisk together the cream and egg. Mix together the almond flour, baking powder, herbs and salt. Stir in the egg mixture until smooth. Stir in the melted butter. Drizzle a bit of oil into a medium sized pan over medium heat. Spoon in a bit of the pancake batter, about 2 Tablespoons per pancake- be careful not to overcrowd the pan! Let the pancakes cook for 2-3 minutes, until the bubbles have burst. Gently flip, and cook the other side for another 1-2 minutes. Lay the finished pancakes on a plate and continue on until all the batter is used. Meanwhile, make the sauce- in a microwave safe bowl, combine all ingredients and microwave on high for 30 seconds. Beat all ingredients together until smooth. Put back into the microwave for 10 second intervals until desired consistency is reached. To serve, drizzle the cream cheese sauce over the pancakes, and top with smoked salmon and fresh herbs.

> Nutrition: 417 calories, 35.8 g fat, 20 g protein, 3 g net carbs

Avocado Breakfast Sandwich

This breakfast sandwich uses an avocado bun- just like the avocado burger- to make a healthy, high fat, low carb breakfast sandwich! Beware, though! This is NOT a to-go breakfast sandwich- it's messy in a good way, but definitely one of those meals you'll want to sit down and eat with a few extra napkins!

Serving: 1

Serving Size: 1 sandwich

Prep Time: 5 minutes

Cook Time: 10 minutes

Ingredients

> 2 strips bacon, cooked

> 1 egg

> 1 avocado, halved

> 1 teaspoon sesame seeds

> 1 slice tomato

> 1 Romaine lettuce leaf

Instructions

Drizzle some oil into a small pan over medium heat. Crack in the egg, and fry to desired doneness. Using one half of the avocado as the base of your bun, top with the tomato and romaine, followed by the egg. Season with salt and pepper. Close the bun, and season with a bit more salt, then top with the sesame seeds. Serve immediately.

Nutrition: 698 calories, 61g fat, 24.1 g protein, 5.5 g net carbs

Lemon Cream Pancakes

Fluffy lemony pancakes are the perfect thing for a weekend morning! The cream cheese sauce compliments the zingy lemon perfectly.

Serving: 2

Serving Size: 1-2 pancakes

Prep Time: 5

Cook Time: 18 minutes

Ingredients

¼ cup almond flour

2 Tablespoons coconut flour

1 teaspoon baking powder

1 teaspoon Stevia

1 egg, beaten

¼ cup almond or coconut milk

1 teaspoon vanilla extract

1 lemon, juice and zest

1 Tablespoon butter, melted

2 Tablespoons coconut oil

For the glaze:

2 tbsp cream cheese

1 teaspoon powdered Stevia

Instructions

Whisk together the flours, baking powder, and Stevia. Beat together the egg, lemon juice and coconut milk with the vanilla extract. Stir in the lemon zest, and then add in the flour mixture, stirring until combined. Stir in the melted butter. Preheat a pan over medium high heat, and drizzle in the coconut oil. Spoon in the mixture, 1-2 dollops at a time. Cook 2-3 minutes, until the bubbles have burst. Gently flip the pancake over, and cook the other side for another 1-2 minutes. Next, make the glaze- In a microwave safe bowl, microwave the cream cheese on high until melted, about 1 minute. Whisk in the powdered Stevia. Drizzle the warm glaze all over the pancakes.

Nutrition: 351 calories, 30.3 g fat, 6.7 g protein, 4 g net carbs

Beef Frittata

Frittatas are an easy, delicious way to use up leftovers! Although frittatas are typically eaten as a breakfast food, they also make a wonderful lunch or dinner as well.

Serving: 1

Serving Size: whole recipe

Prep Time: 5 minutes

Cook Time: 15 minutes

Ingredients

> 1 egg, beaten
>
> 1 Tablespoon heavy cream
>
> 1 serving Beef Fajita Bowl

Instructions

Preheat oven to 350F. Whisk together the egg and the cream. Lay the contents of the Beef Fajita Bowl out into an oven safe ramekin, and pour the egg mixture over top. Bake for 15 minutes, until the egg has set. Serve warm.

> Nutrition: 584 calories, 42 g fat, 39 g protein, 9.7 g net carbs

Cuban Frittata

This frittata is inspired by Cuban sandwiches and is loaded with ham and cheese! Make a big batch and keep it in the fridge to use for breakfast sandwiches or on top of salads.

Serving: 4

Serving Size: ¼ frittata

Prep Time: 5 minutes

Cook Time: 25 minutes

Ingredients

> 4 eggs, beaten
>
> 1 cup heavy cream
>
> ½ lb ham, cooked and diced
>
> 1 cup mozzarella, shredded
>
> 1 tomato, diced

Instructions

Preheat oven to 350F. Whisk together the egg and the cream. Mix in the rest of the ingredients. Bake for 25 minutes, until the egg has set. Serve warm.

Nutrition: 282 calories, 21.6 g fat, 17.7 g protein, 3 g net carbs

Soups and Salads

Creamy Tomato Soup

This soup tastes just like the classic tomato soup you enjoyed growing up, but with much more beneficial fat to keep you in ketosis! Serve with a Low Carb Grilled Cheese for an extra comforting meal!

Servings: 6

Serving Size: about 1 ½ cups

Prep Time: 10 minutes

Cook Time: 40 minutes

Ingredients:

> 2 14.5 oz cans crushed tomatoes (about 4 cups)
>
> 1 cup chicken stock
>
> ½ onion, diced
>
> 1 clove garlic, minced
>
> 2 teaspoons salt
>
> 2 teaspoons pepper
>
> 1 teaspoon nutmeg
>
> 1 teaspoon thyme
>
> 1 cup cream
>
> ¼ cup butter

Instructions:

Melt the butter in a large pot over medium high heat. Add in the onion, garlic, salt, pepper, nutmeg, and thyme. Sauté until the onions are soft and fragrant, about 3 minutes. Add in the tomatoes and stock, and bring to a boil. Reduce heat to low and simmer 20 minutes. Using an immersion blender, puree until smooth. Stir in the cream and simmer another 20 minutes. Serve warm.

Nutrition: 135 calories, 10.1 g fat, 2.5 g protein, 6 g net carbs

Cream of Leek Soup

This soup is a French classic, and very comforting! Serve alongside a piece of crusty Low Carb Baguette for a classic French experience!

Servings: 6

Serving Size: about 1 ½ cups

Prep Time: 10 minutes

Cook Time: 40 minutes

Ingredients:

     1 leek, whites only, chopped

     ½ onion, diced

     1 clove garlic, minced

     4 cups chicken stock

     1 Tablespoon thyme

     1 cup cream

     ¼ cup butter

     1 teaspoon salt

     1 teaspoon pepper

     ½ cup gruyere, shredded

Instructions:

Melt the butter in a large pot over medium high heat. Add in the leek, onion, garlic, salt, pepper, and thyme. Sauté until the leeks and onions are soft and fragrant, about 5 minutes. Add in the stock, and bring to a boil. Reduce heat to low and simmer 20 minutes. Using an immersion blender, puree until smooth. Stir in the cream, and simmer another 20 minutes. Stir in the cheese. Serve warm.

     Nutrition: 175 calories, 14.5 g fat, 4.3 g protein, 3 g net carbs

Cream of Mushroom Soup

Mushrooms are incredibly low carb and high flavor, making them a great ingredient to incorporate into your keto meals! This soup is full of rich cream, parmesan cheese, and coconut oil for a great hit of fat.

Servings: 2

Serving Size: about 1 ½ cups

Prep Time: 10 minutes

Cook Time: 0 minutes

Ingredients:

     8 oz cremini mushrooms, sliced thinly

     1 stalk celery, chopped

     ½ onion, chopped

     1 Tablespoon coconut oil

1 Tablespoon thyme, chopped

1 teaspoon dried thyme

½ Tablespoon salt

½ Tablespoon pepper

½ cup vegetable stock or chicken stock

1 cup cream

3 Tablespoons parmesan cheese, grated

Instructions:

Preheat a medium sized pot over medium heat. Add in the coconut oil, mushrooms, celery, onion, thyme, salt and pepper. Sauté 2 minutes, until soft and fragrant. Add in the stock, and bring to a boil. Reduce heat to low, and simmer 30 minutes. Stir in the cream, and continue cooking another 10 minutes. Stir in the parmesan cheese. Taste, and season with salt and pepper. Serve hot, or transfer to an airtight container and store in the fridge for up to 3 weeks.

Nutrition: 222 calories, 15.6 g fat, 7.8 g protein, 11 g net carbs

Creamy Cauliflower and Seafood Chowder

This chowder is rich, creamy, and perfectly flavorful! This is a great way to use up leftover fish recipes like Red Pepper Cod!

Serving: 6

Serving Size: about ¾ cup

Prep Time: 5 minutes

Cook Time: 30 Minutes

Ingredients

4 slices bacon, diced

½ onion, diced

2 Tablespoons butter

1 Tablespoon olive oil

3 cloves garlic, minced

1 teaspoon paprika

1 teaspoon thyme

2 cups chicken stock

½ head cauliflower, chopped

1 cup heavy cream

¼ lb cooked white fish

3 scallops, cooked and diced

¼ lb shrimp, diced

¼ lb cooked crab meat, shredded

1 tomato, diced

Instructions

Preheat a large pot over medium heat. Drizzle in the olive oil, and melt in the butter. Cook the bacon bits for about a minute in the butter. Add the onion and garlic, along with the paprika and time, and sauté for a minute longer, until soft. Add in the cauliflower and stock, and bring to a boil. Reduce heat to low, and simmer 20 minutes. Using an immersion blender, puree until smooth. Add in the fish, tomato, and cream. Simmer another 5-10 minutes. Serve warm.

Nutrition: 540 calories, 52 g fat, 28 g protein, 7 g net carbs

Nicoise Salad

This salad seems complicated, but all of the individual components can be prepared in advance. The tuna can be cooked up to a day in advance and sliced right before serving, as can the hard boiled eggs. The dressing can be made up to a week in advance, as well. Cook the green beans in advance and keep them in an airtight container - you may want to do this in batches. Green beans make an excellent low carb count snacking option, and a wonderful addition to most salads!

Serving: 1

Serving Size: whole recipe

Prep Time: 5 minutes

Cook Time: 20 Minutes

Ingredients

1 8 oz ahi tuna steak

6 green beans

4 cherry tomatoes

2 eggs

¼ cucumber, sliced

1 cup kale, chopped

2 Tablespoons Dijon mustard

¼ cup olive oil

1 teaspoon dried thyme

Instructions

Bring a pot of water to a boil. Boil the eggs for about 6 minutes, to hard boil. Allow to cool fully before peeling. Pat the tuna dry, and season with salt and pepper. Preheat a small pan over medium high heat. Drizzle a bit of olive oil, and sear the ahi for about 1 minute per side. Transfer the seared ahi to a cutting board, and allow to cool fully before slicing. Bring another pot of salted water to a boil, and blanch the beans for about a minute. Drain, and transfer to an ice bath until ready to use. Next, whisk together the mustard, thyme and olive oil in a large bowl. Taste, and season with salt and pepper as needed. Toss the kale in the dressing, then transfer to a plate. Slice the ahi, and lay on top of the greens. Lay the beans, cucumber and tomato on top. Peel the eggs, slice them in half, and lay them on top of the salad. Serve immediately.

Nutrition: 273 calories, 20g fat, 23g protein, 2g net carbs

Italian Chopped Salad

This chopped salad is so easy to throw together, and super versatile! Add in your favorite marinated meats and veg to make this your own! This salad will keep in the fridge for up to 5 days, so make a big batch and have it on hand for snacking or fast lunch options.

Serving: 2

Serving Size: half recipe

Prep Time: 15 minutes

Cook Time: 0 minutes

Ingredients

> 12 Romaine leaves, chopped
>
> 2 oz prosciutto, sliced into ribbons
>
> 2 oz salami, chopped
>
> ¼ cup artichoke hearts, chopped
>
> ¼ cup olives
>
> 1 jalapeno, sliced
>
> 1 Tablespoon olive oil
>
> 1 Tablespoon lemon juice or white wine vinegar
>
> 1 Tablespoon Italian herbs

Instructions

In a large bowl, whisk together the olive oil, lemon juice and herbs. Toss in the rest of the ingredients, making sure everything is well mixed. Season with salt and pepper. Serve immediately, or store in an airtight container in the fridge for up to 5 days.

Nutrition: 469 calories, 44g fat, 14g protein, 4g net carbs

Cilantro Lime Shrimp and Avocado Salad

This salad is summer in a bowl! The creamy avocado stands up nicely to the tangy shrimp.

Serving: 1

Serving Size: whole recipe

Prep Time: 5 minutes

Cook Time: 5 Minutes

Ingredients

> 6 shrimp, deveined and peeled
>
> ½ lime, juice and zest
>
> 1 Tablespoon avocado oil
>
> ½ teaspoon garlic powder
>
> 2 Tablespoons cilantro, finely chopped
>
> ½ avocado, diced
>
> 1 teaspoon salt
>
> 1 jalapeno, diced
>
> 3 green onions, finely sliced
>
> 3 cherry tomatoes, cut in half

Instructions

Preheat a medium sized pan over medium high heat. Whisk together the lime juice, zest, avocado oil, garlic powder, and cilantro. Toss the shrimp in the marinade, and transfer to the pan. Cook about 1 minute per side, until the shrimp are opaque and firm. Mix the green onions, avocado, jalapeno and tomatoes together, and season with salt. Top with the shrimp. Serve immediately.

> Nutrition: 529 calories, 35.6 g fat, 26g protein, 5g net carbs

Scallop and Mushroom Salad with Goat Cheese Vinaigrette

This combo may seem a bit weird, but it works! The creamy scallops juxtapose nicely with the salty, fatty bacon and meaty mushrooms, and the creamy, tangy goat cheese vinaigrette brings it all together.

Serving: 2

Serving Size: half recipe

Prep Time: 5 minutes

Cook Time: 15 Minutes

Ingredients

> 6 scallops
>
> 2 slices bacon, diced
>
> 1 Tablespoon butter

1 cup mixed mushrooms, sliced

1 Tablespoon thyme

2 oz goat cheese

2 Tablespoons olive oil

1 cup arugula

½ lemon, juiced

Instructions

Preheat a medium pan over medium high heat. Cook the bacon bits with the butter, then remove from the pan and set aside. In the same pan, sauté the mushrooms with the thyme and a pinch of salt until soft and fragrant, about 3 minutes. Remove from the pan and set aside. Next, pat the scallops dry and season with salt and pepper. In the same pan, sear the scallops for about 2-3 minutes per side. Remove from the pan and set aside. Turn off the heat, and whisk the goat cheese, olive oil and lemon juice into the flavored butter. Spoon the goat cheese vinaigrette into a large bowl, and toss in the arugula, mushrooms and bacon. Toss well to combine. To serve, lay the dressed arugula onto two plates, and top with 3 scallops each. Serve warm.

Nutrition: 498 calories, 38.8 g fat, 32.7 g protein, 4.4 g net carbs

Egg Salad

This salad is an instant energy booster and a great grab and go lunch! Leftovers will stay good in the fridge for up to five days. Serve on lettuce wraps or with some fresh greens. Would taste good with crackers or Nordic seed bread, too.

Servings: 4

Serving Size: about ¼ cup

Prep Time: 10 minutes

Cook Time: 10 minutes

Ingredients:

8 eggs

½ cup mayonnaise

1 green onion, thinly sliced

1 teaspoon salt

Mustard

Dill pickles

Paprika for garnish

Instructions:

Put the eggs into a medium sized pot filled with water. Bring to a boil, and boil about 10 minutes, until the eggs are hard boiled (can be done up to three days in advance). Allow to cool, peel, and mash lightly in a bowl with the rest of the ingredients. Sprinkle with red paprika for a garnish. Serve immediately, or refrigerate up to 4 days.

Nutrition: 242 calories, 18.6g fat, 11.4 g protein, 8g net carbs

Chicken Salad

Classic chicken salad is a summertime staple. This recipe has celery and pecans for crunch. You can serve it alongside Nordic seed bread or Keto crackers. Roast or bake your chicken the night before, so it's ready for shredding in the morning.

Servings: 4

Serving Size: 1/2 cup

Prep Time: 10 minutes

Cook Time: 0 minutes

Ingredients:

3 cups cold shredded chicken

1/2 cup full fat mayonnaise

1 teaspoon Dijon mustard

Juice from half a lemon

2 stalks celery, sliced

¼ cup chopped pecans

1.5 Tablespoons fresh chopped parsley

1 Tablespoon chopped dill

Salt and pepper to taste

Instructions:

Combine all ingredients in a large bowl except for the chicken and the pecans. Stir thoroughly. Then add the chicken and toss. Finally, add the pecans and toss again. Taste for seasonings and adjust salt and pepper. Serve cold on lettuce or with crackers.

Nutrition: 367 calories, 25g fat, 34g protein, 2g net carbs

Kale Salad

This low carb salad is just the thing to ensure you're getting the vitamins and minerals you need, while still watching your Macros! It's super crunchy, so it will keep in the fridge with the dressing for about a day without going soggy. This salad is great on its own, and goes well with chicken, pork, or steak.

Servings: 1

Serving Size: about 1 ½ cups

Prep Time: 10 minutes

Cook Time: 0 minutes

Ingredients:

- 1 cup kale, chopped
- ¼ red onion, sliced thinly
- 2 radishes, grated
- 2 Tablespoons olive oil
- ½ Tablespoon Dijon mustard
- ½ Tablespoon mayonnaise
- 1 teaspoon thyme
- 1 teaspoon salt
- ½ teaspoon Stevia

Instructions:

In a large bowl, whisk together the olive oil, Dijon, mayonnaise, thyme, salt and Stevia to make a dressing. Toss in the rest of the ingredients, and mix well. Serve immediately, or keep in an airtight container in the fridge for up to two days.

Nutrition: 322 calories, 30.9 g fat, 2.9 g protein, 9 g net carbs

Warm Zucchini and Goat Cheese Salad

This fabulous salad is low protein, high fat and amazingly flavorful!

Servings: 1

Serving Size: whole recipe

Prep Time: 10 minutes

Cook Time: 30 minutes

Ingredients:

- ½ zucchini, sliced
- 1 Tablespoon olive oil, divided
- 1/2 cup basil, chopped
- 1 handful parsley, chopped
- 1 teaspoon Italian herbs (basil, oregano, parsley)
- 1 clove garlic, minced

½ Tablespoon white wine vinegar

¼ cup sun dried tomatoes

2 oz goat cheese

¼ cup walnuts

Instructions:

Preheat the oven to 375F. Toss the zucchini in one Tablespoon of olive oil and season with salt, pepper, and the Italian herbs. Bake in the oven for 10 minutes. Meanwhile, whisk together the garlic, herbs, white wine vinegar, and second Tablespoon of olive oil. Toss the rest of the ingredients in, and mix well. Serve immediately.

Nutrition: 395 calories, 35.5 g fat, 14.8 g protein, 6 g net carbs

Green Goddess Dressing

This dressing is high fat and high flavor! Perfect for topping on any salad, or using as a dip for veggies!

Servings: 4

Serving Size: ¼ cup

Prep Time: 10 minutes

Cook Time: 0 minutes

Ingredients:

2 avocados

¼ cup olive oil

1 Tablespoon thyme

1 Tablespoon white wine vinegar

1 teaspoon salt

Instructions:

In a blender or food processor, combine all ingredients until smooth. Store in an airtight container in the fridge for up to a week.

Nutrition: 316 calories, 32 g fat, 2 g protein, 2 g net carbs

Thai Coconut Dressing

This dressing is full of coconut milk and exotic flavor! Perfect for dressing on top of Asian style salads, and also works great as a marinade for chicken or pork!

Servings: 4

Serving Size: ¼ cup

Prep Time: 10 minutes

Cook Time: 0 minutes

Ingredients:

- 1 avocado
- 2 cans coconut milk
- 3 red chilis, minced
- 1 clove garlic, minced
- Handful cilantro, chopped
- 1 teaspoon ginger, minced
- 3 green onions, chopped

Instructions:

In a blender or food processor, combine all ingredients until smooth. Store in an airtight container in the fridge for up to a week.

Nutrition: 247 calories, 25 g fat, 2.6 g protein, 3.8 g net carbs

Asian Nut Dressing

This dressing is spicy, creamy, and super flavorful! It works well on Asian style salads as well as a marinade for beef, chicken or pork.

Servings: 4

Serving Size: ¼ cup

Prep Time: 10 minutes

Cook Time: 0 minutes

Ingredients:

- ½ cup almond butter
- ½ cup coconut milk
- 2 limes, juice and zest
- Handful cilantro, chopped
- 3 green onions, chopped
- 4 red chilis, minced
- ¼ cup sesame oil

Instructions:

In a blender or food processor, combine all ingredients until smooth. Store in an airtight container in the fridge for up to a week.

Nutrition: 205 calories, 21.9 g fat, 1.3 g protein, 1 g net carbs

Cilantro Lime Dressing

This zingy dressing is perfect for Steak and Avocado Salad, but will work on any Southwest inspired salad creations!

Servings: 4

Serving Size: ¼ cup

Prep Time: 10 minutes

Cook Time: 0 minutes

Ingredients:

> ½ cup avocado oil
>
> 4 limes, juice and zest
>
> 2 cups fresh cilantro, chopped
>
> 1 jalapeno, chopped

Instructions:

In a blender or food processor, combine all ingredients until smooth. Store in an airtight container in the fridge for up to a week.

> Nutrition: 60 calories, 3.9 g fat, 1g protein, 4 g net carbs

Lemon Thyme Vinaigrette

This dressing is classically French and really yummy! Use it to on a simple green salad, or as a marinade for fish!

Servings: 4

Serving Size: ¼ cup

Prep Time: 10 minutes

Cook Time: 0 minutes

Ingredients:

> ½ cup olive oil
>
> 4 lemons, juice and zest
>
> 4 large stems thyme, chopped
>
> 1 Tablespoon Dijon mustard

Instructions:

In a blender or food processor, combine all ingredients until smooth. Store in an airtight container in the fridge for up to a week.

> Nutrition: 60 calories, 3.9 g fat, 1g protein, 2 g net carbs

Pork Chopped Salad

Using leftover pork chops, you can create this fun, easy salad very quickly! Switch up the ingredients to really make this meat-filled salad your own!

Serving: 1

Serving Size: whole recipe

Prep Time: 15 minutes

Cook Time: 0 minutes

Ingredients

> 2 cooked pork chops, 1" thick (4 oz each)
>
> 1/4 cup kale, chopped
>
> 3 cherry tomatoes, halved
>
> 1 egg, hardboiled
>
> ½ cucumber, sliced
>
> 2 Tablespoons olive oil
>
> 1 Tablespoon white wine vinegar
>
> 2 teaspoons Dijon mustard
>
> 1 teaspoon thyme
>
> 1 teaspoon salt
>
> 1 teaspoon pepper

Instructions

Start by slicing the pork chop thinly, and setting aside. Next, whisk together the olive oil, vinegar, mustard, thyme, salt and pepper in a large bowl, and add in the kale. Toss well to combine. Mix in the cherry tomatoes, cucumber and pork slices. Slice the peeled hard boiled egg in half, and toss it into the salad. Serve immediately, or keep in the fridge for up to 24 hours.

> Nutrition: 681 calories, 57.9 g fat, 29 g protein, 9 g net carbs

Avocado and Chicken Salad

This rich, creamy salad can be eaten on its own, or wrapped in lettuce for a healthy, hand-held option! Switch up the seasoning to suit your own tastes - if you like things on the spicier side, add jalapeno or hot sauce! If you like an herbier salad, add in your favorite fresh or dried herbs!

Serving: 1

Serving Size: whole recipe

Prep Time: 5 minutes

Cook Time: 0 minutes

Ingredients

1 avocado, diced

4 oz chicken breast, cooked and sliced

1 Tablespoon coconut oil

2 teaspoons salt

1 Tablespoon lime juice

1 teaspoon lime zest

Instructions

Mix together all ingredient in a bowl, making sure to mash the avocado and chicken together to make a creamy bind. Taste, and adjust seasoning as needed. Serve immediately, or enjoy within 4 hours.

Nutrition: 663 calories, 55 g fat, 28 protein, 6 g net carbs

Asian Salad

This super simple salad is made with Asian Nut Dressing and super fresh ingredients. If you wish, you can add a piece of chicken or pork on top!

Servings: 2

Serving Size: ½ recipe

Prep Time: 10 minutes

Cook Time: 10 minutes

Ingredients:

2 servings Asian Nut Dressing

¼ cup bean sprouts

¼ carrot, grated

¼ red pepper, sliced thinly

1 avocado, diced

3 green onions, thinly sliced

1 cup shiitake mushrooms

2 Tablespoons sesame oil

Instructions:

Preheat oven to 375F. Toss the mushrooms in the sesame oil, and lay out on a baking sheet. Roast for 10 minutes. Meanwhile, toss together the rest of the ingredients. Make sure the dressing has fully coated each piece. When the mushrooms are done, toss them in right away. Serve immediately, or keep in an airtight container for up to 3 days.

Nutrition: 579 calories, 55.4 g fat, 5 g protein, 9 g net carbs

Lemon Thyme Salmon Salad

This salad is so lovely and delicate, and the perfect lunch for a warm summer day!

Serving: 2

Serving Size: 1 fillet fish

Prep Time: 5 minutes

Cook Time: 25 minutes

Ingredients

2 4 oz pieces salmon

1 Tablespoon olive oil

1 teaspoon thyme

1 teaspoon nutmeg

½ head cauliflower, cut into florets

4 green beans

½ tomato, cut into wedges

1 egg, hardboiled and cut in half

½ green pepper, sliced into strips

2 cups arugula

2 servings Lemon Thyme Vinaigrette

Instructions

Preheat oven to 350F. Brush the oil over the fish, and season with the thyme, nutmeg and a pinch of salt. Bake 25 minutes. Meanwhile, bring a large pot of salted water to a boil, and cook the cauliflower florets for 3 minutes, to blanche. Transfer to an ice bath. Cook the green beans in the same water for 1 minute, and then transfer to an ice bath. Toss the arugula with the dressing, and lay onto two plates. Place one half of the hardboiled egg onto each plate, followed by a few tomato wedges, the green beans and cauliflower. Top with the fish. Serve immediately.

Nutrition: 402 calories, 21.1 g fat, 41.7 g protein, 9.1 g net carbs

Baja Style Halibut Salad

This salad is bright and fresh and full of color! Leftover fish can be used in lettuce wraps to make Fish Tacos.

Serving: 2

Serving Size: 1 fillet fish

Prep Time: 5 minutes

Cook Time: 25 minutes

Ingredients

> 2 4 oz pieces of halibut

> 1 Tablespoon olive oil

> 1 teaspoon oregano

> 1 teaspoon garlic powder

> 1 teaspoon salt

> 2 cups arugula

> 1 tomato, diced

> ½ bell pepper, diced

> 1 jalapeno, diced

> ¼ red onion, sliced

> 1 avocado, diced

> 2 servings Cilantro Lime Dressing

Instructions

Preheat oven to 350F. Brush the oil over the fish, and season with the oregano, garlic, and a pinch of salt. Bake 25 minutes. Toss the arugula with the dressing, and lay onto two plates. Top with the remaining veg. Top with the fish. Serve immediately or keep leftovers in an airtight container in the fridge for up to two days.

> Nutrition: 740 calories, 40 g fat, 95 g protein, 7 g net carbs

Steak and Avocado Salad

This salad is light and flavorful and full of good fat! Perfect for a cold summer lunch!

Servings: 2

Serving Size: Half recipe

Prep Time: 10 minutes

Cook Time: 15 minutes

Ingredients:

> 1/4 lb flank steak, cut into strips

> 1 Tablespoon olive oil

> 1 Tablespoon jalapeno powder

1 teaspoon salt

¼ red onion, sliced

1 avocado, diced

½ tomato, diced

1 serving Cilantro Lime Dressing

Instructions:

Preheat a large pan over medium heat. Toss the steak in the olive oil and jalapeno powder, and fry until fully cooked- about 3 minutes. Transfer to a bowl with the rest of the ingredients, and toss well to combine. Serve immediately. Could also be wrapped in lettuce leaves with Monterey Jack cheese and salsa to create lettuce wraps.

Nutrition: 663 calories, 44 g fat, 50 g protein, 7 g net carbs

Pork and Poultry

Jerk Chicken

Jerk Chicken is deliciously flavorful and full of good fat! Enjoy over cauliflower rice for a Keto friendly Caribbean experience!

Serving: 4

Serving Size: 1 chicken thigh

Prep Time: 5 minutes

Cook Time: 45 minutes

Ingredients

4 chicken thighs, bone in skin on

3 Tablespoons allspice

½ Tablespoon ginger

2 cloves garlic, minced

½ onion, diced

2 scotch bonnets, minced

1 teaspoon cinnamon

1 Tablespoon thyme

¼ cup dry white wine

2 cups chicken stock

2 Tablespoons coconut oil

Instructions

Preheat the oven to 375F. Combine the allspice, ginger, cinnamon and thyme together, and rub into the chicken. Preheat a Dutch oven on the stove over medium high heat, and melt in the coconut oil. Add the onion, garlic, and scotch bonnets, and sauté 1 minute. Add in the chicken and stock, and cover. Transfer to the oven, and cook 40 minutes.

Nutrition: 524 calories, 33.9 g fat, 44 g protein, 5 g net carbs

Thai Chicken Coconut Red Curry

This is such a fragrant and easy dish, where you can make substitutions depending on what you have. You can use shrimp, beef, or pork instead of the chicken. Try yellow or green curry paste instead of the red. Use any combination of fresh Keto vegetables you prefer.

Serving: 4

Serving Size: ¼ recipe

Prep Time: 10 minutes

Cook Time: 20 minutes

Ingredients

1 Tablespoon olive oil

2 Tablespoons red curry paste (or yellow or green)

13.5 ounce can of full fat coconut milk

½ cup chicken broth

1/8 teaspoon Stevia

1 Tablespoon fish sauce

1 1b boneless skinless chicken cut into 1" pieces

3 cups assorted bite-size cut fresh vegetables (green peppers, broccoli,

cauliflower, onion, bok choy, tomatoes, zucchini, etc.)

1 Tablespoon thinly sliced fresh basil (optional)

Squeeze of fresh lime

Instructions

Put your large skillet or wok on medium heat. Heat the olive oil. When warm, add the curry paste and stir fry with a wooden spoon for 1 ½ - 2 minutes until fragrant. Pour in entire can of coconut milk and the chicken broth. Raise the temperature to medium-high. Bring to a simmer. Then stir in the Stevia (no more than 1/8 teaspoon or to taste) and the fish sauce until well blended. Add the meat and all of the vegetables and stir to coat everything in the curry. Simmer uncovered for 5-7 minutes until the chicken is cooked through. Remove from heat. Stir in the basil and a squeeze of fresh lime. Could also add sliced spring onion and a sprinkle of fresh finely chopped cilantro.

Nutrition: 310 calories, 26 g fat, 14 g protein, 7 g net carbs

Indian Butter Chicken with Roasted Cauliflower

If you live in a cold climate, there is nothing more warming or comforting than Indian food! You can find the garam masala at Asian stores or online. This recipe is packed with chicken, butter, and spices. It's delicious. Use ghee to increase your fat intake.

Servings: 6

Serving Size: 1/6 recipe

Prep Time: 30 minutes

Cook Time: 30 minutes

Ingredients

1 2/3 lbs boneless chicken thighs

1 tomato, cored

1 yellow onion

2 Tablespoons ginger

2 garlic cloves, peeled

1 Tablespoon tomato paste

1 Tablespoon garam masala seasoning

½ Tablespoon ground coriander (cilantro)

½ Tablespoon chili powder

1 teaspoon salt

¾ cup heavy cream

3 oz butter or Indian ghee

For Cauliflower:

1 lb cauliflower, chopped into bite size pieces

½ teaspoon turmeric

½ tablespoon coriander seed

½ teaspoon salt

¼ teaspoon black pepper

2 oz melted butter

Instructions

In a blender or food processor, blend the tomato, onion, ginger, garlic, tomato paste, and the spices – garam masala, coriander, chili powder, and salt. Blend until smooth. Add the heavy cream and stir in. Pour into a bowl and add the cut up chicken until well coated. Cover with plastic wrap and marinate in the fridge for at least 20 minutes. You could marinate for several hours to infuse the flavor. When ready to cook, heat up a large frying pan over medium high heat with 1 ounce of the butter. Add the chicken to the pan and fry on each side for several minutes. Then pour the rest of the marinade over the chicken, together with the other 2 ounces of butter. Turn heat down to medium and let simmer for 15 minutes until chicken is fully cooked. For the cauliflower, preheat your oven to 400F. Spread the chopped cauliflower over a foil cookie sheet or baking tray. Sprinkle the seasonings and butter over. Bake for 15 minutes. Serve the butter chicken over the cauliflower and garnish with fresh cilantro and plain unsweetened yogurt.

Nutrition: 592 calories, 52g fat, 24g protein, 6g net carbs

Chicken Avocado Pesto Pasta

This is a quick and easy dinner recipe that from start to finish is on the table in 30 minutes. It uses zucchini 'zoodles' to mimic pasta!

Serving: 2

Serving Size: half recipe

Prep Time: 15 minutes

Cook Time: 15 minutes

Ingredients

2 zucchinis, spiralized or cut into ribbons

8 oz chicken breast, sliced

1 Tablespoon oregano

1 Tablespoon garlic powder

1 Tablespoon coconut oil

1 avocado

2 Tablespoons extra virgin olive oil

1/2 cup water

1/2 cup basil

salt and pepper to taste

Instructions

In a blender or food processor, blend together the avocado, olive oil, water, and basil. Set aside. In a medium pan over medium high heat, melt the coconut oil. Add in the chicken slices, oregano and garlic powder, tossing frequently and cooking until done, about 8 minutes. Add in the avocado mixture and zucchini noodles, tossing well to combine. Cook until heated through, about 7 minutes.

Nutrition: 440 calories, 40g fat, 36g protein, 3g net carbs

Chicken Kababs

Kababs are delicious, and make a great summer treat when grilled on the BBQ! Serve them on their own with a dipping sauce (such as Green Tahini) or on top of greens for a complete meal!

Serving: 4

Serving Size: 1 skewer

Prep Time: 10 minutes

Cook Time: 30 minutes

Ingredients

> 4 3 oz boneless skinless chicken thighs, chopped into chunks
>
> ¼ red onion, sliced into chunks
>
> ½ bell pepper, sliced into chunks
>
> 1 Tablespoon salt
>
> 1 Tablespoon pepper
>
> 1 Tablespoon paprika
>
> 1 teaspoon cumin
>
> 3 Tablespoons olive oil

Instructions

Preheat the oven to 350F. Toss all ingredients together in a bowl, making sure the oil coats everything well. Using four skewers, skewer the meat and veggies evenly onto each skewer. Bake for 30 minutes, until the meat is cooked through and the veggies are soft.

> Nutrition: 270 calories, 17.2 g fat, 25 g protein, 2 g net carbs

Chicken Kale Wrap

This is a super simple recipe to throw together using leftover cooked chicken and a few simple ingredients! It makes a great lunch, or a quick weeknight dinner.

Serving: 1

Serving Size: 1 wrap

Prep Time: 5 minutes

Cook Time: 30 minutes

Ingredients

> 2 large kale leaves
>
> 4 oz chicken breast, cooked and sliced

¼ red pepper, sliced

2 Tablespoons tahini

Instructions

Start by washing and drying the kale leaves, and laying them out on a piece of parchment, so they overlap in the middle. Lay the chicken and pepper slices over top, and drizzle liberally with tahini. Season with salt and pepper, and roll the kale to make a wrap. Serve immediately, or keep wrapped in the parchment in the fridge for up to 24 hours.

Nutrition: 415 calories, 32.1g fat, 26.3 g protein, 5.3 g net carbs

Goat Cheese Stuffed Chicken Breasts

These chicken breasts are elegant and delicious! They can be served hot or cold, and make a great addition to salads.

Serving: 2

Serving Size: 1 chicken breast

Prep Time: 15 minutes

Cook Time: 30 minutes

Ingredients

2 6 oz chicken breasts

6 oz goat cheese

1 Tablespoon cream

1 Tablespoon dried thyme

1 Tablespoon smoked paprika

1 Tablespoon butter

Instructions

Preheat the oven to 350F. Slice the chicken breast open like a book, and place it between two pieces of plastic wrap. Pound lightly to flatten slightly, and transfer the flattened breast to a baking sheet lined with parchment. Continue on with the second breast. Next, beat together the goat cheese, cream, thyme and paprika with a bit of black pepper. Spoon the mixture evenly into the center of each breast, and roll them up. Next, beat together the butter with a bit more pepper, paprika and thyme, and spread the mixture all over the outside of the chicken to coat. Bake the chicken in the center of the oven for 30 minutes. Allow to rest 10 minutes, then slice into medallions.

Nutrition: 646 calories, 44.5 g fat, 55.9 g protein, 3 g net carbs

Beef and Lamb

Beef Stuffed Tomatoes

This Middle Eastern classic is a fun dinner or lunch option! Serve it with a side of greens or on top of cauliflower rice.

Serving: 2

Serving Size: 1 tomato

Prep Time: 5 minutes

Cook Time: 25 minutes

Ingredients

> ½ lb ground beef
>
> 1 Tablespoon olive oil
>
> 1 teaspoon thyme
>
> 1 teaspoon paprika
>
> 1 clove garlic, minced
>
> ½ onion, diced
>
> 2 large red tomatoes

Instructions

Hollow out the centers of the tomatoes by removing the core and the soft insides. Preheat the oven to 375F. Preheat a pan over medium high heat, and drizzle in the olive oil. Add in the onion with a pinch of salt and the spices, and sauté for about a minute. Add in the beef, and cook until done, about 3-4 minutes. Spoon the mixture into the hollowed out tomatoes, and place them onto a baking sheet lined with parchment. Bake 18-20 minutes, until the tomatoes have softened and blistered slightly. Serve warm. Keep leftovers in an airtight container for up to four days.

> Nutrition: 350 calories, 15.5g fat, 36g protein, 5 g net carbs

Greek Lamb Burger

This lamb burger combines classic Greek flavors, giving you a fun international twist on a basic burger! This is a bun less burger, so make sure you've got your knife and fork (and appetite!) ready!

Serving: 2

Serving Size: 2 Patties

Prep Time: 5 minutes

Cook Time: 15 minutes

Ingredients

> 1 lb ground lamb

1 cup shredded romaine lettuce

2 teaspoons salt

1 teaspoon white pepper

1 Tablespoon coconut oil

1 cup Greek yogurt

1/4 English cucumber, diced

1 Tablespoon of fresh dill

1 clove garlic, minced

1 teaspoon salt

Instructions

In a large bowl combine the ground lamb, paprika, sea salt and pepper and form 4 patties. Heat a pan on medium heat and add the coconut oil. Once the coconut oil has melted place the burger patties in the pan and cook for about 5 minutes per side. Meanwhile peel and shred the cucumber and then combine it with all of the other ingredients to make the Tzatziki sauce. To serve, top one patty with the tzatziki and lettuce, and top with the second patty. Serve immediately.

Nutrition: 542 calories, 40g fat, 36g protein, 5g net carbs

Lamb Chops with Buttery Mustard Sauce

Lamb and mustard are a match made in heaven! Serve alongside asparagus or a fresh salad with light dressing.

Serving: 2

Serving Size: 1 chop

Prep Time: 5 minutes

Cook Time: 25 minutes

Ingredients

2 6 oz lamb chops

4 Tablespoons butter

1 stem thyme

3 Tablespoons Dijon mustard

1 Tablespoon salt

1 Tablespoon pepper

Instructions

Preheat oven to 350F. Season the lamb chops with salt and pepper, and lay on a baking sheet lined with parchment. Bake for 20 minutes, until cooked through. Melt the butter in a saucepan over medium high heat.

Add the mustard and thyme. Cook for 30 minutes, stirring occasionally. Remove the thyme stem, and spoon the sauce over the lamb chops.

Nutrition: 429 calories, 27g fat, 25g protein, 9g net carbs

Walnut and Pork Stuffed Lamb Tenderloin

Lamb tenderloin is a sophisticated showpiece dish that is perfect for entertaining! The walnut stuffing is savory, fatty, and complements the lamb perfectly. Serve this masterpiece of a dish with a side of Butter Tossed Asparagus for a beautiful keto-friendly masterpiece! Leftovers keep really well as well, and make a great addition to sandwiches and salads.

Servings: 6

Serving Size: 1 piece

Prep Time: 10 minutes

Cook Time: 45 minutes

Ingredients:

12 oz lamb tenderloin

1 cup walnuts, chopped

2 oz ground pork

1 Tablespoon thyme

1 Tablespoon butter

1 Tablespoon salt

1 Tablespoon pepper

1 teaspoon nutmeg

Instructions:

Preheat oven to 350F. In a pan over medium high heat, melt the butter and add the pork, thyme, nutmeg, salt and pepper. Cook 2-3 minutes, until the pork is cooked. Add in the walnuts, and cook another 2-3 minutes. Let cool fully. Next, make an incision down the length of the tenderloin, and roll your knife through the middle of the tenderloin to open it up. Fill the center of the lamb with the walnut and pork mixture, and seal it back up. Using some butcher twine, tie the tenderloin to keep the stuffing in place. Season the lamb with salt and pepper, and lay it on a baking sheet lined with parchment. Bake in the oven for 35-40 minutes. Let rest for 15 minutes. Slice into medallions and serve.

Nutrition: 800 calories, 66.6 g fat, 45.5 g protein, 0.2 g net carbs

Beef Kababs

Kababs are delicious, and make a great summer treat when grilled on the BBQ! Serve them on their own with a dipping sauce (such as Green Tahini) or on top of greens for a complete meal.

Serving: 4

Serving Size: 1 skewer

Prep Time: 10 minutes

Cook Time: 30 minutes

Ingredients

> ½ lb flank steak, chopped into chunks
>
> ¼ red onion, sliced into chunks
>
> ½ bell pepper, sliced into chunks
>
> 1 Tablespoon salt
>
> 1 Tablespoon pepper
>
> 1 Tablespoon paprika
>
> 1 teaspoon cumin
>
> 3 Tablespoons olive oil

Instructions

Preheat the oven to 350F. Toss all ingredients together in a bowl, making sure the oil coats everything well. Using four skewers, skewer the meat and veg evenly onto each skewer. Bake for 30 minutes, until the meat is cooked through and the veg are soft.

> Nutrition: 219 calories, 15.7 g fat, 16g protein, 2 g net carbs

Basic Burger Patties

The burger patty recipe that works for any burger! Make a bunch of these, and keep them wrapped individually in the freezer! They can be thawed and baked in a 375F oven for 15 minutes, making it quick and fast to have a great burger anytime!

Serving: 12

Serving Size: 1 patty

Prep Time: 15 minutes

Cook Time: 30 minutes

Ingredients

> 6 lbs ground beef
>
> 2 Tablespoons salt
>
> 1 Tablespoon garlic powder
>
> 2 teaspoons cayenne
>
> 3 eggs

Instructions

Preheat oven to 350F. In a large bowl, combine all ingredients well. For 12 equal size patties, and press them onto a baking sheet lined with parchment. Bake for 25-30 minutes, until fully cooked. Serve immediately with your preferred toppings, or allow to cool and wrap individually in plastic wrap to freeze. If frozen, enjoy within 2 months.

Nutrition: 437 calories, 15.2g fat, 70 g protein, 0.2 g net carbs

Keto Chinese Beef and Broccoli

This quick dish couldn't be easier or more flavorful. It's packed with delicious, light Asian flavors, crunchy broccoli, and hearty beef. In 30 minutes or less, you'll have a quick dinner on the table that kids will like, too.

Serving: 4

Serving Size: ¼ of bowl

Prep Time: 15 minutes

Cook Time: 10 minutes

Ingredients

 1 lb beef (sirloin or skirt steak)

 1 or 2 heads of broccoli, cut into small florets

 2 cloves garlic, minced

 1 Tablespoon ginger

For marinade:

 1 Tablespoon soy sauce

 1 Tablespoon sesame oil

 ½ teaspoon salt

 ¼ teaspoon black pepper

For sauce:

 2 Tablespoons soy sauce

 1 Tablespoon fish sauce

 2 teaspoons sesame oil

 ¼ teaspoon black pepper

Instructions

Slice the beef into ¼" thick pieces. Marinate in the marinade ingredients. Heat up a pot of water until boiling and briefly cook broccoli until crunchy and tender. Drain and set aside. Heat up a wok over medium heat using 1 ½ Tablespoons of ghee or olive oil. Add the marinated beef and spread the beef over the bottom of the pan and cook until the edges are crispy. Flip beef over and finish cooking. Add broccoli and cook another several minutes, then add the sauce ingredients. Toss everything to combine with sauce. Could garnish with toasted sesame seeds and sliced green onion.

Nutrition: 273 calories, 17 g fat, 24 g protein, 3 g net carbs

Beef Fajita Bowl

Hungry for Mexican food? Then you'll love making this yummy Beef Fajita Bowl. Leftovers can be made into wraps or a salad, so you actually get three meals in one, only cooking once! Perfect for summer.

Servings: 4

Serving Size: 1 portion

Prep Time: 15 minutes

Cook Time: 15 minutes

Ingredients

> 1 lb steak, sliced into strips
>
> 2 teaspoons olive oil
>
> 2 green bell peppers, chopped
>
> 1 onion, chopped
>
> 1 clove garlic, minced
>
> 1 teaspoon chili powder
>
> 1 teaspoon ground cumin
>
> ½ teaspoon paprika
>
> ½ teaspoon salt

Instructions

Place your 12" skillet on medium heat and add 1 of the teaspoons of olive oil. When pan is warm, add steak and saute until half cooked, about 5-6 minutes. Then add second teaspoon of olive oil and the peppers, onion, and garlic. Saute several minutes, then add the chili powder and cumin and paprika. Cook until steak is completely cooked and the veggies are crisp tender, about another 4-5 minutes. Sprinkle with salt. Divide amongst four bowls and serve hot with salsa, sour cream, and fresh cilantro. As an option, you could add some chopped Thai red chilis for some more heat.

Nutrition: 360 calories, 12 g fat, 48 g protein, 11 g net carbs

Beef Fajita Lettuce Wraps

Using leftovers from the Beef Fajita Bowl, these fun little wraps are the perfect way to satisfy any taco cravings! They make a very portable lunch, dinner or snack, and are a snap to make! You can leave the fajita filling cold for a refreshing, easy lunch, or heat it up and build your fajitas one by one- the choice is up to you!

Serving: 1

Serving Size: 4 wraps

Prep Time: 15 minutes

Cook Time: 2 minutes

Ingredients

> 1 serving Beef Fajita Bowl
>
> 4 large leaves iceberg or Romaine lettuce
>
> 2 Tablespoons salsa, for dipping (optional)
>
> 2 Tablespoons guacamole, for dipping

Instructions

If you prefer your fajita filling to be hot, microwave covered on high for 2 minutes. If not, move on to the next step. Spoon the filling into the lettuce leaf, folding the base slightly to keep everything inside. Spoon the salsa and guacamole on top, and dive in! Serve immediately.

> Nutrition: 513 calories, 37 g fat, 34 g protein, 9 g net carbs

Lettuce Wrapped Lamb Burgers

These lettuce wrapped burgers are a convenient way to bring your bun less burger to work or school for a quick, easy, portable lunch! Using leftover lamb burgers and tzatziki sauce, the crispy romaine lettuce holds it all together, while the addition of sliced bell peppers adds a bit of color and interest to the meal!

Serving: 1

Serving Size: 2 burgers

Prep Time: 15 minutes

Cook Time: 1 minute

Ingredients

> 1 serving Greek Lamb Burger
>
> 1 serving of Tzatziki (from same recipe)
>
> 4-6 large iceberg lettuce leaves
>
> ¼ red bell pepper, finely sliced

Instructions

Warm the burger patties by microwaving on high for 1 minute. Next, lay two or three pieces of lettuce out evenly, and spoon the tzatziki sauce over it. Top with the burger patty and pepper slices, and fold the lettuce leaves over to create a wrap. Do the same with the second burger, and remaining lettuce leaves, tzatziki and peppers. Serve immediately.

> Nutrition: 513 calories, 37 g fat, 34 g protein, 9 g net carbs

Steak and Avocado Taco Cups

Yummy grilled steak and diced avocado make a great Southwest style filling for these crispy taco cups! You'll never miss taco shells again, once you've had these!

Serving: 1

Serving Size: 4 tacos

Prep Time: 15 minutes

Cook Time: 5 minutes

Ingredients

   1 hard boiled egg, chopped

   ¼ lb flank steak, sliced

   1 diced avocado

   1 Tablespoon lemon juice

   2 teaspoons salt

   1 Tablespoon olive oil

   2 oz Monterey Jack Cheese, shredded

   2 Tablespoons salsa

Instructions

Season the steak with salt and pepper. Over medium heat, preheat a skillet with the olive oil. Sear each side of the steak for about 3 – 5 minutes, cooking to medium rare. Take the steak out and let rest for at least 10 minutes before slicing. Toss the avocado with lemon juice in a bowl. Mix in the egg and toss in the steak. Season with more salt and pepper. Preheat the oven to 375F. Lay the cheese into 4 even piles on a baking sheet lined with parchment, and bake 5 minutes until the cheese has started to melt and bubble. Allow the cheese to cool slightly, and then carefully pick up each mound and place it into a muffin tin to cool for another 10-15 minutes, until cool and hardened. Spoon the salad into each cup. Top with salsa. Serve immediately.

   Nutrition: 650 calories, 53 g fat, 40 g protein, 6 g net carbs

Cheese Stuffed Meatballs

Think of these like little meaty fat bombs! These meatballs are perfect when you just want a little something, but also work really well as an appetizer or main. Make a big batch and freeze them, for an easy meatball fix anytime!

Serving: 4

Serving Size: 3 meatballs

Prep Time: 10 minutes

Cook Time: 25 minutes

Ingredients

     1 ½ lbs ground beef

     4 oz cheddar cheese, shredded

     4 Tablespoons parmesan cheese, shredded

     ½ teaspoon salt

     ½ teaspoon pepper

Instructions

Preheat the oven to 350F. Mix all ingredients together in a bowl. Roll out 12 equal sized balls. Lay the balls onto a baking sheet lined with parchment, and bake 25 minutes until the meatballs are browned and cooked through. If freezing, allow to cool fully and store in an airtight container for up to three months. To reheat from frozen, allow to thaw in the fridge overnight and bake 20 minutes at 350F. Serve warm.

     Nutrition: 440 calories, 28 g fat, 46 g protein,2 g net carbs

Cheese Stuffed Burgers

These burgers are rich, and full of gooey cheese! Serve in a lettuce wrap, or on their own topped with tomato, onion and pickles for a decadent burger experience!

Servings: 4

Serving Size: 1 patty

Prep Time: 10 minutes

Cook Time: 35 minutes

Ingredients:

     1 lb ground beef

     1 Tablespoon onion powder

     ½ Tablespoon garlic powder

     1 teaspoon cayenne powder

     1 Tablespoon salt

     1 Tablespoon pepper

     4 cups cheddar cheese, shredded

Instructions:

Preheat oven to 350F. Mix the beef and spices together, and form into four patties. Press ¼ cup cheese into the center of each patty, forming the meat around it. Bake in the oven for 20 minutes. Serve warm or keep in an airtight container in the fridge for 8 days.

     Nutrition: 681 calories, 44.7 g fat, 63.1 g protein, 3.7 g net carbs

Beef Vindaloo

Beef Vindaloo is a spicy, tomato based Indian stew that is rich in flavor. Serve with Cauliflower Rice!

Servings: 2

Serving Size: 1 cup

Prep Time: 60 minutes

Cook Time: 25 minutes

Ingredients:

> ½ lb flank steak, cut into chunks
>
> 1 Tablespoon olive oil
>
> ¼ cup butter or ghee
>
> 2 stalks celery, chopped
>
> ¼ onion, chopped
>
> 3 cloves garlic, minced
>
> 1" piece ginger, minced
>
> 2 tomatoes, chopped
>
> 1 teaspoon red wine vinegar
>
> 2 teaspoons cayenne pepper
>
> 4 red chilies, minced (optional)
>
> 1 cup beef stock
>
> 1 cup heavy cream

Instructions:

Mix together the olive oil, garlic, ginger, vinegar, cayenne and chilies. Add in the beef, and mix well. Let sit for 20 minutes, or overnight. Heat a large pot over medium heat. Add in the butter or ghee, and sauté the tomatoes and onion until soft- about 5 minutes. Add in the beef and marinade, and toss well to combine. Cook 3 minutes. Add the beef stock, and bring to a boil. Reduce heat to low, and simmer 20 minutes. Stir in the cream, and cook 10 minutes longer. Serve warm or keep in an airtight container in the fridge for up to 7 days.

> Nutrition: 436 calories, 30.4 g fat, 35 g protein, 3.5 g net carbs

Beef Stew

This stew is warm and hearty, and really yummy!

Servings: 4

Serving Size: 1 cup

Prep Time: 10 minutes

Cook Time: 55 minutes

Ingredients:

> 1 lb flank steak, cut into chunks
>
> 1 Tablespoon olive oil
>
> 1 Tablespoon thyme
>
> 1 Tablespoon salt
>
> 4 cups beef stock
>
> 2 Tablespoons butter
>
> 1 carrot, chopped
>
> 2 stalks celery, chopped
>
> 1 14.5 oz can diced tomatoes
>
> ¼ onion, chopped
>
> 2 cloves garlic, minced
>
> 2 Tablespoons Worcestershire sauce
>
> ½ cup red wine (optional)
>
> 1 cup heavy cream

Instructions:

Preheat a large pot over medium heat. Drizzle the oil, and brown the beef on all sides- about 4 minutes. Remove from pan and set aside. In the same pot, melt in the butter and sauté the vegetables with the salt, until soft - about 3 minutes. Add in the herbs. Return the beef back to the pot. Add the stock and Worcestershire sauce and wine. Bring to a boil, then reduce heat to low. Simmer 25 minutes. Stir in the cream, and simmer another 15 minutes. You could also make this in a crockpot! After browning the beef, add the rest of the ingredients (except cream) to the crockpot and cook on low 4-6 hours. Turn heat off, let sit for 30 minutes to cool down, then add the heavy cream.

> Nutrition: 450 calories, 30.4 g fat, 35 g protein, 4.5 g net carbs

Seafood

Red Pepper Cod

This easy, classic recipe is perfect for a quick weeknight meal! The cooked cod will last for up to a day in the fridge - so you may want to make another piece, just to have it available. Serve with sautéed vegetables, a salad, or on top of zucchini noodles for a decadent weeknight dinner!

Serving: 1

Serving Size: 1 piece

Prep Time: 10 minutes

Cook Time: 35 minutes

Ingredients

    ½ red pepper, diced

    1 Tablespoon olive oil

    1 teaspoon red pepper flakes

    ½ lemon, sliced into three equal sized medallions

    1 6 oz fillet cod, preferably Ocean Safe certified wild caught

    1 teaspoon dried oregano

    1 teaspoon dried thyme

    1 teaspoon salt

    1 teaspoon pepper

Instructions

Preheat the oven to 375F. Toss the pepper with the olive oil and a pinch of salt, and transfer the mixture into an ovenproof baking dish. Bake for 20 minutes, until soft. Transfer the roasted pepper to a blender or food processor, and puree until smooth. Next, lay the cod onto a baking sheet lined with parchment. Preheat oven to 350F. Lay the lemon wheels onto a baking sheet lined with parchment, and place the fish on top. Season the fish with the salt, pepper, thyme, red pepper flakes and oregano, and spoon the pureed pepper over top. Bake 12 minutes. Turn the broiler on to high, and broil for 5 minutes. Serve immediately.

    Nutrition: 336 calories, 16.2 g fat, 40 g protein, 6g net carbs

Sea Bass with Prosciutto and Herbs

This recipe is restaurant quality, and so easy to prepare! Eat it on its own for a luxuriously simple dinner, or pair it with zucchini noodles or sautéed spinach.

Serving: 1

Serving Size: 1 piece

Prep Time: 15 minutes

Cook Time: 25 minutes

Ingredients

    3 oz sea bass fillet, preferably wild caught

    ½ lemon, sliced into three equal sized medallions

    1 teaspoon dried oregano

    1 teaspoon dried thyme

    1 teaspoon salt

1 teaspoon pepper

2 Tablespoons olive oil

4 cherry tomatoes

¼ cup basil, chopped finely

3 stalks asparagus

1 Tablespoon butter, melted

1 oz prosciutto, cut into thin ribbons

Instructions

Preheat the oven to 375F. Lay the lemon wheels onto a baking sheet lined with parchment. Brush the fish with 1 Tablespoon of olive oil, and lay it on top of the lemon wheels. Toss the asparagus and tomatoes in the remaining Tablespoon of oil, and arrange it around the fish. Season everything with the salt, pepper and dried herbs. Toss the butter, prosciutto, and basil together, and lay it on top of the fish. Bake for 25 minutes. Serve warm.

Nutrition: 586 calories, 16.2 g fat, 40 g protein, 6g net carbs

Thai Coconut Cod

This fabulously creamy, spicy fish dish goes perfectly on top of cauliflower rice! If you prefer a bit more spice, feel free to add as many chilies as you like; if you're unsure of the heat level, start with one chili - you can always add more at the end! Leftovers keep well for up to two days in the fridge, and can be reheated by microwaving on high for 2 minutes.

Serving: 2

Serving Size: half recipe

Prep Time: 10 minutes

Cook Time: 15 minutes

Ingredients

2 6 oz pieces cod

1 Tablespoon coconut oil

1/2 can coconut milk

1 handful cilantro, finely chopped

8 large basil leaves, chopped

2 green onions, finely sliced

1 clove garlic, minced

1" piece ginger, grated

4 red chilis, finely sliced (optional)

1 Tablespoon sesame seeds

For the cauliflower rice:

½ cup riced cauliflower

½ can coconut milk

Instructions

Preheat the oven to 350F. Season the cod with salt and pepper, and lay it onto a baking sheet lined with parchment. Bake in the oven for 20 minutes, until flakey. Meanwhile, drizzle the coconut oil into a small saucepan, and add the green onion, ginger, garlic and chilies. Sauté for 30 seconds, and then add the coconut milk. Taste, and season with salt. Add the cilantro and basil, and reduce heat to low. Simmer 20 minutes. While the cod is in the oven and the coconut sauce is simmering, combine the remaining half can of coconut milk with the cauliflower rice in a microwave safe bowl. Cover, and microwave on high for 4 minutes. Season with salt and pepper, and fluff with a fork. To serve, spoon out the coconut rice onto a plate, and place the fish on top. Spoon the sauce over everything. Garnish with sesame seeds

Nutrition: 482 calories, 34 g fat, 42.5 g protein, 5g net carbs

Thai Coconut Cod Lettuce Wraps

This recipe is perfect for lunch, snacks, or a cold dinner on a hot day! These fabulously portable wraps are the perfect make-ahead thing to pack for a workday lunch or snack, and also make a fun addition to a summer day picnic!

Serving: 1

Serving Size: 3 wraps

Prep Time: 15 minutes

Cook Time: 0 minutes

Ingredients

1 serving Thai Coconut Cod

6 large pieces iceberg lettuce

3 large basil leaves

Handful cilantro, torn

4 red chilis, sliced (optional)

Instructions

Lay the iceberg leaves out two at a time, so they overlap each other slightly. Flake ⅓ of the fish into the first lettuce wrap. Add 1 basil leaf and a few cilantro leaves, as well as the chilies if you're using them. Fold the lettuce around the fish to create a bundle. Secure with a toothpick, or wrap in parchment to keep the wrap secure. Continue on with the next set of ingredients, until all three wraps are finished. Keep in the fridge for up to 24 hours.

Nutrition: 592 calories, 46 g fat, 35 g protein, 6g net carbs

Crab Stuffed Cucumbers

These make an excellent snack, but can also be served as an hors d'oeuvres or a supplemental dish at a brunch or lunch.

Serving: 4

Serving Size: 2 pieces

Prep Time: 15 minutes

Cook Time: 0 minutes

Ingredients

> 1 cucumber
>
> ½ cup cream cheese, softened
>
> 2 Tablespoons butter, softened
>
> 1 Tablespoon heavy cream
>
> 1 teaspoon paprika
>
> 1 small handful fresh dill, chopped (plus more for garnish)
>
> ¼ cup crab meat, picked through and shredded (canned is fine)
>
> 1 teaspoon salt
>
> 1 teaspoon pepper
>
> 1 lemon, zest only

Instructions

Slice the cucumber into about 8 medallions, each roughly 1 ½" thick. Using a small spoon, carefully scoop out some of the middle, making sure to leave the base intact. Mix together the rest of the ingredients. Spoon the mixture into the cucumber rounds, and garnish with dill. Serve immediately, or keep in an airtight container in the fridge for up to 24 hours.

> Nutrition: 179 calories, 17.4 g fat, 3.1 g protein, 3 g net carbs

Salmon with Beurre Blanc

Beurre Blanc is a classic French sauce that is tangy, creamy and deliciously keto friendly! This restaurant quality fish goes beautifully with asparagus or greens. Make sure your chunks of butter are very cold in order to allow the sauce to emulsify properly.

Serving: 4

Serving Size: 1 fillet of fish

Prep Time: 15 minutes

Cook Time: 20 minutes

Ingredients

    4 3 oz fillets salmon

    2 Tablespoons olive oil

    ½ lemon, juice and zest

    ¼ cup dry white wine

    ¼ cup heavy cream

    ¼ cup cold butter, cut into chunks

    1 Tablespoon fresh dill, chopped

Instructions

Preheat the oven to 350F. Lay the salmon onto a baking sheet lined with parchment paper, and season with salt and pepper. Bake 15 minutes, until the fish is fully cooked. Allow to rest while you prepare the beurre blanc. Preheat a small pan over medium high heat. Add in the wine and lemon juice, and cook until it has almost completely evaporated. Whisk in the cream, and reduce heat to low. Whisk in the cold butter, one chunk at a time, whisking well until it's completely incorporated into the cream. Continue on, until all the butter has been mixed in and a thick, white sauce has formed. Whisk in the dill and lemon zest, and remove the sauce from the heat. Leftovers will keep in an airtight container in the fridge for up to three days.

    Nutrition: 330 calories, 28 g fat, 18 g protein, 1g net carbs

Spinach Stuffed Cod

These stuffed cod rolls look fancy, but they're so easy to make and can be rolled in advance for quick heating and serving! Serve them with asparagus, broccoli, peppers or greens!

Serving: 4

Serving Size: 1 fillet of fish

Prep Time: 15 minutes

Cook Time: 25 minutes

Ingredients

    4 3 oz fillets cod

    1 cup spinach

    1 Tablespoon olive oil

    1 clove garlic, minced

    1 lemon, juice and zest

    1 Tablespoon thyme

    1 teaspoon salt

    1 teaspoon pepper

4 strips bacon

Instructions

Preheat the oven to 350F. Preheat a medium pan over medium heat. Drizzle in the oil, and add in the garlic, spinach and salt and pepper. Sauté the spinach for a minute or so, and squeeze in the lemon. Continue sautéing until the spinach has wilted down. Set aside. Make an incision into the cod, and slice either side to open up the fillets like a book. Spoon the spinach mixture evenly into the center of each fillet, and fold it back up to cover the filling. Tie a bacon strip around the fillet, to keep it in place. Lay the wrapped fillets onto a baking sheet lined with parchment. Bake 15-20 minutes, until the fish is opaque and flakey. Serve immediately. Leftovers will keep in an airtight container in the fridge for up to three days.

Nutrition: 407 calories, 13.7 g fat, 65.6 g protein, 1g net carbs

Parmesan Crusted Halibut

This parmesan-almond crust is perfect for any type of fish, and also works well on chicken. Halibut is buttery, soft, and really decadent! If you choose to go for a slightly less expensive option, cod makes a great substitute.

Serving: 4

Serving Size: 1 fillet of fish

Prep Time: 15 minutes

Cook Time: 20 minutes

Ingredients

4 3 oz fillets halibut

1 egg, beaten

¼ cup almond flour

3 Tablespoons parmesan

1 teaspoon garlic powder

1 teaspoon thyme

1 teaspoon salt

1 teaspoon pepper

1 Tablespoon olive oil

Instructions

Preheat the oven to 350F. In a bowl, combine the almond flour, parmesan, garlic, thyme, salt and pepper. Coat each fillet in the egg, and toss into the almond flour mixture. Lay on a baking sheet lined with parchment, and drizzle the oil over top. Bake for 20 minutes. Serve immediately. Leftovers will keep in an airtight container in the fridge for up to three days.

Nutrition: 266 calories, 14.8 g fat, 30 g protein, 1.2 g net carbs

Crab Stuffed Avocado

This stuffed avocado is creamy and sophisticated! Eat it for a light lunch or dinner, on top of greens.

Serving: 2

Serving Size: ½ avocado

Prep Time: 5 minutes

Cook Time: 0 minutes

Ingredients

> 4 oz crab meat, cooked and picked through
>
> 2 Tablespoons mayonnaise
>
> 1 teaspoon salt
>
> 1 teaspoon pepper
>
> 1 teaspoon paprika
>
> 1 avocado, halved

Instructions

Mix together the crab, mayo, and seasonings. Spoon into the avocado halves. Serve immediately.

> Nutrition: 319 calories, 25.7 g fat, 9.4 g protein, 6 g net carbs

Fish Tacos

Using leftover Baja Style Halibut Salad, you can easily make these fish tacos for a quick, easy cold lunch! Perfect for a hot day!

Serving: 1

Serving Size: 4 tacos

Prep Time: 5 minutes

Cook Time: 0 minutes

Ingredients

> 1 serving Baja Style Halibut Salad
>
> 8 large pieces iceberg lettuce
>
> 2 Tablespoons salsa (optional)

Instructions

Flake the fish and mix with the salad. Lay out 1-2 pieces of lettuce to create a wrap, and spoon ¼ of the mixture into the center. Wrap to form a little taco. Continue until all ingredients have been used. Serve with salsa.

> Nutrition: 740 calories, 40 g fat, 95 g protein, 7 g net carbs

Cod Bruschetta

This gorgeous white fish is the perfect vehicle for a combination of tomatoes, prosciutto and herbs! This restaurant quality meal would be great served alongside asparagus or greens.

Serving: 2

Serving Size: 1 fillet

Prep Time: 5 minutes

Cook Time: 25 minutes

Ingredients

> 2 4 oz pieces cod
>
> 1 tomato, diced
>
> ½ onion, diced
>
> 2 Tablespoons olive oil
>
> 1 Tablespoon Italian Herbs
>
> 4 oz prosciutto, chopped
>
> Handful fresh parsley, chopped
>
> 1 teaspoon salt
>
> 1 teaspoon pepper

Instructions

Preheat oven to 350F. Toss together all ingredients, except the fish. Lay the fish onto a baking sheet lined with parchment, and spoon the bruschetta mixture over top. Bake 25 minutes. Serve warm.

> Nutrition: 341 calories, 18.2 g fat, 28.4 g protein, 3.5 g net carbs

Desserts and Drinks

Keto Bulletproof Coffee

Boost your coffee's fat content and make your breakfast amazing by enjoying a cup of this delicious Keto friendly Bulletproof Coffee.

Serving: 1

Serving Size:

Prep Time: 5 minutes

Cook Time: 0

Ingredients

> 1 cup black coffee

1 Tablespoon grass-fed unsalted butter

1 Tablespoon coconut or MCT oil

½ Tablespoon heavy cream

½ teaspoon vanilla extract

Instructions

Mix everything together by hand or in a blender. Serve warm or cold! You can substitute almond extract for the vanilla or leave it out.

Nutrition: 255 calories, 28.5 g fat, 0 g protein, 1.0 g carbohydrates

Almond Butter Bulletproof Coffee

This slightly sweet version of Bulletproof Coffee is a super fast and easy way to get your morning caffeine kick, along with a good dose of fat! Prepared Almond Butter Fat Bombs are added to regular coffee to make this nutty, creamy coffee.

Serving: 1

Serving Size:

Prep Time: 10 minutes

Cook Time: 0

Ingredients

1 cup coffee

1 Almond Butter Fat Bomb

Instructions

Brew your coffee as you normally would. Using your blender, blend together the coffee and a Fat Bomb. Drink your coffee hot, or add ice cubes for iced coffee.

Nutrition: 300 calories, 31g fat, 7g protein, 4g net carbs

Chocolate Smoothie

Keto smoothies are having their moment in the spotlight, and it's easy to see why! Creamy, thick and delicious, they are the perfect treat for snacking or breakfast! This chocolate smoothie is so thick and creamy, it'll remind you of a chocolate milkshake! Enjoy it extra cold to really get a satisfying experience!

Servings: 1

Serving Size: whole recipe

Prep Time: 5 minutes

Cook Time: 0 minutes

Ingredients:

1 Tablespoon chia seeds

1 egg yolk

1 Tablespoon almond butter

1 Tablespoon cocoa butter

¼ cup heavy cream

1 Tablespoon cocoa powder

1 teaspoon Stevia

½ cup ice

1/4 teaspoon chocolate essence (unsweetened) or ¼ teaspoon vanilla extract

Instructions:

Pour the ice and cream into the bottom of the blender, to prevent the other ingredients from sticking to the bottom. Add in the rest of the ingredients, and blend on high until smooth. Serve immediately.

Nutrition: 575 calories, 44 g fat, 34 g protein, 3 g net carbs

Vanilla Smoothie

This creamy vanilla shake is the perfect thing to jump start your day!

Serving: 1

Serving Size: whole recipe

Prep Time: 5 minutes

Cook Time: 0 minutes

Ingredients

1 cup coconut milk

1 Tablespoon coconut oil

½ Tablespoon vanilla extract

1 teaspoon Stevia

Instructions

Combine all ingredients in a blender until smooth. Serve immediately.

Nutrition: 669 calories, 70.8g fat, 5.5 g protein, 4 g net carbs

Strawberry Cow Smoothie

This smoothie is refreshing, sweet and fun! When your body adjusts to the keto lifestyle, your taste buds naturally adjust to find foods naturally sweeter. In the beginning, feel free to use a bit of Stevia if you like, but you may find you don't need it!

Serving: 1

Serving Size: whole recipe

Prep Time: 5 minutes

Cook Time: 0 minutes

Ingredients

    ½ cup frozen strawberries

    ½ cup full fat coconut milk

    1 cup ice

Instructions

Pour the coconut milk into the bottom of the blender to prevent the other ingredients from sticking. Add in the rest of the ingredients, and puree until smooth. Serve immediately.

    Nutrition: 301 calories, 28.6 g fat, 2.8 g protein, 9 g net carbs

Golden Milk Smoothie

Golden Milk is all the rage these days, and this smoothie is definitely full of benefits! Turmeric has been touted as the newest superfood, and has been proven to cleanse the liver and organs for optimal health. Enjoy this smoothie very cold.

Serving: 1

Serving Size: whole recipe

Prep Time: 5 minutes

Cook Time: 0 minutes

Ingredients

    1 Tablespoon turmeric

    1 cup coconut milk

    1 teaspoon Stevia

    1 cup crushed ice

Instructions

Puree all ingredients together until smooth. Serve immediately.

    Nutrition: 460 calories, 25.3 g fat, 1.7g protein, 1.4 g net carbs

Almond Butter Smoothie

This is a filling and yummy smoothie you can have for breakfast or as a quick snack to up your fat intake. It's super low carb and delicious!

Serving: 2

Serving Size: about 1 cup

Prep Time: 5 minutes

Cook Time: 0 minutes

Ingredients

> 2 Tablespoons almond butter
>
> 1 1/2 cups almond milk
>
> 1 Tablespoon hemp seeds

Instructions

Start by pouring the almond milk into the blender to avoid the ingredients sticking at the bottom. Add in the rest of the ingredients. Turn the blender on, starting at a low speed and increase as needed. Add extra water if you desire your smoothie more on the liquid side. Pour into a cup and serve immediately. Place any leftover smoothie into an airtight container, and enjoy within 24 hours.

> Nutrition: 483 calories, 34.6g fat, 5.5g protein, 4g net carbs

Pink Power Smoothie

This smoothie is full of good fat, and a great flavor and color! Keep any leftovers in an airtight container in the fridge for up to 24 hours so you can enjoy a quick pick me up later on!

Serving: 2

Serving Size: half recipe

Prep Time: 5 minutes

Cook Time: 0 minutes

Ingredients

> 1/2 cup raspberries
>
> 1/2 Tablespoon lemon zest
>
> 1 cup coconut milk
>
> 1 Tablespoon flaxseeds

Instructions

Start by pouring the coconut milk into the blender to avoid the ingredients sticking at the bottom. Add in the rest of the ingredients. Turn the blender on, starting at a low speed and increase as needed. Add extra water if you desire your smoothie more on the liquid side. Once it looks even, pour into a cup and serve immediately. Pour any leftover smoothie into an airtight container and enjoy within 24 hours.

> Nutrition: 310 calories, 29.9g fat, 3.8g protein, 9g net carbs

Raspberry Chia Pudding

Chia pudding is so versatile, and really easy to prep in advance! Because chia seeds get better as they expand in liquid, this pudding will continue to thicken and sweeten as it sits in the fridge. The best part is, it's good for up to a week in the fridge, so if you're a really big fan of it you can make enough to last you all week, and indulge as needed.

Serving: 2

Serving Size: about 3/4 cup

Prep Time: 5 minutes

Cook Time: 5 minutes

Ingredients

> 1 cup almond milk
>
> 1/2 cup chia seeds
>
> ¼ cup frozen raspberries
>
> 1 Tablespoon flaxseeds
>
> 1 Tablespoon hemp seeds

Instructions

Combine all ingredients together, mixing well so the raspberries crush a bit. Store in an airtight container overnight. Enjoy leftovers within 7 days.

> Nutrition: 642 calories, 50 g fat, 15.9 g protein, 8g net carbs

Raspberry Chocolate Fudge

This rich, chocolaty fudge is the perfect thing to hit the spot when you're craving something sweet. Best of all, it's virtually carb and protein free and high fat, which can help kick start your ketosis.

Serving: 16

Serving Size: 1 piece

Prep Time: 2 minutes

Cook Time: 10 Minutes

Ingredients

> ½ cup raw cacao powder
>
> 2 Tablespoons unsweetened dark chocolate, shaved
>
> 2 Tablespoons Stevia
>
> ½ cup coconut oil
>
> ¼ cup raspberries, mashed lightly

¼ cup almond milk

Instructions

Mix all ingredients together until well combined. Prepare a 10" baking dish with parchment paper or plastic wrap, and carefully spoon the fudge mixture into the center. Using a spatula, spread the mixture evenly into the baking dish, and cover with plastic wrap. Refrigerate for an hour, and cut into 16 equal pieces. Store wrapped in the fridge for up to one month.

Nutrition: 74 calories, 8.1g fat, 0.6g protein, 0.9g net carbs

Strawberry Chia Pudding Popsicles

Popsicles are such a sweet, refreshing treat! These popsicles have extra fat and protein from coconut milk and chia seeds, and are sweetened naturally with fruit (although you can use a bit of Stevia if you like).

Serving: 6

Serving Size: 1 popsicle

Prep Time: 4 hours, including freezing time

Cook Time: 0 minutes

Ingredients

2 cups coconut milk

¼ cup chia seeds

¼ cup frozen strawberries, thawed

Instructions

Mash together the berries and chia seeds. Stir in the coconut milk. Transfer the mixture to 6 popsicle molds, and freeze for at least 4 hours. Popsicles will last in the freezer for up to 8 weeks.

Nutrition: 277 calories, 24.9 g fat, 5 g protein, 3 g net carbs

Almond Butter Cookies

These cookies are reminiscent of childhood – soft and chewy – while staying extremely low carb and high fat! What more could you want?

Servings: 10

Serving Size: 1 cookie

Prep Time: 5 minutes

Cook Time: 10 minutes

Ingredients:

¾ cup almond butter

¼ cup powdered Stevia or erythritol

1 egg yolk

¼ teaspoon cinnamon

Instructions:

Preheat oven to 350F. In a medium sized bowl, beat together all ingredients until smooth. Roll the cookie dough into 1-1 ½" balls, and lay them out onto a baking sheet lined with parchment. Press each ball down with a fork, to form the final cookie shape. Bake 10-12 minutes, until golden brown and fragrant. Let the cookies cool completely before serving. Store cookies in an airtight container at room temperature for up to a week.

Nutrition: 98 calories, 10 g fat, 4 g protein, 1.4 g net carbs

Snacks and Sides

Butter Tossed Asparagus

The old adage is true - butter DOES make it better! This asparagus dish is loaded with delicious fat and flavor and makes the perfect side dish.

Servings: 2

Serving Size: 5 pieces

Prep Time: 0 minutes

Cook Time: 15 minutes

Ingredients:

10 spears fresh asparagus

2 Tablespoons butter

1 Tablespoon olive oil

2 large stems thyme

1 teaspoon salt

1 teaspoon white pepper

Instructions:

Bring a large pot of salted water to a boil. Toss in the asparagus spears, and boil for 1 minute to blanch. Drain, and transfer to an ice bath. Set aside. Preheat a large pan over medium heat. Drizzle in the oil and add the butter and whole thyme stem. Cook until the butter has melted fully and has started to foam, about 2 minutes. Add the blanched asparagus spears to the foaming butter, and toss well to coat. Cook for 1-2 minutes, tossing well the entire time. Serve immediately.

Nutrition: 186 calories, 18.7 g fat, 2.8 g protein, 2 g net carbs

Caramelized Onions

These caramelized onions are low carb, relatively high fat, and make a great addition to pizzas, burgers, or anything else you can come up with.

Servings: 8

Serving Size: 1 Tablespoon

Prep Time: 10 minutes

Cook Time: 65 minutes

Ingredients:

> 4 onions, sliced thinly
>
> ½ lb butter
>
> 1 Tablespoon salt

Instructions:

Melt the butter in a pan over medium heat. Add in the onions and the salt. Toss well with tongs until the onions start to cook down. Continue to cook, stirring occasionally, for about an hour, until the onions are brown and soft. Transfer to an airtight container and keep in the fridge for up to 4 weeks.

> Nutrition: 225 calories, 23.1 g fat, 0.9 g protein, 3 g net carbs

Curry Mayonnaise

Curry Mayo is a great option to mix up flavors! Use this mayo on burgers or in the Egg Salad or Chicken Salad as a substitute.

Servings: 8

Serving Size: 1 Tablespoon

Prep Time: 5 minutes

Cook Time: 0 minutes

Ingredients:

> ¼ cup mayonnaise
>
> 1 Tablespoon curry powder

Instructions:

Whisk ingredients together until smooth. Store in an airtight container for up to 5 weeks.

> Nutrition: 45 calories, 5 g fat, 0 g protein, 0 g net carbs

Green Tahini

This tahini is enhanced with greens for additional nutritional value and a hit of color! Use this sauce as a dip for veggies, a dressing for salads, or as a replacement for mayo.

Servings: 8

Serving Size: 1 Tablespoon

Prep Time: 5 minutes

Cook Time: 0 minutes

Ingredients:

- 2 Tablespoons tahini paste
- 2 cloves garlic
- 2 teaspoons salt
- 1 Tablespoon olive oil
- 1 lemon, juice and zest
- ¼ cup water
- ¼ cup fresh kale

Instructions:

In a blender or food processor, combine all ingredients until smooth. Taste and adjust seasoning as needed. Store in an airtight container for up to a month.

Nutrition: 43 calories, 3.9 g fat, 0.7 g protein, 0.3 g net carbs

Cheesy Fondue

Fondue is one of the best snacks for sharing. By using low carb veggies like celery and red peppers, you (and your friends!) can enjoy this high fat, low carb treat.

Serving: 4

Serving Size: 2 pieces pickles, 2 pieces pepper, 3 pieces celery, ¼ fondue sauce

Prep Time: 10 minutes

Cook Time: 30 Minutes

Ingredients

- 1 cup cheddar cheese, shredded
- 1 cup gruyere cheese, shredded
- ¼ cup dry white wine
- 1 cup heavy cream
- 1 teaspoon garlic powder
- 1 teaspoon salt
- 1 teaspoon cayenne (optional)
- 3 stalks celery, chopped into 12 equal sticks
- ½ red bell pepper, sliced into 8 thin strips
- 4 pickles, cut in half lengthwise

Instructions:

In a medium sized saucepan, melt the cheeses and wine together over medium heat. Stir in the cream and spices, mixing well to combine. Transfer the finished sauce to a fondue pot, and keep warm. Arrange the veggies and bread onto a plate. Using fondue forks, dip the veggies into the cheese sauce and eat immediately.

Nutrition: 376 calories, 32 g fat, 19.5g protein, 4.4 g net carbs

Green Bean Fries

Have a craving for fries, but no potatoes on the Keto Diet, so what do you do? Try these delicious green bean fries smothered in a cheesy herbed mixture. Yummy!

Serving: 4

Serving Size: 8 Pieces

Prep Time: 10 minutes

Cook Time: 10 Minutes

Ingredients

> 24 green beans
>
> 1 egg
>
> ½ cup parmesan
>
> 1 teaspoon garlic powder
>
> 1 teaspoon Italian herbs
>
> 1 teaspoon salt

Instructions

Preheat oven to 400F. Fill a small pot with water up to three quarters. Bring the water to a boil. Blanch the beans for 2 minutes, and immediately drain and transfer them to an ice bath. Next, beat the egg in one bowl, and combine the dry ingredients in another bowl. Prepare a baking sheet lined with parchment. Bread each bean by dipping it first into the egg, then into the cheese mixture. Lay the prepared beans on the baking sheet, and bake for 15 minutes until crispy. Store any leftover beans in an airtight container at room temperature, and enjoy within 4 days.

Nutrition: 113 calories, 6g fat, 9g protein, 2g net carbs

Seed Crackers & Guacamole

This excellent seed cracker recipe is delicious and makes a perfect snack! You can also have these crackers with soup, as a snack, or to put in a work lunch.

Serving: 4

Serving Size: About 3 crackers, with 2 Tablespoons guac

Prep Time: 10 minutes

Cook Time: 45 Minutes

Ingredients

 1/4 cup chia seeds

 1/4 cups sesame seeds

 1/4 cups sunflower seeds

 1/2 Tablespoon Italian herbs

 1/2 teaspoon salt

 1 cup water

 1 egg

 1/2 mashed avocado

 Juice of half a lime

 Pinch of sea salt

Instructions

Preheat the oven to 350F. Combine the seeds, herbs, salt and egg in a bowl, and allow the mixture to sit for 5 minutes. Line a baking sheet with parchment paper and spread the seed mixture evenly until flat. Bake for 30 minutes. While still warm, cut the seed mixture into 12 equal sized squares. Flip the crackers over, and bake for another 15 minutes. While the crackers are baking combine all the guacamole ingredients in a bowl and mash until smooth.

 Nutrition: 280 calories, 24g fat, 8g protein, 3g net carbs

Celery and Almond Butter

There are many wonderful flavors and textures in this simple and easy snack! The crispy green crunch of celery pairs perfectly with creamy nutty almond butter.

Serving: 1

Serving Size: 8 pieces celery, 2 Tbsp almond butter

Prep Time: 2 minutes

Cook Time: 0 Minutes

Ingredients

 2 stalks celery

 2 Tablespoons almond butter

Instructions

Cut the celery into 8 equal sized sticks and dip into the almond butter. For a more portable snack, spread the almond butter into the cavity of the celery stalk, and pack in an airtight container for up to 24 hours.

Nutrition: 230 calories, 18g fat, 8g protein, 4g net carbs

Salted Macadamias

Nuts are a great way to get a quick dose of fat. These nuts are SO easy to do, and so delicious! Once you've figured out the basic recipe, it's easy to season these nuts with any herbs or spices.

Serving: 1

Serving Size: whole recipe

Prep Time: 5 minutes

Cook Time: 5 Minutes

Ingredients

> 1/4 cup Macadamia nuts
>
> 1 Tablespoon coconut oil
>
> 1 teaspoon sea salt

Instructions

Preheat oven to 350F. Toss the macadamia nuts in the oil and salt. Lay onto a baking sheet, and bake 5 minutes, making sure not to burn the nuts. Allow to cool fully.

Nutrition: 224 calories, 22g fat, 3g protein, 1g net carbs

Nordic Seed Bread

This bread is said to have been invented by the Vikings, and has recently gained new popularity. This variation uses flax, pumpkin seeds, walnuts, macadamia nuts, and almonds. You can swap out the nuts or change the proportions according to your taste; just avoid higher carb nuts like cashews and pistachios.

Servings: 12

Serving Size: 1 piece

Prep Time: 10 minutes

Cook Time: 30 minutes

Ingredients:

> 1 cup almonds
>
> 1 cup walnuts
>
> 1 cup ground flax seeds
>
> 1 cup pumpkin seeds
>
> 1 cup sesame seeds

½ cup ground macadamia nuts

½ cup sesame seeds

5 eggs

½ cup coconut oil

2 teaspoons salt

Instructions:

Preheat oven to 325F. In a large bowl, whisk together the eggs, oil and salt. Add in the seeds, and mix well to combine. Next, press the mixture into a loaf pan lined with parchment. Bake for 1 hour, and allow to cool fully before slicing. Slice the bread into 12 equal sized pieces, and wrap individually. Keep leftover pieces individually wrapped at room temperature for up to 4 weeks.

Nutrition: 369 calories, 31.5 g fat, 10 g protein, 5 g net carbs

Almond Butter Fat Bombs

With a nutty flavor and lots of good fats, these Fat Bombs are one bite snacks you'll really enjoy. You'll need mini muffin tins or muffin cups to make these!

Servings: 6

Serving Size: 1 Fat Bomb

Prep Time: 5 minutes

Cook Time: 5 minutes

Ingredients:

¼ cup almond butter

¼ cup coconut oil

2 Tablespoons cocoa powder

¼ cup Stevia or erythritol

Instructions:

With a mixer or by hand, mix together the almond butter and a coconut oil. Microwave for about 30-45 seconds to soften, then stir until smooth. Add the cocoa powder and the sweetener, then stir those in and mix well. Pour into either silicone or mini muffin tins lined with papers. Stick in the fridge until firm.

Nutrition: 189 calories, 19.1 g fat, 3.2 g protein, 1.4 g net carbs

Mediterranean Fat Bombs

Most Fat Bombs focus on sweet - these are definitely savory and also have a high salt content to help replenish any lost electrolytes.

Servings: 6

Serving Size: 1 piece

Prep Time: 10 minutes

Cook Time: 5 minutes

Ingredients:

> ½ cup cream cheese
>
> ¼ cup butter
>
> 1 teaspoon dried oregano
>
> 1 teaspoon dried thyme
>
> 1 teaspoon dried basil
>
> 1 teaspoon garlic powder
>
> 5 pieces of sundried tomatoes, sliced
>
> 3 olives, sliced
>
> ¼ cup parmesan cheese, grated
>
> ½ teaspoon salt
>
> 1 teaspoon pepper

Instructions:

Beat together the butter and cream cheese until smooth. Beat in the rest of the ingredients, making sure everything is evenly mixed. Prepare a baking dish with a bit of coconut oil. Spoon the mixture in, and spread it evenly throughout the dish. Refrigerate for an hour, up to 6 weeks. Cut into 6 equal pieces.

> Nutrition: 155 calories, 15 g fat, 3 g protein, 1.2 g net carbs

Tahini Sauce

Tahini Sauce is a flavor-packed sauce made with sesame paste (also known as tahini). This thick, creamy, dairy free sauce is the perfect dip for veggies, but can also be used as a dressing in lettuce wraps, a sauce for meat, or salad dressing! Double or even quadruple the tahini recipe and keep some on hand in the fridge to use as needed- it will easily last for up to two weeks in an airtight container!

Servings: 1

Serving Size: 20 veggie sticks, with about ¼ cup tahini

Prep Time: 10 minutes

Cook Time: 0 minutes

Ingredients:

> 1 Tablespoon tahini paste
>
> 1 teaspoon chopped parsley

1 Tablespoon lemon juice

¼ cup water

½ Tablespoon salt

1 clove garlic

¼ cup olive oil

½ cucumber, cut into 8 equal pieces

1 stalk celery, cut into 8 equal pieces

Instructions:

In a blender or food processor, combine the tahini, parsley, lemon juice, water, salt, garlic and oil until smooth. Transfer to an airtight container, and store in the fridge for up to two weeks. Serve with veggie sticks.

Nutrition: 555 calories, 58.5 g fat, 4 g protein, 8 g net carbs

Baked Brie

This baked Brie recipe is savory, comforting, and nice for special occasions. For added decadence, serve with Nordic seed bread and sliced low carb veggies like celery, cucumber, or peppers.

Servings: 2

Serving Size: ½ wheel

Prep Time: 5 minutes

Cook Time: 10 minutes

Ingredients:

6 oz Brie cheese

½ oz walnuts

½ oz pine nuts

½ oz pecans

1 clove garlic, minced

2 teaspoons smoked paprika

4 stems thyme

1 Tablespoon salt

1 Tablespoon pepper

1 Tablespoon olive oil

Instructions:

Preheat the oven to 375F. In a medium sized bowl, combine the nuts, garlic, herbs, paprika, salt, pepper and oil. Lay the cheese onto a baking sheet lined with parchment, and spoon the nut mixture over top, so it completely covers the cheese. Bake for 10 minutes, until the cheese is melted and the nuts are fragrant and toasted. Any unfinished cheese can be wrapped and kept in the fridge for up to a month.

Nutrition: 501 calories, 44 g fat, 21 g protein, 3.4 g net carbs

Spicy Mayo

This spicy mayo makes a wonderful burger topper, and is also a great dip for veggies, fried pickles, onion rings, or anything else you can think of! Make a big batch and keep in the fridge!

Servings: 12

Serving Size: 2 Tablespoons

Prep Time: 10 minutes

Cook Time: 10 minutes

Ingredients:

3 cups mayonnaise

6 Tablespoons hot sauce or sriracha

Instructions:

Whisk the two ingredients together until smooth. Keep in the fridge for up to 8 weeks.

Nutrition: 90 calories, 10 g fat, 0 g protein, 0 g net carbs

Chapter 9:
Keto Tips and FAQs

In the previous two chapters, you received two separate 4-week meal plans, plus 100 recipes to get you started on the Keto Diet. But I want to make sure I've covered absolutely everything in this book, so in this chapter, I'm going to answer some frequently asked questions, as well as supplying you with even more tips and tricks to sustain the Keto Lifestyle long term. Let's get started!

Keto Diet FAQ

Q: Is It Okay to Be in Ketosis for a Long Time, Like Two Years or Longer?

A: Yes! While being in a state of ketosis was originally designed to see our human ancestors through annual six-month winters with limited food resources, there is absolutely no medical or scientific evidence to back up the claim that long term ketosis is harmful for the body in any way. It is a restrictive diet that may be difficult mentally to keep up long term, but it doesn't have any physical long term negative side effects. Get regular medical check-ups at least every six to eight months. Monitor your blood and breath using Keto Monitors. You'll be just fine!

Q: Is It Okay to Cycle In and Out of Ketosis?

A: Yes, it is! As stated previously, our human ancestors would usually go into a ketosis metabolic state every single winter. You don't want your insulin levels to get too low. You can incorporate intermittent fasting as part of the Keto Diet as well. To cycle out of ketosis, gradually increase your carbohydrate count. The only downside to cycling in and out of ketosis is that you'll experience Keto Flu type symptoms each time you go back into ketosis. But it's fine to kick yourself out of ketosis for a period of time. Don't be surprised if you don't feel good or gain some weight back, though! Being out of ketosis comes with its own side effects.

Q: How Can I Be a Vegetarian and Go Keto at the Same Time?

A: Just because you're vegetarian doesn't mean you should find the Keto Diet too restrictive and not try it. You'll still follow your Macros, but you'll get your protein predominantly from nuts, eggs, and dairy items. Other sources include vegetarian 'meat' sources like tempeh, tofu, and seitan. You'll also need to take supplements, like Vitamins D3, DHA & EPA, and the minerals of iron and zinc. You will need to watch your carbs as a vegetarian, because it can be tempting to eat too many. Eat lots of good low-carb veggies, especially spinach, kale, broccoli, cauliflower, and zucchini. Also, consume plenty of plant based oils, especially coconut oil, MCT oil, olive oil, avocado oil, and red palm oil. There are plenty of vegan 'dairy' options you can purchase as well. Read your food labels and purchase the products that have the most proteins and good fats.

Q: How Long Before I See Better Health and Weight Loss?

A: Within the first month! The quicker you can get into ketosis, the quicker you'll see better health and weight loss. For some people, jumping in feet first is a welcome challenge. They'll start the meal plan, get cooking, and start feeling the effects within a few days. But for most of us, easing into such a restrictive diet takes a little more time. The longer you're in ketosis, the more benefits you'll experience.

Q: Will There Be Kidney Stones on the Keto Diet?

A: Your liver gets all the credit for producing ketones, but your kidneys play an important role in this diet, too. Your body is 70% water, so you really do need to stay ultra hydrated on this diet. If you don't, that increases the amount of uric acid in your body, producing kidney stones and gout. Remember, this is not Atkins! It's a medium protein diet, not a high protein diet. The fats are really what you want to be consuming. Follow the meal plan guidelines in the previous chapters and balance your good fats. Drink lots of water with lemon in it. The citrates in lemon keep calcium molecules from sticking together, thus preventing kidney stones. If you're still concerned, take oral potassium citrate tablets to decrease the likelihood of kidney stones.

Q: Why Am I Losing Muscle On This Diet?

A: Your muscles are one of the places on your body where extra glycogen is stored. So, when you switch to a very low carb diet, within a few days your body starts searching for any leftover glycogen to be used as energy. That's why you start losing muscle. After just four weeks of being in ketosis on the diet, your muscle glycogen counts will drop to about half. This makes sense from a historical standpoint, too; when your human ancestors went into ketosis in the winter, that was to conserve muscle energy, not expend it. This diet is excellent for those looking to lose weight and overcome a number of ailments. But if you're seeking a high intensity workout or are an athlete, then consult a nutritionist to keep your muscles in peak physical condition.

Tips for Ketogenic Diet Success!

Up until now, you've read dozens of tips and tricks on how to change your eating habits to the Keto Diet lifestyle! You've cleaned out your cupboards and replaced carbohydrates with plenty of good fats. You've started on a meal plan, learned to cook new recipes, and transitioned after the first four weeks.

But in order to have success on the Keto Diet for a long time, we've got some more helpful information for you.

Keto Diet on a Wallet Diet

How do you both save money and save carbohydrates while staying in ketosis? There are many ways to stick to a financial budget. One tip is to purchase your pantry items in bulk. You can keep a price book to compare the prices in stores between things like olive oil, nuts and seeds, chicken broth, and baking ingredients. Purchase large food storage containers to store your bulk purchases in your pantry.

Shop around at different stores. You can find inexpensive herbs, spices, and vegetables at ethnic markets. Things like coconut milk, curry pastes, soy sauce, teriyaki sauce, and a huge fish selection are at Asian markets. Their prices are usually much lower than American supermarkets. Don't forget to compare online prices, too. You could score amazing deals off Amazon.com.

Your freezer can also help you save money. Buy meats or fish in bulk, then individually package them in plastic bags and store in the freezer. You can put butter in the freezer, too!

Buy generic store brands instead of national brands, which spend millions of dollars a year on marketing. Generic canned tomatoes, frozen vegetables, and baking items are much less expensive.

Fall Back Keto Foods

Yep, we all get tired in the evening and just want to whip up a quick batch of pasta and sauce. It's so easy … and it's not Keto friendly. Always have Keto safe fall back foods to keep in the back of your mind, for the times you're too tired and your blood sugar is too low to think.

Try these ones:

- Hard boiled eggs
- Cottage cheese
- Nuts or seeds
- Slice of cheese
- Keto Fat Bomb
- Easy smoothie

Meal Prepping

You want to know the real secret to cooking fast, easy meals? Take care of the meal prep beforehand! You can marinate meats, slice or dice veggies, defrost foods, and put together dry baking mixes before you do your actual cooking. I keep plastic containers of cooked shredded chicken, sliced celery, and diced onions in my fridge. I eat those three foods all the time. That way, it's easy to throw together a quick salad or soup. Choose the foods that you eat frequently, and prepare them to keep in your fridge or pantry. That makes cooking much faster.

Family Keto Fun

How about converting your family to also eat on the Keto Diet with you? It's much easier to not eat any bread when nobody in the house is eating it, either. It also cuts down on meal preparation time, since you're not making two dishes. For kids, you can turn it into a game to see what foods they can eat, too. The Ketogenic Diet works whether you are single or you have a family. When you have a family situation, then here are tips to make the transition:

- Sit down with your family members and tell them the new diet you're going to be on
- Have everyone together, as a family, decide on the meals that look good from those provided in this book
- Create a new grocery list based on those meals and shop for those ingredients with family members
- Try out these new meals and recipes, starting with easy ones pretty much everyone loves (omelets, burgers, salads, etc.)

Jump Around

Getting some sort of daily movement or exercise into your schedule will only help your body along your Keto Diet journey. It's excellent to see your weight loss, and the tendency is to just leave it and enjoy that natural weight loss. But you are a human being that was designed to walk and enjoy all the benefits of daily moving around. There are many places to start a simple walking routine: in nature, in a city downtown, inside a shopping mall or galleria, or in neighborhoods.

Put Together a Recipe Collection

Get some more recipe books! For those of you on a budget, you can get a library card and read the cookbooks. You can also buy used books online at Amazon.com or Barnes and Noble. There are many helpful Keto Dieters on the internet who share their experiences and their recipes, too. Put together your own collection, with your own cooking notes. It will give you a much greater variety and help you explore more of what this diet is all about.

Show Off Your Progress

One of the best things about eating the Keto Diet is you'll physically see such a change in your body. I encourage you to celebrate and show off your progress! Post your pictures on social media, treat yourself to new clothes, and reward your hard work with (non-food) items that bring you joy.

You'll be much happier and have more energy to enjoy and do the things you want with the people you love.

Conclusion:
Your Food, Your Health

In many ways for me, this Ketogenic Diet book has been part instruction manual and part memoir. I've shared with you my personal health challenges that brought me to this diet many years ago.

It's meant a lot to me to see and experience the changes in my own life that have come from a healthier body. It helped my issues with diabetes, which honestly scared me. I don't have any fear about health issues anymore. That's an extraordinary reward that the Keto Diet has bestowed on me. How would you like to be that way, too?

To Be Read Again and Again

There's plenty of books out there you'll read to the last page, put down, and never pick up again. That's not what this book is designed for. It's a guide and a manual for you to read over and over. Reread the chapters on Macros, benefits, and troubleshooting. Really think about the meal plans and the recipes. Pay attention to the bevy of amazing tips and tricks sprinkled throughout the previous pages.

This book is excellent for those who are just starting out and have barely heard of the Keto Diet. It will help you. It's also designed for Keto Dieters who are having issues getting what they want out of the diet, whether that's weight loss or health. I'm very proud of my 30-minute fast meal plan, because I'm super busy myself and knew others are, too. And finally, I wrote this so that the Keto Diet doesn't become just another nutritional fad project in your life. But that it takes root and grows as its own part of your lifestyle, sustaining itself and giving you plenty of rewards and benefits along the way.

What you eat is so important. You don't need a health scare to tell you how important; you know it already.

So, let's eat the good stuff your body can use for a different form of energy. One that will give so much back to you every day of your life!

If you have taken away 1 single useful thing of value or learnt something that you thought was nice and helpful, could you please help a friend out and leave a review over on amazon?

It's totally great that you are sharing with folks about the book and this will then help more folks to know about what you know too!

Thank you so much!

Appendix

Grocery List for Each Meal Plan

Here is a grocery list for you! It's split into two-week lists, so that you only have to shop every other weekend. You also get grocery lists for both meal plans. Buying in bulk saves you time and money, so do that whenever you can.

Before we get started with the lists, you'll want to stock your pantry with Keto approved ingredients. These form the basis for almost every recipe! Every two weeks, you'll go through the following list and make sure you have enough. If not, add the restocked item to the grocery list:

Restock the Pantry Every Two Weeks with the Following:

Black coffee	Cinnamon
Coconut milk (cans)	Ground cumin
Container chicken broth	Cayenne pepper (dried)
Container coconut oil	Chili powder
Container cocoa powder	Italian herbs
Container almond milk	Oregano
Stevia	Thyme
Vietnamese fish sauce	Nutmeg
Almond flour	Ginger
Vanilla extract	Allspice
Bottle lemon juice	Turmeric
Container almond butter	Garam Masala
Container mayonnaise	Garlic powder
Container Dijon mustard	Onion powder
Container olive oil (buy several!)	Fennel seed
Container heavy cream (buy several!)	Ground coriander (cilantro)
Coconut flakes	Chopped pecans
Salt and pepper	Almonds
Paprika and smoked paprika	Walnuts

Macadamia nuts	Sunflower seeds
Ground flax seeds	Hemp seeds
Pumpkin seeds	Chia seeds
Sesame seeds	

Basic Meal Plan Grocery List:

First 2 Weeks:

Produce & Fresh Herbs:

7 avocados	1 bunch arugula
5 green bell peppers	Fresh cilantro, parsley, basil, and dill
2 red bell peppers	4 jalapenos
3 limes	2 Scotch bonnets
6 lemons	1 bunch green onions
3 bunches celery	1 package bean sprouts
Container cherry tomatoes	1 small carrot
6 tomatoes	Fresh spinach
36 green beans	Garlic cloves
Package shiitake mushrooms	1 leek
Package cremini mushrooms	10 spears asparagus
3 red onions	2 zucchinis
6 yellow onions	1 head broccoli
2 radishes	3 heads cauliflower
2 cucumbers	Jar of artichoke hearts
2 heads Romaine lettuce	Jar green olives
2 heads iceberg lettuce	Jar sundried tomatoes
2 heads kale	Small package raspberries

Meat & Seafood:

1 lb steak

    1 lb ground pork

    8 lbs ground beef

    1 lb ground lamb

    2 6 oz lamb chops

    2 4 oz pieces salmon

    2 packages bacon

    6 shrimp

    4 3 oz cod fillets

2 4 ounce pieces of halibut

1 8 oz ahi tuna steak

1 whole chicken

8 large chicken breasts

3 lbs boneless chicken thighs

4 pork chops

Package prosciutto

2 ounces salami

Eggs & Dairy:

3 one dozen egg cartons

    3 packages butter

    Package gruyere

    Package shredded parmesan

Package shredded cheddar

Package block cream cheese

Container plain Greek yogurt

6 oz goat cheese

Other:

2 14.5 ounce cans crushed tomatoes

    Jar salsa

    Jar dill pickles

    Package frozen strawberries

    Package frozen raspberries

    Container avocado oil

Bottle sesame oil

MCT oil

White wine vinegar

1 bar unsweetened dark chocolate

Thai red/yellow/green curry paste

Bottle white wine

Second 2 Weeks:

Produce & Fresh Herbs:

9 avocados

3 green bell peppers

1 red pepper

2 lemons

7 limes

Container cherry tomatoes

5 regular tomatoes

Garlic cloves

3 red onions

5 yellow onions

1 bunch green onions

24 green beans

1 jalapeno

2 Scotch bonnets

8 red Thai chilis

Fresh basil, dill, cilantro, and parsley

Package white mushrooms

Package cremini mushrooms

3 asparagus stalks

5 zucchinis

1 cucumber

1 carrot

2 bunches celery

Bunch arugula

1 head iceberg lettuce

2 heads kale

1 head Romaine lettuce

1 leek

2 heads broccoli

3 heads cauliflower

Small package raspberries

Meat & Seafood:

4 lbs flank steak

1 lb skirt steak

1 lb ground beef

2 lbs smoked salmon

½ lb ham

1 cup ground pork rinds

Large package bacon

1 oz prosciutto

2 6 oz pieces cod

4 3 oz halibut fillets

3 oz fillet of sea bass

½ lb white fish

9 scallops

¼ lb shrimp

¼ lb crab meat

4 chicken thighs, bone in skin on

13 large chicken breasts, boneless, skinless

Eggs & Dairy:

4 one dozen egg cartons

4 packages butter

Gruyere

Package block cream cheese

Package shredded mozzarella

Package shredded cheddar

Package shredded Parmesan

Package shredded Monterey Jack cheese

2 lbs goat cheese

Other:

Bottle white wine

Bottle red wine

Package frozen strawberries

Package frozen raspberries

Bottle avocado oil

Bottle sesame oil

White wine vinegar

Red/yellow/green curry paste

Container beef stock or broth

1 14.5 oz can diced tomatoes

2 14.5 oz cans crushed tomatoes

Bottle Worcestershire sauce

Jar tahini paste

Jar salsa

Soy sauce

Cocoa butter

Bottle of hot sauce or sriracha

30-Minute Fast Meals Grocery List:

First 2 Weeks:

Produce & Fresh Herbs:

7 avocados

Package cherry tomatoes

7 regular tomatoes

2 red onions

4 yellow onions

4 green bell peppers

2 red bell peppers

2 radishes

6 lemons

3 limes

3 jalapenos

4 Thai red chilis

Garlic cloves

2 bunches green onions

Package white mushrooms

2 packages cremini mushrooms

Package shiitake mushrooms

1 package bean sprouts

Fresh basil, dill, cilantro, and parsley

Package fresh raspberries

10 green beans

2 zucchinis

2 cucumbers

1 carrot

2 bunches celery

3 heads Romaine lettuce

1 head iceberg lettuce

3 bunches kale

1 bunch arugula

3 heads broccoli

2 heads cauliflower

Meat & Seafood:

2 lbs ground beef

1 lb ground pork

1 lb ground lamb

1 lb steak

1 lb skirt steak

1 lb flank steak

2 6 oz lamb chops

4 oz smoked salmon

4 4 oz cod fillets

4 4oz pieces of halibut

2 4 oz salmon pieces

1 8 oz ahi tuna steak

6 shrimp

6 slices bacon

6 oz prosciutto

2 oz salami

6 large chicken breasts, boneless skinless

Eggs & Dairy:

2 one dozen egg cartons

5 packages stick butter

Package shredded mozzarella

Package shredded parmesan

2 packages block cream cheese

Container Greek yogurt

Other:

Package frozen strawberries

2 packages frozen raspberries

Jar sundried tomatoes

Jar green olives

Jar artichoke hearts

Container tahini paste

Bottle sesame oil

Cocoa butter

Bottle fish sauce

Cacao powder

Soy sauce

Second 2 Weeks:

Produce & Fresh Herbs:

7 avocados

Package cherry tomatoes

7 regular tomatoes

2 red onions

4 yellow onions

4 green bell peppers

2 red bell peppers

2 radishes

6 lemons

3 limes

3 jalapenos

4 Thai red chilis

Garlic cloves

2 bunches green onions

Package white mushrooms

2 packages cremini mushrooms

Package shiitake mushrooms

1 package bean sprouts

Fresh basil, dill, cilantro, and parsley

Package fresh raspberries

30 green beans

2 zucchinis

2 cucumbers

1 carrot

2 bunches celery

3 heads Romaine lettuce

1 head iceberg lettuce

3 bunches kale

1 bunch arugula

3 heads broccoli

2 heads cauliflower

Meat & Seafood:

2 lbs ground beef

1 lb ground pork

1 lb ground lamb

1 lb steak

1 lb skirt steak

1 lb flank steak

2 6 oz lamb chops

4 oz smoked salmon

4 4 oz cod fillets

4 4oz pieces of halibut

2 4 oz salmon pieces

1 8 oz ahi tuna steak

6 shrimp

6 slices bacon

6 oz prosciutto

2 oz salami

6 large chicken breasts, boneless skinless

Pork rinds

Eggs & Dairy:

3 one dozen egg cartons

5 packages stick butter

Package shredded mozzarella

Package shredded parmesan

2 packages block cream cheese

Container Greek yogurt

½ lb goat cheese

Other:

Package frozen strawberries

2 packages frozen raspberries

Jar sundried tomatoes

Jar green olives

Jar artichoke hearts

Container tahini paste

Bottle sesame oil

Cocoa butter

Bottle fish sauce

Cacao powder

Soy sauce

Recipe Index

Pork and Poultry

Beef and Lamb

Beef Fajita Bowl

Beef Fajita Lettuce Wraps

Lettuce Wrapped Lamb Burgers

Steak and Avocado Taco Cups

Cheese Stuffed Meatballs

Cheese Stuffed Burgers

Beef Vindaloo

Beef Stew

Seafood

Red Pepper Cod

Sea Bass with Prosciutto and Herbs

Thai Coconut Cod

Thai Coconut Cod Lettuce Wraps

Crab Stuffed Cucumbers

Salmon with Beurre Blanc

Spinach Stuffed Cod

Parmesan Crusted Halibut

Crab Stuffed Avocado

Fish Tacos

Cod Bruschetta

Desserts and Drinks

Keto Bulletproof Coffee

Almond Butter Bulletproof Coffee

Vanilla Smoothie

Strawberry Cow Smoothie

Golden Milk Smoothie

Almond Butter Smoothie

Pink Power Smoothie

Raspberry Chia Pudding

Raspberry Chocolate Fudge

Strawberry Chia Pudding Popsicles

Almond Butter Cookies

Snacks and Sides

Butter Tossed Asparagus

Caramelized Onions

Curry Mayonnaise

Green Tahini

Cheesy Fondue

Green Bean Fries

Seed Crackers & Guacamole

Celery and Almond Butter

Salted Macadamias

Nordic Seed Bread

Almond Butter Fat Bombs

Mediterranean Fat Bombs

Baked Brie

Spicy Mayo

The Step By Step Guide To Intermittent Fasting On The Ketogenic Diet

Keto Diet For Beginners

Will Ramos

The Step By Step Guide
To Intermittent Fasting On The Ketogenic Diet

Chapter 1: Getting To Know Each Other

How would you like to take your Ketogenic Diet to the next level?

Just like in a video game, where you receive new bonuses and rewards for becoming more proficient, so the Keto Diet has its own way to 'level up' so that you can gain excellent new benefits.

You've probably been enjoying your Keto Diet for at least a few months by this point. You've finally been able to wrap your mind around understanding which foods you can – and can't – eat. It's not been an easy journey, especially when that yucky Keto Flu made you didn't feel well as your body changed from a carbohydrate metabolic state to a ketosis metabolic state.

However, you've made it through! So, congratulations. It's not easy making such a large transition to eating an entirely new way. Especially because the Keto Diet is, for all intents and purposes, such a High Fat Low Carb (HFLC) diet that it's quite restrictive!

Mastering the basics is just Step One of a much larger journey, and one that I hope you'll continue to find success with as you become more advanced and more knowledgeable.

The Keto Diet will give you so many rewards, amongst them:

- A smaller number on that weight loss scale!
- Increased health, coming from all those Keto benefits
- Better energy
- An overall increased sense of well-being, from how you sleep to stabilizing your blood sugar to prevent mood swings

How you feel in your body impacts every single other area of your life. Being on the Keto Diet, you've already experienced some of these rewards or maybe all of them.

So, are you ready to experience even more rewards?

In this book, we'll show you how!

Leveling Up Your Keto Diet

You've also learned that Ketogenic Dieting is definitely a lifestyle change. You've been shopping for new ingredients, cooking new meals, bypassing the carbohydrates on restaurant menus, and perhaps also incorporating an exercise plan as well. Every diet benefits with a little physical movement.

But there is still one more additional way to level up your Keto Diet, and that's the main topic we'll cover in the following pages.

It's going to take your diet to a new level that you never thought possible, simply because it's not covered in many beginning Keto Diet articles and books.

You don't want to just do the same old, same old Keto dieting that you have been.

That's when it's time to take on a new challenge!

Introducing Intermittent Fasting

What is this new challenge of which I speak?

It's called Intermittent Fasting, or IF, for short. We'll go greatly in-depth in this book as to how it affects your body at a cellular level, how it's best integrated into the Keto Diet, how it helps your body stay in ketosis, how it's a useful tool to get into ketosis quickly, and why you should try it.

You'll receive really amazing answers to the above questions. By the time you get to the grocery list and the last page, you'll be armed with all the tools, tips, and tricks you need to successfully level up your Ketogenic Diet by using Intermittent Fasting.

But This Book Contains So Much More …

This book isn't just about the Keto Diet and it isn't just about Intermittent Fasting, either. It's designed and written to provide you with all kinds of interesting information to help, including:

- The what's what of Intermittent Fasting
- All the science behind Intermittent Fasting and what makes it tick
- How Intermittent Fasting integrates with the Keto Diet
- The ten things that will help make Intermittent Fasting easier
- Why you want to go for Intermittent Fasting
- What to watch out for while you're fasting
- How to deal with these 2 main problems of Intermittent Fasting with ease
- What you want to know before you start Intermittent Fasting
- A complete, detailed 28-day guide to being both on the Keto Diet and Intermittent Fasting at the same time
- A 7 Day Meal Plan for being on the Keto Diet and doing a Fast at the same time
- All the recipes to go with those 7 days to save you the hassle
- A grocery list for the 7 days to give you the low down on what to best get
- Plus, all the instructions you need to create your own meal plans for continued and prolonged success

Your body will change after you've added Intermittent Fasting to your Keto Diet!

My Ketogenic Story

There are so many hidden carbohydrates (including all kinds of sugars) lurking in the foods you eat, that even someone who appears healthy on the outside can suffer from unexpected and severe health problems on the inside.

That's exactly what happened to me. I was a hale and healthy male athlete in my teens! I was playing sports, getting outside a lot, didn't carry any extra weight, and my BMI was totally normal. If you saw me, you'd have no idea that I was secretly unhealthy. I sure didn't know.

So, imagine my total surprise when I was suddenly diagnosed with diabetes.

Wait, what?

Yeah, whatever stereotypes you think about the average diabetes sufferer, that surely wasn't me. But suddenly, it was. I now had a disease that radically changed my relationship with food. I'd always exercised frequently, that I just didn't think it was necessary or important to care about what was on the plate. I just burned all those calories, anyway.

But diabetes has nothing to do with calories, being thin, exercising, or sports. That was eye-opening. I was thrown for a loop and struggled with my life into my early adulthood, trying everything I could think of to lessen my symptoms and get my diabetes under control. It took longer than I want to admit (especially to you!) to finally realize there was this incredible link between diet and health. Hey, I was a teenager okay?

Yet, once I recognized this link, my whole outlook changed immediately. I started with the Atkins Diet, which was popular at the time, then shortly thereafter started exploring the Keto Diet. This was around the early 2000s. The Ketogenic Diet sounded weird and extreme to me, with its ridiculously high fat contents and ridiculously low carb contents, but hey – I was already experimenting, so why not?

Well, needless to say, that Keto Diet experiment turned into a full tilt obsession as soon as my diabetes numbers started looking healthier. The more I ate this diet, the better my numbers got. Each doctor visit I was improving. I read everything I could get my hands on, including all about the nutrition, the science, the practical application, the recipes, and the meal plans. I absorbed this knowledge even better than a sponge, because my own health was at stake!

My experiments and personal field tested knowledge paid off. You might not believe me, but it's the truth:

The diabetes is gone. A long gone memory by this point.

And, I've been on the Ketogenic Diet for fourteen years.

My Keto Diet story doesn't just end there, though. I also include Intermittent Fasting into my weekly schedule. I spend five days a week eating in 6-hour windows, and I fast for the remaining 18 hours. On the other two days, I stretch my eating windows to 10 hours, fasting for 14 hours. That gives my body a chance to better absorb the good fats, high quality proteins, and extremely low carbohydrate Macro counts that I stick to!

Intermittent Fasting has taken my diet into places that I never thought it could do. My energy is as high as it was when I was in my early twenties, but at least now I have the wisdom to go with it! It's like the best of both worlds – the body of a 20-year-old and the wisdom of a 40-year-old! My energy allows me to accomplish all the big goals that I have in my life, that cover all areas: work, family, personal relationships, health and fitness, and time spent doing fun things, too.

Honestly, I've been on the Keto Diet with Intermittent Fasting for so long, that I don't spend a lot of my time thinking about my diet. It all comes naturally. Since I see such tangible results, that motivates me to stay on it.

I changed the metabolic process in my own body, I'm in ketosis 100% of the time, and I've never been healthier. On the inside and the outside this time.

On the Intermittent Fasting Fast Track

When you incorporate Intermittent Fasting into your Keto Diet, then you'll not only level up your diet, you'll be on the fast track towards a better, healthier you. This book will definitely take you into a whole different way of eating that you've probably never tried before. It's work, but it's good work, the kind that gets results. A lot of work is mindless, boring, and just repeats itself over and over, never getting anywhere.

But eating the Keto Diet and incorporating Intermittent Fasting?

That's a plan that gets you somewhere. It gets you there fast, too. All you've got to do is learn about it and why it works so well. That is what the next chapter will help you with!

Chapter 2:
The Not So Secret Weapon To The Keto Diet

The Ketogenic Diet has taken on such popularity in such a short period of time because people get results! You just read about the results I got while I was on it, and I have absolutely zero regrets with it. There's not a single day where I've woken up and decided to try another way of eating – not even for one day!

That's the kind of results you're looking for, too. A diet you'll never regret and always see results from. That was also the kind of motivation I saw in my personal life that's inspired me to create this Keto Diet book for you.

I want you to look, feel, and live just as happily as I do on this Keto lifestyle.

It really is that simple.

Before we go into the details about Intermittent Fasting, I wanted to spend time talking about the Keto Diet. You can try Intermittent Fasting without the Keto Diet, but then you won't get all the extraordinary benefits that you do from being in ketosis. So, I strongly recommend that you get into ketosis and stay there while you're on your Intermittent Fasting cycles.

Prepare yourself! We're going to delve past the simple food items sitting in your fridge right now and examine them at a molecular level.

It is time for lots and lots of nutrition science!

All About Macros

Being in ketosis is all dependent on consuming the right types of nutrients, the right amounts, and eating those nutrients from the right sources. Let's start with the right types of nutrients. There are three main Macronutrients, nicknamed Macros for short, that you need to diligently keep track of when you're staying in ketosis on Keto Diet.

1. Fats
2. Proteins
3. Carbohydrates

For those of you who've been on the Keto Diet for even a few months, it is clear why these three nutrients are important. They each provide nutrition and energy to your cells that you can't get without consuming them.

These three Macros seem pretty self-explanatory. Fats are things like oil and animal fats. Proteins come from meat, and carbohydrates are found in every slice of cake. But it's not that simple. Fats can be good fats or bad fats, which is explained later in this chapter. Protein could be animal and that's the most popular source, but there are plant proteins as well. Some carbohydrates are starches, while many are actually sugars, and there are several sugar groups.

So, it's not as easy as it looks to tell what actually is a Macro that's good for you, and what's not. If you consume too much of the bad fats, you'll develop health problems. If you don't get enough fats, you won't stay in ketosis and experience weight gain as well as all the other ketosis benefits. It's just really important that you read about these Macros in-depth and understand how they're processed in your body.

Macro #1: Fat

Now we get to the fun part of nutrition science! We're going to talk about fat, the most important Macro on the Keto Diet, and also the most misunderstood, falsely accused, misaligned, and just plain hated.

"Fat" is just a short term nickname for the fatty acids that are present in fats. Fatty acids are long chains of molecules with different chemical components that are various combinations of three atoms: carbon, hydrogen, and oxygen.

There are two types of fats that are lurking in the foods present at your grocery store or served at restaurants:

- Good Fats
- Bad Fats

Basically, the good fats give you amazing energy, improve your good cholesterol, benefit insulin levels, and control your blood sugar. The bad fats do the opposite. They contribute towards weight gain, raise your bad LDL cholesterol levels, create inflammation, block your arteries, and contribute towards other chronic conditions.

How do you know which fat is your friend and which is your enemy? Read on below to tell the difference.

Good Fats:

- Saturated Fats – The fatty acid molecules are saturated with hydrogen atoms, thus giving these good fats they're name. You can find saturated fats in animal products like meats and dairy. On the Keto Diet, you want to be consuming naturally occurring saturated fats from animals, only.
- Monounsaturated Fats – These fatty acid only have one double bond that links carbon atoms to hydrogen atoms. These fats don't have as many calories as the saturated fats, so you'd want to eat more of them. They do protect against cardiovascular disease, though. Saturated fats come from animal sources, while monounsaturated fats come from plant sources – nuts, avocados, olive oil, etc.

- Natural Polyunsaturated Fats – The processed version of these fatty acids is very bad for you, but the naturally occurring version is great! They're called different names like Omega-3 and Omega-6 fatty acids. You can get your Omega-3 and Omega-6 from walnuts, spinach, eggs, chia seeds, salmon, broccoli, and pumpkin seeds. All those foods are Keto Diet friendly, so eat up!

Bad Fats:

- Processed Saturated Fats – In addition to naturally occurring saturated fats, these fats can also be created in a laboratory and put into processed foods. That's why they go on the naughty list. Only get your saturated fats from animal sources like meat, dairy, eggs, and seafood.
- Processed Polyunsaturated Fats – The natural version is good, but the processed polyunsaturated fats aren't good. As long as you avoid corn oil, soybean oil, margarine, and those types of foods, you won't be consuming these bad fats. That's why it is important to only buy Ketogenic Diet friendly ingredients and leave these bad fat sources on the shelf.
- Trans Fats – Trans-fatty acids are the worst kinds of fats! These are the bad apples that spoil the bunch, because there are so many sources of good fats. But you've got to stay away from these ones. They were created by the food industry and aren't found in naturally occurring sources from animals or plants. They're like a Frankenstein laboratory experiment gone wrong! If you eat even a small amount of trans fats, your bad cholesterol levels will rise and you'll be more prone to disease. Trans fats are mostly found in fried or processed foods. Beware!

After learning about the differences between the good fats and bad fats, it becomes pretty obvious that you should only stick to natural animal or plant sources for your fat intake. Being in ketosis on the Keto Diet is all about consuming the right nutrients from the right sources in the right percentages. Enjoy the good fats, of which there are so many, and you'll not have to worry about all the negative side effects that go with eating the bad fats!

Macro #2: Protein

Together with the good fats, protein is one of your body's primary sources of fuel! You can either eat animal proteins, such as meat, fish, eggs, and seafood, or plant protein that's found in nuts, beans, and quinoa. Your brain requires massive amounts of protein for all of its processing and daily functions. Protein is very similar to a general handyman, repairing and rebuilding your tissues, making enzymes for better digestion, making hormones (which is what it also does in your brain), and contributes towards building many new cells in your body for things like your muscles, skin, blood, cartilage, and bones. Together with being a fuel source, you can see why it's very important for your body.

What about protein's different sources? Those complete protein sources that are totally used by the body with no waste come from the following foods:

- Beef
- Poultry

- Eggs
- Fish
-

- Dairy protein
- Legumes (beans, peas)

Did you notice most of these foods are Keto Diet friendly? In addition to only consuming a moderate amount of protein, you're also eating it from the correct sources! That equals less amino acids leftover to turn into glucose and store in your cells. Win-win!

Macro #3: Carbohydrates (Sugars)

What about carbohydrates? This is the big "no no" category on the Keto Diet, so hopefully you've been watching your carb counts and keeping them nice and low. When we talk about carbs, we're talking about the three distinct atoms of carbon, hydrogen, and oxygen. The word "carbohydrate" contains these three words. "Carbo" for "carbon," "hydr" for "hydrogen," and "ate" for "oxygen." By themselves, these are three very harmless elements and are the building blocks of life.

But when combined into carbohydrate molecules, these three atoms become a group of sugars, starches, and cellulose (plant sugars) called saccharides. Your body can process four chemical groups of saccharides: the monosaccharides, disaccharides, oligosaccharides, and polysaccharides. It is the fourth group, the polysaccharides, that are processed by the body and then stored as energy in your cells.

Sugars are even less complex carbohydrates than the saccharides. They come in many forms, including:

- Sucrose (table sugar) – This is the regular sweet white or brown sugar you can purchase in stores that's also found in so many food items, especially baked goods. Table sugar comes from the stems of the sugarcane plant and the roots of the sugar beet. It also contains cellulose plant sugars.
- Fructose (fruit sugar) – This is what gives fruits like strawberries, cherries, bananas, and apples their characteristic sweetness. It is also present in some natural sweeteners like honey and agave. Fructose is a monosaccharide sugar. It can also bond to glucose and form sucrose. Fructose is easily made into syrups, like the high fructose corn syrup that's so prevalent in foods these days.
- Cellulose (plant sugar) – Cellulose is a polysaccharide sugar that's found in plant cell walls and certain vegetable fibers. Some of your favorite vegetables have really high amounts of cellulose, which is why they're not allowed on the Keto Diet. That includes potatoes, carrots, and corn. Humans can't digest cellulose, so it's usually broken down into its smaller glucose molecules and – you guessed it – stored in your cells for future energy.
- Lactose (milk sugar) – People who are lactose intolerant can't digest milk sugars, which are disaccharides made up of galactose and glucose. Cows' milk is too high in lactose sugar (carbohydrates) to have on the Keto Diet. Dairy cheeses have smaller amounts of lactose.
- Glucose (blood sugar) – Glucose is probably the most important sugar of all, because it is such an important energy source. It's also the simplest sugar, being just a monosaccharide. Glucose is made by plants when they photosynthesize, so that's it's primary source in your diet. Glucose is absolutely key when it comes to your normal body functioning.

It's impossible to eliminate all sugars and carbohydrates from your diet – nor would you want to! Carbohydrates provide fuel, contribute towards stabilizing your blood sugar, and are also frequently found in many fibrous foods like seeds, nuts, legumes, and vegetables.

It is when you eat too many carbohydrates, but especially glucose (which is found in regular sugar, fructose and cellulose), that things start to go haywire. Your health will start to take a turn for the worst, and you'll also notice the weight gain, too.

How Your Body Processes These Macros

The Keto Diet, like every other diet, is at the core a meal plan. It is based on how your body actually processes the different nutrients that you eat. A meal plan filled with lots of carbohydrates, sugars, fats, and high in protein is going to be processed by your cells in a certain way.

It's extremely important to understand the science behind how your body processes these Macros (protein, carbohydrates / sugars, fats) every single time you eat them. I know it's easy to forget that, after you've eaten your dinner, all those nutrients are now sitting in your stomach. So then, it's your cells' job to process those nutrients.

But in this case, those Macros are not each processed alike, because they are used by your body in completely different ways and for different functions.

So, what is exactly happening in your body when you eat these nutrients? Let's take a look at each one and answer that question:

1. Processing Good Fats

You read above about the fatty acids that are found in the good fats from animal and plant sources. How does your body process these complex fatty acid molecules?

After you eat good fats, your cells break them down into both glycerol and those fatty acids. This process is called lipolysis. Both the glycerol and those fatty acids are released into your blood and travel through your bloodstream to your liver.

That's where those same fatty acids can then be either broken down directly and used for that day's energy, or they can enter into a new multiple step process called gluconeogenesis, which turns those fatty acids into glucose. Amino acids are combined with the fatty acids to manufacture glucose. Then the glucose is used the same way as other carbohydrates are processed, which is explained below.

What about extra fats? Are those used as energy, like glucose, or are they stored, like excess protein and carbohydrates?

The answer is yes: those fats are stored. They are stored as triglycerides in fat cells called adipocytes. Those cells can expand, but they do have a limit. In addition, that stored fat can also be stored in your muscles to provide extra energy for when you need it. When you're doing moderate intensity exercising, your muscles open up those stored fat cells and use that energy to meet your fuel needs.

A recent study published in February 2014 reported that eating polyunsaturated fats led to an increase in lean muscle tissue. Stick to the natural sources for these fatty acids, and you can help your body meet not just weight loss goals, but fitness ones as well!

2. Processing Protein

After you eat your protein serving, it is digested in the stomach and absorbed by the intestines. Then it goes directly to your liver, where the nitrogen and the amino acids are broken down and separated. Your amino acids are sent to your muscles for fuel. There are nine essential amino acids in protein, and if all of those are present, then your body uses them all up happily. However, any excess protein that's not used by your body is then turned into either glucose (sugar) or fat and sent to your cells for energy and storage purposes.

That's right. If you eat too much protein, it is stored and causes you to gain weight!

3. Processing Carbohydrates

How does your body process the glucose sugars found in carbohydrates? It's done many times a day. As soon as the glucose from the sugars enters your stomach, enzymes and your pancreas start to break down the molecules. Your pancreas also releases insulin to deal with this influx of glucose, which contributes to your blood sugar rising. The insulin helps bring your glucose levels down.

The reason you don't want to completely eliminate glucose from your diet (and just subsist on completely carbohydrate free foods) is because you could go the opposite way and develop hypoglycemia. This is when your glucose levels dip too low. Go even lower, and you could pass out. Sometimes people who give blood have a tendency to faint. This is because they've lost too much glucose blood sugar. Your brain cells can only get energy from glucose, so don't cut out carbohydrates completely!

So, you want to make sure that even though you're keeping your carbohydrate counts extremely low, that you aren't eliminating them from your diet entirely! Sugar is not just sweet, it is a treat. A little goes a long way towards stabilizing your blood sugar.

Your Macro Percentages

The USDA Nutritional Guidelines clearly state you should be consuming 5% of your daily calories from fats, 35% of your daily calories from proteins, and 35% of your daily calories from carbohydrates. It seems like the wisest choice to be on such a balanced diet, right?

It's not. The Macros on a Ketogenic Diet are vastly different.

You should be consuming 70% of your daily calories from those good fat sources, 19% of your proteins from natural animal and plant sources, and 5% - 8% of your carbohydrates from healthy sources.

It looks like this:

70% FATS – 19% PROTEINS – 5% CARBOHYDRATES

These are the Macros that you should track, and the proper percentages that you need in order to get into ketosis and stay in that metabolic state.

There are many online Ketogenic Macro calculators, and I encourage you to calculate your exact Macro percentages. They change depending on many factors in your physicality, including your height, weight, current age, gender, and BMI.

As a general guideline when reading about the contents of these Macros on a food label, you should look for these quantities:

MEN:
208g FATS – 125g PROTEINS – 31g CARBOHYDRATES

WOMEN:
167g FATS – 100g PROTEINS – 25g CARBOHYDRATES

For men, this adds up to 364 total grams of food per day, and for women, it adds up to 292 total grams of food per day. These are the Macros that you should be tracking each day that you're on the Ketogenic Diet.

Macros are so important that we'll be discussing them throughout the rest of this book. Make sure you've gone to the online calculator to find your exact percentages and daily grams. When we add Intermittent Fasting to the Ketogenic Diet, it only works if you're watching your nutrients closely!

What About My Daily Calories?

Ever since calories were discovered by Nicolas Clement in 1824 as a unit of heat energy, they've been at the center of dieting. On average, a moderately active 175 pound male should be eating 2,800 calories per day, and the moderately active 125 pound female should be eating 2000 calories per day.

If you eat as many calories as you're burning, then you won't lose weight. However, when you're in ketosis, it doubles the rate of fat burning and you'll use more calories than you would to burn the same number of grams of fat!

In essence, you'll burn more calories on the Keto Diet just by burning the large amount of good fats that you are consuming.

Also, and we'll discuss this concept more throughout this book, it's not just about the number of calories you're burning. It's about two additional factors:

1. The types of calories – whether from fats, proteins, or carbohydrates
2. The amount of time between consuming calories

With factor number two, the amount of time between consuming calories, that's when a new concept called Intermittent Fasting comes into play. You can consume more calories per feeding time at your meal and lose weight compared to somebody who's consuming fewer calories but eating more frequently.

Pretty fascinating stuff, which flies in the face of conventional wisdom. What is conventional wisdom?

"Cut Calories and You'll Lose Weight!"

Not necessarily.

This is such a prevalent mind-set, though, that we'll go into the scientific evidence that supports Intermittent Fasting.

Suffice it to say, for now you can safely ignore the calorie counts of foods and concentrate instead on their Macronutrients. Stick to the Macros, and you'll kick your body into a ketosis metabolic state.

Getting into Ketosis

How do you get into ketosis?

By changing the percentages of those three Macros: fats, proteins, and carbohydrates.

Unfortunately, our American current dietary guidelines as established by the USDA have nothing to do with how your body actually processes Macros. So, in essence, you are surrounded by carbohydrates, sugars, starches, excess bad fats, and too much protein. You can witness this for yourself when you go to the grocery store, try to order a meal in a restaurant, or simply drive past all the places to buy food, including convenience stores and coffee shops.

Above, you read that excess nutrients from all three Macros are stored on your body. Why isn't it used more effectively? Your body has this magnificent and very effective way of storing what's not needed. Waste and toxins are removed on a daily basis, but nutrients like carbohydrates are not. Those carbs are stored in your body until they are needed. What time are they needed? That depended on times of food shortage and scarcity.

Your body doesn't realize that it is the 21st century and you have plenty of food sources that are readily available. There's little chance of going hungry year round.

That wasn't the case 30,000 years ago or even earlier. Every year brought with it cold winters and months of food scarcity. You had to store extra weight, or otherwise you were in danger of starving. So, the excess proteins and excess carbohydrates were completely essential human survival. This is a good thing for the history of the human species, but what about when you don't want to carry that excess storage anymore? That's why we're trying to switch metabolic states.

A metabolic state is a series of smaller processes that take those Macros from your foods and use them for energy in your body. There are two types of metabolic states:

1. Carbohydrate Metabolic State
2. Ketosis Metabolic State

In the first one, carbohydrates are your primary source of fuel. Remember that those carbohydrates contain plenty of glucose. Some of that glucose is processed by your body and used as energy by your cells.

But most of the rest is stored.

We see that carbohydrate storage as gained weight. It's not so much that you're becoming heavier. You're actually becoming more 'sugary'! That weight comes from too much sugar.

In the second metabolic state, ketones produced by your liver are used as your primary source of fuel. With your carbohydrate intake vastly reduced down to about 30 grams per day, that's a pretty drastic loss of those sugars like sucrose, fructose, cellulose, and glucose. Consequently, your body isn't getting the previous fuel source it is been using basically all your life! Without its primary source of fuel (sugars and carbs), your body has to turn to another source for fuel. So, your body has to break down those good fats for energy instead! This is a good thing. Do you know why?

Your body will also be using the stored fat in your cells for energy, too! That means you'll be losing weight.

When your body uses stored fat as energy, that's a process called beta-oxidation since it uses oxygen atoms. When beta-oxidation is complete, the end result is a ketone. This ketone is just another source of fuel for the rest of your cells. When you combine these two processes of beta-oxidation and ketone production into one term, that's ketosis. Your liver becomes a ketone producing factory, converting all the stored fat (i.e. the weight you're desperately trying to lose) to energy. In essence, you're using resources from your own cells for energy.

That translates into fewer pounds on the scale! As well as all the other benefits of being in ketosis that you've read about before.

It's all about staying in ketosis.

Monitoring Ketosis

There is no way to visibly tell on the outside of your body that you're in ketosis. Your eyes don't change color, you don't develop any symptoms, and there's really no indicator that your liver is producing ketones. But, in order for the Ketogenic Diet to really work, especially when combined with Intermittent Fasting, you've got to stay in ketosis. It's very important!

So, you need a way to check that you're in ketosis and then continuously watch it while you're eating high fat, low carb. How do you do that?

You've probably heard of Ketone monitor tools and might even be using them yourself. When you add Intermittent Fasting to the Keto Diet, it is even more crucial that you monitor ketosis. So, you can't skip this step.

If you're not familiar with them, there are three ketosis measuring tools you can purchase either online or from a store like Walmart or Target. They are:

1. Ketone Urine Strips
2. Ketone Blood Monitor
3. Ketone Breath Monitor

First, you'll start with the Ketone Urine Strips. These are the least expensive of the three, and they will give you a quick and accurate reading. You urinate on a stick and then compare the resulting color to the chart on the package. If you're in ketosis, that's excellent. However, these urine strips don't work after you enter ketosis. So, they're just for the beginning stage of entering into the Ketogenic Diet.

The Ketone Blood Monitor measures your ketones in a similar way to a diabetes insulin tester. It takes the reading from a drop of your blood. That makes sense, since glucose (sugars) are carried by the bloodstream to your liver. Ketones are also carried by the bloodstream as a fuel source to the rest of your cells. Measuring this way is very accurate.

A Ketone Breath Monitor is also simple to use and doesn't require that you prick your finger, so I personally recommend it as my favorite way of measuring ketosis! It's like an alcohol breathalyzer. Plug in the monitor, blow into it, and then check to see what color it is. Compare the color against a chart included with the monitor to see how far into ketosis you are. Ketones are present in your breath.

After you enter ketosis, pick one of the second two monitors (Blood or Breath) to test. I'll mention these monitor devices several more times throughout the rest of this book, because it's the most accurate way to truly test whether you're in ketosis. So, invest in the monitor of your choosing and keep it handy throughout your Keto Diet journey!

It's really the best way to gauge your success, too!

Macros, Monitoring, and More

This chapter was all about the basic strong and solid foundations of the Keto Diet:

- Going from a carbohydrate metabolic state to a ketosis metabolic state
- Entering into ketosis through diet
- The three Macros on the Keto Diet: Fats, Proteins, and Carbohydrates
- The types of Macros you should be eating (good fats, naturally sourced proteins, low amounts of plant sugars)
- How those Macros are processed in the body
- The difference between Macro percentages and calories
- Tracking your ketosis through a Keto Monitor device

Just like baking a cake requires its core ingredients and then flavorings are added on top – so, too, are we going to add a new element to the Keto Diet that we'll talk about for the rest of the book:

Intermittent Fasting!

Although it's tempting to think so, it's not just about the foods you can or cannot eat, plus the Macros that you're consuming in the correct percentages on the Keto Diet. Getting your recommended fats and protein percentages, plus restricting carbs is important as the heart of the Keto diet.

Intermittent Fasting is not a necessary part of the Keto Diet, and many dieters choose not to try it.

But we'll go deeply into how Intermittent Fasting affects your body, the nutrition science behind it, several different ways to fast, how to do it properly, answer all of your questions about it, and give you a list of its main benefits.

Fasting boosts the Keto Diet to a whole new level. It gets you into ketosis faster and keeps you there. You can eat more calories than if you weren't fasting. It accelerates weight loss and you don't even need to add lots of exercise to do it. Fasting gives you even more health benefits than just being in ketosis alone.

Intermittent Fasting has such a major impact on how you feel each day, your health, and your overall well-being.

With your Keto Monitor device handy, your personal Macro percentages, and a fasting schedule, success is assured on the Keto Diet!

Chapter 3: We Say IF You Say What?

What is Intermittent Fasting?

It's just what it sounds like – fasting for short periods of time in between eating your Keto Diet friendly meals or snacks.

When you fast, you completely abstain from any food or beverage that contains calories. You're allowed water to stay hydrated.

Intermittent fasting is part of a continuous looping cycle that you'll be on during the Ketogenic Diet.

Every time you're sitting down at the table or grabbing a bite on the go, you're engaged in the feeding state of the cycle.

After you've eaten and you're waiting for the next meal, you're in a fasting state. During the fasting part of the cycle, you could either feel full having just eaten, feel satiated and not hungry at all, feel moderately hungry, feel very hungry, or feel famished. Your entire experience on the Keto Diet will be made up of this continuously looping cycle. You're either feeding or fasting.

To Fast or Not to Fast – That is the Dieting Question

Do you have to fast while on the Keto Diet? Is it a requirement to get the diet to work properly?

Nope, not at all. It's not something that you should be forced into doing! That's just as bad as trying to scarf down disgusting protein shakes, force yourself to go to the gym at 5:00 in the morning, or choke down weight loss pills.

The success of your diet depends a lot on not just physical factors, but psychological ones, too. If your mind is actively working against your ideals with this diet, then naturally it isn't going to work.

However, I really encourage you to try it!

Intermittent Fasting is used in conjunction with the Ketogenic Diet in order to speed up your results, give your body a chance to rest or digest between meals, and to help you lose weight quicker.

There are two basic goals with Intermittent Fasting:

1. Burn even more fat than without it
2. Boost your energy levels

Fasting seems like an odd addition to a diet. If you wanted to accelerate your weight loss, wouldn't you just exercise more? Most of us believe – thanks to diet gurus and the multi-billion dollar health and fitness industry - that losing weight is about eating less and exercising more. It's fewer calories in and more calories burned.

Right?

Well, sort of. It's much more complicated than that. As you read in the previous chapter, you're not necessarily eating less. You're just eating the right types of foods in the correct percentages. Ketosis changes your body's metabolic state, so now you're burning your own stored energy. So, the diet in itself actually causes you to burn more calories, not necessarily by adding exercise.

What makes Intermittent Fasting so special?

It's amazing because of what's happening at the cellular level inside your body when you stop the feeding cycle and go into the fasting cycle.

Cleaning Up With Autophagy

We're constantly learning new things about how our body's cells work. Since the dieting industry is such an enormous business, scientists study exactly how nutrients impact our body, how our body processes nutrients, and the link between nutrition and fuel.

One scientist studies a revolutionary cellular process that's the scientific proof behind why Intermittent Fasting works. Japanese cell biologist Yoshinori Ohsumi discovered this process, which is called autophagy. His work was such a breakthrough, he won the 2016 Nobel Prize in Physiology or Medicine.

What's autophagy – and what does it have to do with Intermittent Fasting?

Autophagy comes from the Greek words for "self-devouring." Sounds a bit gruesome, but it is a natural process that your cells go through all the time. In essence, it is cellular spring cleaning. Your cell can actually disassemble its own unnecessary or non-functioning components and recycle those components. Autophagy is activated when you fast, because it is a natural response to the lack of incoming sufficient fuel sources: good fats, proteins, carbohydrates, or sugars.

Cells that perform autophagy are actually removing their own harmful and toxic components. Those components are responsible for so many bad things that happen to your body as you age, including:

- Skin damage, like wrinkles and sagging skin
- Failing eyesight and hearing
- Memory problems
- Loss of energy
- Increasing aches and pains
- A more sluggish metabolism

- Continual weight gain or stagnant weight that won't come off

The cellular components causing all of these issues are just like old junky clutter hanging on inside your cells. But when you are on the Keto Diet and Intermittent Fasting at the same time, your cells get the message that it is time to clean out all that stuff. It's removed as waste or toxins and some parts are recycled to make your cells run better, faster, more efficient, and ultimately healthier for you. The result is that you feel better, look better, and actually slow down the aging process!

But that's the power of autophagy!

You can absolutely trigger autophagy by just fasting on a regular diet that includes higher carbohydrates. But ultimately, it's the combination of Intermittent Fasting and the high fat fuel source on the Ketogenic Diet that really causes your cells to internally clean house!

Fasting Burns More Fat

Autophagy isn't the only continuous and helpful process going on in your body at the cellular level when you fast intermittently. You actually already fast intermittently each day, by not consuming food all night when you're sleeping. Then you have "breakfast" (breaking the fast) in the morning, stopping that fasting period and starting a new feeding period. Fasting at night gives your digestive processes a chance to rest, while your body is given the opportunity to devote more time towards other processes, like the autophagy mentioned above, using proteins to build or repair tissue, and many other nightly functions.

Let's say that you're not on the Keto Diet, so you're consuming your multiple servings of carbohydrates per day. What happens when you decide to fast and you're not in ketosis?

Your body is using those carbohydrate sugars like sucrose and glucose for energy. But the longer your fast is, the less glucose there is entering your body, so your cells are forced to look elsewhere for a fuel source. Guess where they turn to? That's right – the stored fat energy in your cells. That sounds awfully similar to what happens when you're in ketosis on the Keto Diet, doesn't it?

In essence, the Keto Diet is in its own way a fasting type of diet. You're reducing your carbohydrate intake so greatly that it forces your body to use the stored fat from your cells for energy. Then, adding Intermittent Fasting interspersed with Keto Macro meals causes your body to burn even more fat because you're decreasing your food intake even more. The whole process looks like this:

You Eat Good Fats

|

Fats Enter the Stomach

|

Liver Breaks Down Fats For Energy (Beta-Oxidation)

|

Liver Produces Ketones

|

Ketones Used As Fuel

|

You Stop Eating and Fast for 18 Hours

|

No Additional Glucose or Good Fats Enter the Body

|

Liver Has to Use Stored Fat to Make Ketones

|

Ketones Used As Fuel

The longer you fast in between high fat Keto meals, the more weight that you lose because your liver is using all that stored fat to make ketones. This is the basic relationship between ketones, good fats, stored fat, and glucose.

Silly Myths About Intermittent Fasting

Whenever a trendy new eating plan (or, in this case, fasting plan) comes down the pike, many folks are quick to jump in and start spouting all these untruths. Some of them become very pervasive, especially in the Keto Diet community, because they coincide with a lot of common sense and therefore, must be true.

Not so!

On that note, we're here to provide you with the real deal scientific answers behind any myths about Intermittent Fasting. Let's get them out in the open, so that you go clear-eyed into any future fasting schedule. It's better to be informed than to follow advice that doesn't work, so steer clear of these myths!

Myth #1 – Fasting is Unhealthy or Dangerous

As has been mentioned above, you actually fast every night of your life! Fasting is not unhealthy. It's a natural process that allows your body to rest between feeding times. We live in the most food abundant time in human history. Grocery stores and restaurants serve anything you want to eat, 24 hours a day, 7 days a week. We eat at least three meals a day, plus snacks, desserts, and caloric beverages. Most American packaged foods and restaurant meals are crammed with way too much sugar, salt, bad fats, chemicals, and high carbohydrate amounts. It seems to me that having all this inexpensive food readily available contributes more to health problems than fasting ever could! Consuming high quantities of the "no no" foods is far more dangerous than simply abstaining from eating for a 24-hour time period.

Myth #2 – Fasting Puts Your Body in Starvation Mode

Starvation mode is when your brain and other organs start shutting down because they're completely deprived of any fuel source, whether it's glucose or ketones. However, it's not possible that fasting for up to 36 or even 48 hours at a time creates any long-lasting starvation effects. Why is that? It's because your liver will use the stored fat you already have existing in your cells as the ketones for fuel. Just because you're not taking in new forms of fuel doesn't mean that fuel sources don't exist! In fact, fasting puts your body into fat-burning mode. It's not harmful.

Myth #3 – Fasting Depletes Your Muscles

This seems like it's the case, but it's not true at all. Muscle is functional tissue that you need in order to physically move around. But this stored energy that's used by the liver is made up of free fatty acids. When you fast for a brief period of time, which is 3 days or less, then your body uses the stored fatty acids, not actual muscle tissue. It's only after a prolonged period of starvation, much longer than just 3 days, that your body has to then use muscle tissue for fuel. But short-term Intermittent Fasting does not use muscle tissue, because your body doesn't have to. There's plenty of stored fat to make those ketones for fuel! The kind of short-term fasting we're talking about in this book has nothing to do with your muscles. It's all about using that stored fat.

Myth #4 – Fasting is Unnatural

Contrary to popular belief, our bodies were not originally designed to thrive the best in an abundant food environment. We are extremely adaptable to changing food supply sources. That's why it takes such a short period of time to switch from using glucose as a fuel source to using ketones. It's also why we're so good at storing extra fat on our bodies! Our human ancestors went through food shortage times pretty much every year, especially in the winter. In fact, it would be detrimental for our bodies to not have a back-up contingency plan in place for times of food shortage. We would have quickly died out thousands of years ago if we couldn't survive periods of fasting. Fasting is both natural and biologically safe.

Myth #5 – Fasting Decreases Energy

This is another myth that seems like it should be true. After all, the less we eat, the less energetic we feel, right? But it doesn't make sense from a historical perspective. Let's say it's 30,000 years ago and a human hasn't eaten for a single day. If that person's metabolism decreased after just one day of fasting, then they wouldn't have any energy to go out to hunt or gather more food! After a second day, supposedly that person would be even weaker. If energy continually was lost after fasting, our species would not have survived. We needed energy even after fasting to go out and hunt more food. So, when you're fasting, your metabolism actually goes *up.* You're burning more stored fat as fuel, and that increases your metabolism. It also means your personal energy supply doesn't run out. As long as you've got plenty of stored fat for your liver to turn into ketones for fuel, your metabolism and energy levels will be just fine!

Myth #6 – You Don't Get Enough Calories or Nutrients When Fasting

It's true that during fasting times, you're not eating any of your Macros or calories. But does that mean an Intermittent Fasting schedule completely deprives your body of the foods you need to survive? Nope, not at all! You're not fasting for days and days or even weeks on end. You're just fasting for short time periods, between 18 and 24 hours. You can go a little longer once you get the hang of fasting, but Intermittent Fasting periods are only about three days or less. When you do enter into your feeding time periods after fasting, you'll have plenty of your Macros and calories to eat. We'll go more in-depth about what to eat between fasting in this book. But rest assured, you'll actually be able to eat all of the fat, protein, and carbohydrate grams that you need.

Whew! It's a good thing we got through those myths. They are both sneaky and negative, because they can turn many would-be dieters off from both the Keto Diet and Intermittent Fasting. Fasting is not dangerous, harmful, doesn't use muscle tissue, doesn't kick your body into starvation mode, and doesn't deprive your body of all the nutrients and calories you need.

Fasting is actually a healthy way to stay in ketosis while you're on the Keto Diet. It's just one more trick to get your body to use stored fat to make ketones for fuel.

Fast 1, 2, 3

Now, you may be wondering how exactly do you incorporate Intermittent Fasting with your Keto Diet? There are three types of fasting schedules. Whichever one you decide to go with is entirely up to you, depending on your weekly schedule and what will work best in your life. These three schedules are:

1. 24 to 48 hour Fasting – This is what most people imagine when they think "fasting." You just stop eating for a complete day or two. This is the most extreme way to fast intermittently and is recommended for more advanced Keto Dieters.
2. Eat a Little, Fast a Lot – You reduce your feeding time to a short window that's usually an average of 6 hours in the middle of the day. The other 18 hours, you're fasting and not eating anything at all.
3. Skip a Meal – Many of us skip breakfast, so we're familiar with extending our previous night's fast. You could choose another meal as your fasting period, like lunch or dinner. This is the simplest, easiest, and most common way to fast intermittently.

See, fasting isn't so bad! For those of you who've had early classes or jobs, you've probably skipped breakfast multiple times. You just had no idea you were Intermittently Fasting at the same time. Remember that fasting isn't dangerous or unhealthy. It's just another way to burn stored fat.

In Chapter 6, we'll go through a complete structured day by day guide to including Intermittent Fasting with your Keto Diet. We'll start by skipping a meal every three days, just to get used to fasting. Then we'll introduce smaller eating windows, where you're consuming all of your Macro percentages within a 5-hour timeframe. Then finally, we'll go into the complexities and preparation for your first 24-hour fast. It's a four week schedule that also includes exactly what you'll be eating on the Keto Diet as well.

As a brief disclaimer, I just want to remind you that there's a lot of flexibility with Intermittent Fasting. You might find that just skipping a meal every three or four days does it for you because your schedule right now is so busy. Or, you might find that eating in a smaller window of time is the way to go, plus you see the weight loss and energy benefits. For some of you, longer fasting is a welcome challenge and you want to see just how far it can take you. All of these scenarios are great. In other words, there is no set and perfect Intermittent Fasting schedule that will fit every person and every lifestyle.

The only thing that every person must do while both fasting and feeding on the Keto Diet?

You guessed it. Staying in ketosis!

That's why you need to be monitoring your ketones using the Breath Monitor or Blood Monitor. Neither Intermittent Fasting or the Keto Diet will give you the weight loss and health benefits you're looking for, if you don't stay in ketosis.

Other than staying in ketosis, your Intermittent Fasting schedule is yours to customize to your lifestyle.

Intermittent Fasting is a way to boost your Keto Diet foundational basics, so that you're increasing the rate at which your liver produces ketones for fuel. The more stored fat is used for fuel and the longer you're in ketosis, the more weight you'll lose and the more health benefits you'll receive!

We've already discussed a couple of introductory benefits in this chapter, including:

- Increased weight loss
- More stored energy burned for fuel
- Increasing autophagy, which is cellular spring cleaning
- Boosting your metabolism, which burns even more stored fat

But when it comes to the benefits of Intermittent Fasting, that's just the beginning. Read on to the next chapter to discover even more.

Chapter 4:
What's So Good About Intermittent Fasting?

Most diets are all about, well, dieting. And diets equal deprivation. You stop eating the foods you like, you cut back on your calories, you suffer from cravings, you have to force yourself to exercise and you hate it, and you're just generally miserable. Meanwhile, the number on the scale never budges and you actually feel not just worse, but heavier and with even less energy than when you began this so-called miracle diet!

Ugh, it's enough to turn anyone off and rightfully so.

But the Keto Diet together with Intermittent Fasting provide so many benefits and in such a short period of time, that you'll wonder why you ever even considered a different eating plan. Below are the ten biggest and most noticeable benefits from fasting on the Keto Diet, plus a bonus benefit that I think you'll really love!

10 Benefits of Intermittent Fasting on the Keto Diet

1. A Powerful Combination for Weight Loss

When you decide to switch from the regular 3 meals plus snack Keto Diet and instead group your meals together into a much shorter window, that kickstarts your body into a state of significant weight loss! A research article published by the Department of Kinesiology and Nutrition at the University of Illinois in Chicago discovered that overall body weight decreased on restricted feeding schedules. Over a 12 week time period, the participants ate between 10:00 am and 6:00 pm, then fasted until the next day at 10:00 am. While these people were not counting their calories on the Keto diet, on average they lost up to 2.6% of their body weight.

Other studies have shown people who combine the two (Keto and Intermittent Fasting) lose twice as much weight as those who do the fasting, but not the Keto. They're both good on their own, but like a superhero duo team, when they get together, that's when the real results happen!

In short, the science backs up the experiences for those who've been on the Ketogenic Diet and now incorporate Intermittent Fasting – it helps you lose even more weight.

2. Intermittent Fasting Increases HGH

What's HGH (human growth hormone), and why is it a good thing that Intermittent Fasting increases it? Just like other well known hormones such as testosterone and estrogen, HGH is a natural substance. It's produced by your pituitary gland and goes straight to your liver for metabolism. HGH is a 'monitoring' hormone that affects many processes in your body, including:

- Muscle and bone growth
- Sugar and fat metabolism
- Body fluids
- Overall body composition
- Cell regeneration and reproduction
- Slowing down aging
- Recovering from both disease and injury

When you don't have enough HGH, then that increases body fat, a lower lean body mass, and even decreased bone mass. In short, it's a good thing when HGH is increased. If you fast for just a 24 hour period, you can potentially increase your HGH production naturally by 1300% if you're female and 2000% if you're male. That's plenty to give you all those above benefits all their own.

When you lose fat by being on the Keto diet, and then add Intermittent Fasting, which boosts HGH, that's a recipe for anti-aging!

3. Fast Muscle Gain with Intermittent Fasting

As you read about above, one of the myths with Intermittent Fasting is that you'll not only lose weight, you'll lose muscle, too. You'll feel weaker because your cells will attack your muscles and consume them for energy, rather than nutrients. Thank goodness this is just a myth, because that would be a terrible side effect of fasting, making it completely not worth your time or effort!

But in fact, the opposite is true. Fasting helps you gain muscle, precisely because you're manufacturing more of the HGH talked about in the last benefit. It increases muscle mass. Not to mention the fact you're also on the Ketogenic Diet at the same time. So, you are eating about 19% of your calories from protein as your secondary Macro.

Being in ketosis between fasts is an amazing muscle boosting metabolic state for your body. The most popular fasting schedule for bulking up to gain muscle is the 18:6 – fasting for eighteen hours and eating for a six hour period, seven days a week. Just make sure you're eating the full amount of calories to off-set your muscle building. Stick with your Macros and you'll be amazed!

4. Intermittent Fasting Reduces Insulin

As we talked about in Chapter 2 above when just going over the basic scientific evidence behind ketosis, it stabilizes your blood sugar. This in itself is one of the massive benefits of the Keto Diet. But you also get another blood sugar bonus when you add Intermittent Fasting to Keto. You reduce insulin production.

Why is that a benefit? When you eat sugar, those molecules can only enter the fat cells with insulin. Insulin is a hormone, like HGH, but it's made in the pancreas. Insulin not only takes the sugar to the cells, it keeps it there. When you fast, your insulin levels drop, so your fat cells can release all that stored sugar. Now, you can use the stored sugar for energy, instead of having it just sit there.

It's just another and natural way to lose even more weight!

5. Speed Up Cell Repair and Regeneration

You are made up of trillions of cells that are continuously going through their life cycles. As time goes on and you age, it's harder to replace cells, repair cells, and regenerate cells. You see it as aging – the loss of energy, being more susceptible to illness, getting creaky joints and arthritis, failing eyesight, hearing loss, and a host of other symptoms.

But you can definitely help turn back the clock by being on the Ketogenic Diet and intermittently fasting! These two processes definitely increase your stem cell production, and stem cells can magically morph into any cell your body needs. So, those great stem cells can now be used to keep you feeling fit and younger, even down to the cellular level. Just because you can't see it, though, doesn't mean you can't feel it! You definitely will.

6. Keto + Intermittent Fasting = Super Brain

Have you heard about the brain benefits you get on the Keto Diet? They're pretty numerous, since your brain requires and uses so much energy. When you're eating such a high fat and moderate protein diet, both protein and ketones are providing fuel and energy for your brain. Also, your liver enters a state called gluconeogenesis, meaning it produces new glucose from the glycerol in the fatty acids of triglycerides. The liver then sends that glucose to your brain for fuel.

So, that's already happening as an awesome benefit on the Keto Diet. When you add Intermittent Fasting, your brain increases one particular protein called BDNF (brain-derived neurotrophic factor). BDNF interacts with neurons in your central nervous system, supporting them and encouraging the growth of new neurons. In essence, both Keto and Intermittent Fasting together make your brain a super machine, using glucose from fats for fuel and forging stronger neural pathways. You'll think better, remember better, and your recall time will reduce.

7. All Clear for Autophagy

Autophagy was mentioned back in the previous chapter as one of the basics of Intermittent Fasting. But this really is one of those recently discovered benefits backed up by the scientific community that truly supports fasting as a viable body improvement practice.

In essence, autophagy is your cell's completely natural internal car cleaning and tune-up process. When Intermittent Fasting, autophagy is turned on and that gives the signal for your cells to start self-cleaning. Your cells basically take out their old parts, get rid of damaged parts, and then bring in shiny new parts. Now your cells run faster and more smoothly. Autophagy takes part in any cell in your body, so this improves your brain function, digestive system, muscles, bones, and other organs. You'll feel less pain from inflammation, too. Once the old junk is cleared out, that means your cells can function better.

8. Recover Faster from Hard Workouts

Intermittent Fasting can help you recover much faster from a hard workout than if you weren't fasting, or even on the Keto Diet. That's because, as another side effect of such a massive increase in the HGH production in your pituitary gland, muscle protein synthesis takes place quicker.

Oh, and it also helps if you've had a muscle injury, too. This is an amazing bonus for athletes and other active people, who get sprains, pull muscles, and other muscular injuries. Try Intermittent Fasting along with your Ketogenic Diet – and you'll be amazed at how much faster you're able to bounce back on your feet again and get back to the gym or the athletic field.

9. Get into Ketosis Faster

With the rise in popularity of the Keto Diet, many dieters have been looking for ways to get into ketosis even faster than the normal two week time period it usually takes. Also, many dieters experience what's affectionately nicknamed the "Keto Flu," which is a collection of flu-like symptoms that happen in your body when you're switching from that carbohydrate metabolic state to a ketosis metabolic state.

Stick to your Macros, and you'll eventually get into ketosis. But add Intermittent Fasting, and now your liver is using even more stored fat to produce ketones for fuel. That accelerates the rate at which you go into ketosis. Many dieters also report that this bypasses those Keto Flu symptoms. Check your own ketosis using a monitoring tool, and see for yourself just how much quicker you're able to achieve this new metabolic state. The longer you stay in ketosis, with the help of both the Keto Diet and regular Intermittent Fasting, the more weight you'll lose.

10. Can Eat More Calories and Still See Weight Loss

Most diet books you've read have all preached the same boring message of deprivation: cut calories to lose weight. Fewer calories means fewer pounds. Well, when you are consuming your calories from such a high fat / moderate protein / very low carbohydrate Keto Diet and you get into ketosis, your liver will use stored fat to make ketones for fuel. Then, when you add Intermittent Fasting, you can actually eat more calories during your feeding times – and still lose weight! Would you rather eat 1800 calories from three meals a day or 2000 calories within a short 5-hour window?

When I tell you that eating 2000 calories in a short window and fasting the rest of the time will actually help you lose weight faster than eating fewer calories, the choice becomes clear. But those 2000 calories comes from the Macro percentages on the Keto Diet, not 2000 calories from a carbohydrate heavy diet. When you eat plenty of the right kinds of calories and then fast the rest of the time, that's when you've optimized your body for peak weight loss.

Bonus Benefit – You Don't Have to Exercise to See Results!

Most diet books talk about exercising as if it's this magical weight-loss tool that will shed ten pounds a week. Just buy this treadmill, and the weight will drop off! But you know that's not reality. The reality is that exercise is hard. It's the tough way to burn fat and build muscle.

So, as a total bonus that goes along with the Keto Diet and Intermittent Fasting, you don't have to exercise in order to see weight loss results. You certainly can if you want to, especially when meeting personal body goals. But you don't have to. You will still lose weight, because you're actually burning stored fat at a cellular level. Your body is a metabolism machine, and if it can't get the fuel it needs from what you're eating, it will start rummaging around in your energy stores and pull the fuel from there. Less stored energy equals more weight lost. No exercise required!

Positive Change for Your Body

There are numerous other benefits from both the Keto Diet and Intermittent Fasting, but every person is different. Your experience combining these two powerful health tools will be much more profound than simply cutting calories or increasing your exercise or even using the Keto Diet by itself.

Time is on your side when you eat your Keto Macros and practice Intermittent Fasting on a regular basis. The longer you're in ketosis and the more regularly you fast, the more benefits you'll receive. Many dieters have met unbelievable weight loss goals while doing this. This is not a crash diet to just melt off 20 pounds and then go back to eating bread sticks. But who wants to eat a high carbohydrate diet, when you feel so good and look so good staying in ketosis?

Being on the Keto Diet and doing Intermittent Fasting both equal positive change for your body.

Chapter 5:
Troubleshooting for Intermittent Fasting and the Keto Diet

In the previous chapter, you read all about the amazing benefits that you get from not just sticking to your Macros on the Ketogenic Diet, but also adding Intermittent Fasting as an incredible boost for weight loss, health, and many more awesome side effects.

But there are some potential pitfalls and problems that you could encounter while pursuing both a high fat / low carbohydrate diet and trying fasting at the same time. In this chapter, I'll go into some of these and help you through each of them one by one.

For the most part, these common obstacles have rather simple, easy solutions. You'll be able to recover and get back on track towards meeting your health and fitness goals in no time!

Problem #1 – The Weight Won't Budge

You've been following the Keto Diet, you're sticking to your Macros, you're adding a few skipped meals here or there – and still, the weight just won't come off. You've tried adding exercise or counting calories, and still you've yet to see a pound lost. What's happening to your body?

Many Keto dieters with the best of intentions just go as low carb and high fat as they can. But they don't put in the due diligence necessary to make this diet work. It's not a 'cheat day' diet, where you can reach for that piece of bread on a Friday after abstaining from carbohydrates all week!

This diet is all about the numbers, specifically these numbers:

- Your Macro percentages
- Your specific calorie counts
- Your ketosis monitor number

When the weight won't budge, the best and quickest solution is to go back to basics. Follow these steps:

1. Weigh yourself today.
2. Go online, find a Macro calculator, and pull up your exact Macro percentages for fats, proteins, and carbohydrates. Your Macro calculator should also give you the calorie counts required for your specific body. That's your baseline, where you start to build the diet.

3. Follow the 7-Day Meal plan in this book. Even if you've been Keto dieting for months, stick to this short meal plan.
4. Read Chapter 8 to craft your own meal plan.
5. Purchase a Keto Breath or Blood Monitor if you haven't done so already, and track that at least every other day.

After following those five steps, you'll discover the loophole that's preventing you from losing weight. Usually it's too much protein. It's easy to go overboard on the chicken and burgers!

Get back into ketosis as soon as you can, and then add Intermittent Fasting according to the rules in this book. Your weight will start to come off.

Problem #2 – Excess Mineral Loss

When your liver produces ketones for fuel, a lot of sodium is excreted from your body in the process. Since you're not eating large amounts of glucose on the Keto Diet, you're not producing as much insulin. Insulin helps sodium absorb into your body. So without it, you really do urinate out too much salt. Your goal should be between 2000 mg and 4000 mg of salt per day.

Fortunately, salty foods are delicious! Reach for salty cheeses, salted nuts, salted butter, and put a bit of extra salt on vegetables and meats. You are also encouraged to sip on salty chicken or beef broth. Did you know that getting enough sodium will also help with carbohydrate withdrawals? It boosts your electrolytes, too. Salt is great!

You also need to make sure that you're getting enough minerals like magnesium and potassium. Excess mineral loss can cause some nutritional deficiencies. You'll start to feel more lethargic and weaker without knowing why.

The best advice is to take a mineral supplement and to keep replenishing the vitamins and minerals you need. Many Keto Diet approved foods, like salmon, dark leafy greens like kale, and almonds contain high amounts of beneficial minerals.

Problem #3 – Feel Sick When Breaking the Fast

Fasting is easier than you may think. But when you start breaking the fast and re-enter the world of eating, that might pose a bit of a tricky problem.

Sometimes, especially after a longer fast of 24 hours and more, when you break the fast by eating again, you'll feel sick. You'll be nauseous, tired, and just generally out of it, feeling worse after breaking the fast than you did by not eating anything at all. People who fast to the extreme actually experience great difficulties trying to eat food again. It causes a possibly fatal shift in your body's interior balance of fluids and electrolytes. Shorter fasts of 3 days or less aren't as harmful, but they can also possibly make you not feel so good. That's because of the problem above, which is excess mineral loss. Low carbohydrate diets encourage the unhealthy loss of too many essential minerals.

So, the first meal that you have after a fast, especially one that lasts 3 days, should be made up of plenty of mineral rich and Keto Diet approved foods that have been appropriately salted. One example would be grilled salmon with several slices of avocado and a dark leafy green salad with lemon. Eat as much as you can until you feel full, even if you don't have an appetite. Keep drinking lots of water with electrolytes like lemon slices. These foods will fill you up, provide those essential minerals you've excreted during your fast, and keep you in ketosis, too.

Problem #4 – My Metabolism Has Slowed Down

Intermittently Fasting while on the Keto Diet should cause your metabolism to go up. That's because you're using even more stored fat for ketones for fuel. But what if your metabolism is slowing down and your weight loss is more sluggish than it used to be?

This is one of the few problems that really does depend on the calories you're consuming. Eating too few calories can stall your metabolism, slowing both your weight loss and your energy.

The solution is to go back to tracking your Macros, making sure you're eating enough during those feeding time windows between fasts. Keep your calorie counts up. I've always highly recommended that Keto dieters keep an accurate food diary, which you'll use to track everything. It makes it easier to tell if you've made a mistake, too.

Problem #5 – My Weight Loss Has Plateaued

Ah, the dreaded weight loss plateau. Yes, it can happen even if you're on the Keto Diet and Intermittently Fasting at the same time. If you add exercise to the mix, then that increases the likelihood you'll reach a weight loss plateau, because muscle weighs more than fat. For our intents and purposes, a weight loss plateau is losing less than 1 pound per week. There are two key culprits behind a weight loss plateau:

1. Your body decreases its total daily energy expenditure
2. Your calorie deficit decreases, because you don't require as many calories to maintain your new weight

In essence, you've lost some weight and you're happy with it, but your body isn't. Your body believes that if you continue on this route, you'll go into a starvation period and eventually die. So, it pulls out all of its biological tricks to make sure you've stopped losing weight!

The first solution to this problem is to schedule a doctor's appointment. Underlying thyroid issues and other medical problems might be preventing you from having success on this diet. Anything related to auto-immune problems can also either stall or reverse weight loss. Let your doctor know your diet and get your bloodwork done. That'll help rule out any medical problems.

All cleared from the doctor? Then go back to the Keto Diet and start tracking your calories. Just because calories aren't as important on the Keto Diet doesn't mean they're inconsequential! Use an online Keto Diet calculator to see just how many calories from each Macro you should be eating every day. Then track your calories each day.

Also, you'll want to recalculate your Macros each month. That's because your Macro percentages are based on weight – and you're losing weight! Go back to the Macro calculator that you used and get your new percentages based on how you currently weigh. That'll help you bust through your plateau.

It's best to go slowly, so that your body doesn't try new and sneaky ways to keep that weight from continuously dropping right off. Remember that you're biologically designed to not starve yourself, and you need plenty of nutrients even in weight loss phases.

Problem #6 – I'm Hungry!

Your body is hard-wired to not go hungry. So, any attempt to start a fast will be met with loud protests. Your brain will come up with every reason and excuse under the sun for you to break the fast early. You'll feel not just hungry, but hungry for all those foods you're not supposed to be eating while in ketosis – carbohydrates! For some of us, being hungry really alters our moods. Why is that? It's the change in your blood sugar. When your blood sugar is stabilized, that helps regulate the emotional hormones in your brain, which makes you feel calmer and less irritable.

When you first start trying Intermittent Fasting, if you've never done it before, you'll feel the hungriest. So just know, that it does get better over time. You'll learn to feel better and less hungry. It gets easier.

There are a few solutions to quieting the hungry hormones. The first is to make absolutely sure you're getting enough good fats during your feeding times between fasts. Your Fat Macro is the most important, so keep an eye on it and consume as many good fats as you can. That will help keep you satiated between fasts. The second solution is to drink plenty of water with lemon both during the fast and during the windows of time you're feeding, too. Staying extra hydrated helps stave off hunger pangs. You can also sip on salty chicken or beef broth. That will help replenish salt as well, which keeps carb cravings at bay at the same time. You can also try to get more sleep. Sleep deprivation can lead to hunger pangs. Try getting at least seven to eight hours per night. That will help with your weight loss, too!

Problem #7 – I'm *Not* Hungry!

While problem 6 comes from not eating enough of the Fat Macro on the Ketogenic Diet, you could also develop this issue of just not feeling all that hungry when your feeding window time starts. You've just broken your fast and it's time to eat. You've got your Keto recipes to make and food right in front of you … and you're just not interested in eating it. You know you only have a 6 hour window in which to eat this food before you're fasting again, so you start to panic a bit. How are you supposed to get all of your Macro grams into your body when you literally have no appetite at all?

It's okay to not be hungry at the end of an Intermittent Fasting cycle. People who've been doing really well on the Keto Diet and staying in ketosis for weeks and months at a time can become fat-adapted, which means that you need fewer meals to feel satiated. This 'problem' is actually a good thing! It's perfectly fine to just stay on the Keto Diet without including Intermittent Fasting at all. Fasting is simply a way to unlock bonus health benefits. It's not absolutely necessary. The one thing that is necessary is to stay in ketosis.

So, on the day that you're not hungry and it's your feeding window time to eat, just relax. Use the Ketone Breath or Blood Monitor to check your ketone levels and make sure you're in ketosis. Then go about the rest of your day. You might not feel hungry for many hours and your 18 hour fast could turn into a 24 hour fast. That's perfectly fine.

The next time you are hungry, eat a Keto meal. Eat two more Keto meals within a 24-hour timeframe, so that you've met all of your Macro requirements for a single day. Then just stay on Keto without any Intermittent Fasting for several days. This will help your body get back into a regular feeding schedule. Don't worry about your weight loss or gain (if either scenario happens) during this period. Just work on getting your hunger back to a normal state.

Then, you can slowly ease back into Intermittent Fasting by skipping a meal every third day. Every person's body is different, so Intermittent Fasting for longer periods of time might reduce your appetite too much. You want to make sure you're eating enough Macros and calories to get all of your recommended vitamins and minerals, too. Monitor your ketones and, as long as you stay in ketosis, you'll do just fine.

Problem #8 – I Can't Find the Perfect Eating Window of Time

For many of us, our lives are incredibly busy. It can be a difficult challenge to find the balance between times when you're fasting and times when you should be feeding. Luckily, you have a lot of flexibility here. You don't have to follow somebody else's Intermittent Fasting schedule if that doesn't work for you. You don't even have to follow the feeding windows in this book. You can certainly come up with your own schedule.

The only rule of thumb when it comes to finding the best eating window of time, is that your last meal should occur about two to three hours before bedtime. Eating windows of time last around six hours, which gives you eighteen hours of fasting. So, for example, if you go to bed at 11:00 at night, your six-hour feeding window could be between 3:00 pm and 9:00 pm. That's the latest it could be. This is a perfectly fine Intermittent Fasting eating schedule.

Other than that guideline, you're free to come up with the schedule that works for you.

Here are some possible examples:

- Have a full time nine to five job? Try an eating window between 7:00 am and 1:00 pm. Take in most of your calories at breakfast and then the rest at a noon lunch time.

196

- Work a late shift? Schedule your feeding window between 9:00 am and 3:00 pm, in the middle of the day before your shift starts.
- An early riser? Then your eating window can be between 5:00 am and 11:00 am. You'd take in all of your calories in the morning.

Find in your schedule the times when it makes the most sense for you to be eating. Then, make sure you're getting all of the Macro grams for your Fats, Proteins, and Carbohydrates. The rest of the time, you should be fasting.

Problem #9 – I've Fallen into an Eating Rut – Help!

Yes, it can happen to the best of us when the diet is quite restrictive. The Keto Diet eliminates so many foods that you've happily munched on in the past. It's easy to start to feel deprived, especially when you're surrounded by carbs, fruits, candy, snacks, ice cream, pizza, and other tempting nibbles! You really do have to plan out your day according to what and when you're eating. The schedule is also restrictive, too.

So, what do you do if you've fallen into an eating rut, you can't remember the last time you actually ate something that truly satisfied you, you're tired of the same-old cravings, and you're about to run to the nearest bakery and shove your mouth full of donuts?

Wait. Stop!

Breathe. Seriously. Just breathe with me. That's right. It's your hunger pangs and your body's former cravings for glucose that are making you go a little crazy. That's okay. It's totally normal and is always an active discussion amongst Keto dieters. What can you do? Here are a few tips:

- Find recipes for Keto versions of your favorite foods. There are plenty of online recipes and YouTube video recipes that show you exactly how to make Keto pizza, Keto bread, Keto crackers, Keto ice cream, and Keto candy. Just do a bit of searching, and you'll find them!
- Search out Keto communities, either in person or online. You can share your diet woes and get more tips on how to keep this diet new and exciting.
- Explore new flavors from other cultures. There's the most common ones, like Italian, Mexican, Chinese, and French. More unusual cuisines come from Morocco, the Middle East, Scandinavia, the Pacific Islands, Australia, and Cambodia. Just changing up the palate can help you cope with this diet.
- To go with the above tip, keep a very well stocked herb and spice cabinet. That way, you can turn base ingredients like chicken breasts, ground beef, eggs, and pork into new flavor combinations

When you add Intermittent Fasting, that restricts the Keto Diet even more. When you're really struggling with trying to eat enough in a short period of time, then ease off the Intermittent Fasting. Try to rediscover the joys of eating just on the Keto Diet. Then you can slowly re-introduce Intermittent Fasting.

The more deprived you feel, the greater the chance you'll want to reach for the bread and knock yourself out of ketosis. Try to make the Keto Diet more fun – and you'll not only lose more weight, you'll enjoy your feeding times that much more!

Problem #10 – That Fat Macro is Intimidating

Yes, it is! How are you supposed to not just eat 75% of your daily calories in good fats – but consume all those grams in a six-hour window? For some people, it not only sounds intimidating, but a little off-putting. At least you don't have to hook up a feeding tube to do it!

Well, there are two tools in this book to help you get all of your Fat Macro grams:

1. The Structured Guide to Intermittent Fasting in Chapter 6
2. The 7 Day Meal Plan in Chapter 7

Take the guesswork off the table and just follow those two guides. They have the appropriate Fat Macros built in to them, so it's really easy to get started. You can also create your own meal plan using the tips in Chapter 8, and then follow that. There are plenty of Keto Diet meal plans available online or from fellow Keto Dieters. Sticking to a meal plan is the best way to stop counting Fat Macro grams, and just trust that you're getting the amount that you need.

As a super quick guide, here are the top thirteen highest fat foods. They're super healthy for you, too. When you're a few grams short and need more fat, turn to one of these in this list:

1. Butter – 100% fat
2. Olive Oil – 100% fat
3. MCT Oil – 100% fat
4. Heavy Cream – 95% fat
5. Green Olives – 88% fat
6. Macadamia Nuts – 88% fat
7. Cream Cheese – 88% fat
8. Sour Cream – 86% fat
9. Coconut Cream – 86% fat
10. Walnuts – 84% fat
11. Brazil Nuts – 84% fat
12. Almond Butter – 79% fat
13. Avocado – 77% fat

All of these foods are not only delicious, they will help you get in enough of your Fat Macro. Some of them do have a minor carbohydrate count, so don't forget to take that into account with your Macros. Snacks like green olives, macadamia nuts, Brazil nuts, and almond butter with a low carb veggie like celery or cucumber will get you to your Fat Macro number in no time!

It's All About the Numbers

Most of the above ten issues with either the Keto Diet or Intermittent Fasting really come down to the numbers. With this way of eating, it's always a good thing to go back to basics:

- Tracking your Macros in grams
- Tracking your calories
- Monitoring your blood or breath for ketosis
- Sticking to a routine fasting schedule

Many of these issues will soon resolve themselves in less than a week! To prevent further issues going forward, I highly recommend that you keep a daily food diary. It provides you with a wonderful written record – and keeps you accountable when hitting your numbers!

So, we've been talking a lot about the basics of Intermittent Fasting: its benefits, troubleshooting issues, busted its myths, and given you three different ways to fast. How exactly do you do this on a day to day basis? We'll get into the daily schedule in the next chapter!

Chapter 6:
Take It Easy With Some Structured Planning

You've read all about the theories and reasons why you should incorporate Intermittent Fasting into your Keto Diet.

But, how exactly are you supposed to do that from day to day?

In this chapter, we'll do exactly that. We've provided your first four weeks on the Keto Diet with Intermittent Fasting eating and exercising plan. Even if you're a beginner, you can start following this guide on Day One and proceed all the way to Day Twenty-Eight. More advanced Keto Dieters can start anywhere in Week Two or even Week Three, and follow the more advanced steps. By Week Four, you'll be attempting your first extended 48-hour fast. We'll also teach you how to break that fast.

This chapter is the most comprehensive and gives you an incredible amount of information. In essence, it's your own Keto Diet food diary and meal plan all in one! That makes it your new best friend which will be here every step of the way during your first month combining ketosis with fasting. This is where we take theory and incorporate it into your daily life.

Life in the Fasting Lane

We'll start by skipping a meal every three days, just to get used to fasting. Gradually we'll introduce reduced eating windows, where you're consuming all of your Macro percentages within a 6-hour timeframe. Then finally, we'll go into the complexities and preparation for your first 24-hour fast. Once you've gotten the hang of that fast, we'll proceed in Week Four to the 48-hour fast.

As a quick note, this guide is just one way to incorporate Intermittent Fasting into your Keto Diet. You're certainly more than welcome to change up this schedule as you see fit and try a different method. You might find you prefer meal-skipping and just don't have a meal every other day. Or, you might really enjoy the 6-hour eating windows right off the bat and just want to do that because it's easier and fits right into your life! You might find 24-hour or even 48-hour fasts give you amazing results and you won't mind having one each month.

All of these possible scenarios are great! Remember that, as always, the Keto Diet is personal to you and your body. We want you to not only see results with Intermittent Fasting, but to enjoy yourself. It will boost your weight loss and your energy, too. Staying in ketosis for four weeks does magical things to your body!

There's definitely some stuff you need to do as preparation for the Keto Diet journey to come! It helps to have all of your helpful tools assembled before you begin, so that you're fully prepped and ready to go. That includes purchasing a Keto Blood or Breath monitor, buying the necessary cooking implements and kitchen tools for making Keto meals, and investing in a new notebook as your food diary. You'll also want to go online and find a Macro calculator. Fill out the questionnaire and then write the results here:

- Fats: _____ grams
- Proteins: _____ grams
- Carbohydrates: _____ grams
- Total Calories: _____

It's also helpful to set goals. How much weight do you want to lose by the end of these four weeks? Do you have any other Keto Diet goals? Add those to your food diary to help you stay on track.

- Weight Loss goal: _____ pounds in _____ weeks
- Fitness goal: _____

If you're not following the 7 Day Meal Plan in this book, you also want to come up with a meal plan for your first week. Include the recipes that you'll need, too. You'll also want to purchase the ingredients for at least the first seven days of Keto meals, based on your personalized Macros.

You'll notice in Week One there's no exercise plan (yet). That's because we want your body to get used to Intermittent Fasting before we add exercise to it. Let's just focus on your eating plan and eating schedule. There's plenty of time to add exercise later!

Whew! There's a lot to do before Day 1, but these are all the foundational tools you'll need to get through your first week both Keto dieting and Intermittent Fasting. Now you're ready to start and you've laid the groundwork for a successful first month!

Week One

Day 1

Day 1 is going to be a normal, regular day without any major changes to your Ketogenic Diet at all. We're going to ease slowly into Intermittent Fasting. So, for today all you've got to do is cook and eat three regular Keto meals plus a snack / dessert / drink. You can start on Day 1 of the 7 Day Meal Plan in the next chapter. Or, follow your own customized meal plan. You can also eat your meals whenever you want. Make sure you reach your Macros. Track what you ate in your food diary. Monitor either your breath or blood and check for ketosis.

There are no specific guidelines about exactly when you should measure ketone levels. In the morning, ketone concentrations are lower and higher in the evening. Two factors throw off ketone levels: right after exercising and when you're dehydrated.

Going forward, just monitor your ketones at a consistent time every time you do. If you test at 10:00 am today on Day 1, then always test at 10:00 am on future days. You're trying to find your baseline and your normal readings. Then, when it changes, you'll know!

Day 2

Today is your first attempt at Intermittent Fasting! We're going to do a skipped meal, just like in the 7 Day Meal Plan. Many Keto Dieters skip breakfast, because that's an easy meal to skip. A lot of us just aren't hungry in the mornings. Also, skipping breakfast extends your fast from the night before, increasing its benefits. You can skip lunch or skip dinner, too.

Whichever meal you decide to skip, make sure for the remainder of your meals, you're getting in your Macros. This means having extra Macro grams at the other meals than you normally would. How did this first day of fasting go? Were you hungry during the skipped meal period? Or, was it relatively easy? Record your experience.

Day 3

If Day 2 went well by both fasting and adding Macros to other meals, you're welcome to repeat it on Day 3. Pick a meal to skip and increase your Macros for the other meals.

If Day 2 was difficult and you were very hungry between meals, then just go back to a regular eating schedule on the Keto Diet. Cook and eat your three Ketogenic meals just like you normally would.

Day 4

Repeat Day 3. Skip one of your meals as your time spent Intermittent Fasting, and eat your other meals with the increased Macro grams. Check to see that you're in ketosis using a monitoring tool. Track your Macros, your calories, and your Keto monitoring readout in a food diary.

Day 5

No Intermittent Fasting today. You are going to cook and eat your Keto meals as normal, with the Macros spread throughout the day. This gives your body a chance to rest between times of fasting. You may find as you proceed that you become more fat-adapted, which will slowly decrease your hunger. For those of you who like tracking data, you can check your ketones again today. Staying consistently in ketosis will help you lose the weight, too.

Day 6

Today, you'll practice Intermittent Fasting for a longer period of time. You're going to have an eating window of 10 hours, with 14 hours off for fasting. This eating window can start at any time in the morning and continue for the ten hours. For example, you could start it at 8:00 am and continue until 6:00 pm. After your eating window is done, you're not to eat any solid foods or broths until tomorrow. You are allowed to drink some water with lemon slices to keep up your electrolytes.

During your 10-hour eating window is when you'll consume all of your Macros. You can split up the Macros into any meal combination you like. A heavy breakfast, light lunch, and heavy dinner would be an option. Or, any other combination that works for you. Don't forget to snack within those ten hours, so you can reach your Macro counts. Track everything in your food diary, too.

Day 7

Yay, you've got to the end of your first week! Celebrate by weighing yourself. Have you lost any weight yet? A healthy weight loss schedule is up to two pounds per week. How are your energy levels? Are you doing well with the Intermittent Fasting times? Did you prefer the skipped meals or the 10-hour window? Tweak and adjust as the schedule goes forward.

Today, you'll want to repeat Day 6 by doing another 10 hour window. It has to be the exact same time as yesterday, to make sure you're getting the full fourteen-hour fasting cycle. So, if you started your ten hour window at 8:00 am yesterday, you'll start it at 8:00 am today. Again, get all of your Macros in your eating window. When it stops, that's when it's time to fast.

Week Two

Day 8

After several days of skipped meals and two days of 10-hour eating windows, it's time to shorten your eating window and increase your fasting time. What time did your 10-hour eating window end yesterday? Count forward sixteen hours, and that's when your 8-hour eating window should start today. For example, if you ended your 10-hour window at 6:00 pm last night, you'll start your 8-hour eating window at 10:00 am today, and it will end at 6:00 pm. That's sixteen hours of fasting, consuming nothing but water with lemon slices for electrolytes. You'll want to eat all of your Macros in your shorter 8-hour window. That includes breakfast, lunch, dinner, and your snack / dessert / drink.

Day 8 is also a good time to plan out meals for Week Two. Find recipes for those meals with the included Macros, and go shopping for your ingredients to restock your kitchen. Also, monitor your ketones again. Are you staying in ketosis? If so, great! If not, adjust your Macros, follow the troubleshooting tips in the previous chapter, and get back into ketosis.

Day 9

The 8-hour feeding window from yesterday is repeated today, at the exact same time you started it yesterday. Eat all of your Macros in the 8 hours. If you're having a bit of a challenge consuming enough of your Fat Macros in a shorter time frame, try taking some MCT oil. Start with a small amount, like a teaspoon, since it does cause nausea in some people. A 1 Tablespoon serving has 100 calories and 14 grams of good fats.

Day 10

Repeat your 16 hour Intermittent Fasting / 8 hour Keto Dieting routine today as well. Just make sure you're consuming all of your daily Macros in those 8 hours. If you're having difficulty, it's okay to go back to a regular Keto eating schedule. Adjust the eating window time, too, if it's not working out. If it is working out, great! After trying fasting for ten days, your body does start to change.

Day 11

Today is the day to not only continue on your 16 hour fasting / 8 hour eating plan, but to try incorporating some exercise into it. You don't have to, but getting exercise is wonderful for your body and has so many benefits. You'll sleep better, too. Since your body is adjusting to a fasting schedule, don't overdo it on your workouts. A gentle 30 minute routine to get your heart rate up is usually all it takes. Just like yesterday, eat your Macros within the 8 hours. Track and record your experience.

Day 12

Today, we're going to shorten our eating window by one more hour, thus increasing our fasting window. You'll now be fasting for 17 hours and eating for 7 hours, and we'll repeat that cycle for several days. When was the end of yesterday's eating window? Count forward 17 hours, and that's when your 7 hour time frame begins. Now, you'll be eating all of your Macros in a 7 hour period. Take your mineral supplements and gently increase your MCT oil dosage as well. Get plenty of water during fasting periods. You can add 30 minutes of exercise, but not if you are feeling weak or struggling with this eating routine. Give your body time to adjust.

Day 13

How did yesterday go when eating for just 7 hours during the day? The time goes by quick! By now, you should be able to tell when you're staying in ketosis even during those fasting times. It's pretty noticeable! You'll feel it if you knock yourself out.

Repeat your 7-hour eating window schedule from yesterday. You can add exercise, too. Eat and track your Macros, making sure you're also getting your recommended calories. As eating windows get shorter, many Keto Dieters reduce the number of meals to two, plus a snack or Keto beverage. Eating twice a day works out for a lot of people, so give it a try!

Day 14

Congrats – you've reached the end of the second week. You went from a 10-hour window down to a 7-hour eating window, increasing your fasting time by three hours! That's three extra hours your body is spending pulling fuel sources from existing fat cells rather than relying on incoming fuel sources from your meals. You also added exercise, which burns even more fat in your cells. You've started to super-charge the Keto Diet effects by fasting.

It's time to assess the week. How did you do on your increased Intermittent Fasting? Was it easy to add exercise to it? Have you been tracking your Fats, Proteins, and Carbohydrates each day?

Weigh yourself to see if you've lost more weight. If so, excellent! If not, then the troubleshooting tips in the previous chapter can help you. In addition to sticking to your 7-hour eating window today, check your ketones again using your monitor. Intermittent Fasting helps bump you into ketosis faster than simply cutting carbs. So, that's a noticeable change this week.

Week Three

Day 15

Day 15 begins with a new eating plan for this week, but now it's going to be based on a new eating window of just 6 hours. That's 18 hours spent fasting the rest of the time. Count forward from yesterday one additional hour, and that's when your fast should begin. You can adjust and tweak your fasting schedule during Days 15 and 16 to see which is the best 6-hour timeframe for you. But by Day 17, your routine should be consistent. Consistency with your feeding/fasting cycles is key to getting all the benefits from doing this.

You're also going to do your first 24-hour fast this week, so plan for that in your schedule. Go shopping for your Keto Diet ingredients and restock your cupboards. Make sure you have plenty of mineral rich foods for the day after your fast, and keep a good supply of salty broths on hand, too.

Day 16

Today is the second day of your new 6-hour eating window and 18 hour fast. Eat all of your Macros inside of those 6 hours, and track them in your food diary. Are you feeling more energy? Many Keto Dieters enjoy such a short eating window, since it really makes the effects of fasting noticeable. You can add some exercise to your schedule as well. Start with 30 minutes and gradually increase, depending on your fitness goals and how well you're doing on your fasting / feeding cycles. It's okay to cut back on your fitness if you're feeling weak or sluggish in any way.

Day 17

Continue with your 6-hour feeding / 18-hour fasting schedule today. Get in as many Macros as you can within those short six hours. Add your exercise to your routine, too. Make any adjustments like necessary. During fasting times, you should only be drinking water with a bit of lemon for electrolytes.

Day 18

Today is all about preparing for tomorrow's 24-hour fast. It's imperative that you eat all of your Macros in their 6-hour feeding window today. Abstain from exercising, to give your muscles a chance to fully rest today and tomorrow. Check that you're in ketosis, too. If you're not, don't do the fast. Try a few more days of 18-hour fasts before you attempt a longer one. Once you're in ketosis, you can do a 24-hour fast.

Day 19

Today is your first 24-hour Intermittent Fasting day! Count 24 hours from the beginning of yesterday's fasting time and don't eat anything during that whole time. For example, if your 6-hour eating window ended at 6:00 pm yesterday, you're not to eat anything until 6:00 pm today.

Break your fast gently with some MCT oil and eat mineral rich foods like salmon, dark greens, avocado, nuts, and olives. Don't worry about getting in all of your Macros, but do stop all eating at least two hours before bed-time. Abstain from exercise today, too.

Day 20

Time to return back to your 6-hour feeding / 18-hour fasting cycle. How did yesterday's extended fast go? Make sure to rehydrate yourself today with plenty of water. Today, you do want to eat all of your Macros just like you did on Day 18, even if you're not hungry. You're helping your body refuel itself with good fats. If you want to return to your exercise routine, you can as long as you feel up to it. Don't overdo it, though!

Day 21

Day 19's extended 24-hour fasting time was quite a challenge, but you got through it and did great! That's cause for celebration, and you can weigh yourself again, too. How close are you to meeting the weight loss goals you set before your monthly challenge began? If you've lost at least 5 pounds, then it's a good idea to go back to an online Macro calculator. Recalculate your Macros based on your new weight.

How is the 6-hour eating window going for you? If you prefer the 7-hour or the 8-hour timeframes, it's perfectly fine to return to those schedules instead! The important thing is to stay in ketosis. Check it again today using the Breath or Blood Monitor.

Week Four

Day 22

This week has an advanced 48-hour multi-day fasting time period that takes up Days 24 and Day 25. You're welcome to try it! Many of you have already experienced extraordinary health benefits just by doing the Intermittent Fasting so far, and we know you love a challenge! If at any point, you're feeling overwhelmed or sick or not enjoying the process in any way, it's okay to return to a normal Keto Diet schedule.

This is the beginning of the week, so it's a good idea to plan out your meals, shop for the ingredients, and stock your kitchen in preparation. Remember to purchase the mineral supplements and mineral-rich foods you'll need on Day 26 to break your fast. As for today, just continue on your 6-hour eating window like you did yesterday.

Day 23

Today is about preparing for your multi-day fast, which begins tomorrow. Eat all of your Macros within your 6-hour window, tracking them to make sure you've eaten enough good fats. Take note of the time your 6-hour window ends. You'll count 48 hours in advance, and that's when you can break your fast. Abstain from exercising today and throughout the fast as well. You can take light walks, but just don't be too strenuous on yourself.

Day 24

Fast all day today! Drink water, take a mineral supplement, and satisfy any hunger pangs with a small teaspoon of MCT oil. It's 100% good fats, and it won't affect either you being in ketosis or take away the benefits of the fast.

Day 25

Fast all day today as well. Drink water, take another mineral supplement, and you can have another teaspoon of MCT oil during the fast. Fast until it's been 48 hours since your Day 23 eating window ended. Break your fast with a low carb meal that includes mineral-rich foods like salmon, dark greens, and avocado. Don't try to get in your complete Macros before bed-time.

Day 26

Ease back into your 18-hour fast / 6-hour eating window today. Eat your full Macros during those six hours. How did your 48-hour fast go? You can check your ketones to see how well you did! For most of you, staying in ketosis while fasting has really boosted its benefits!

Day 27

Repeat Day 26 with your normal 6-hour eating window. Today, though, you've given your body enough of a chance to rest from the effects of the 48-hour fast. So, you can add back in your regular exercise routine. Eat and track your Macros.

Day 28

Many congrats to you for getting through an amazing month of Keto Dieting and Intermittent Fasting! You can weigh yourself again and enjoy the results from your hard work. Go back to your food diary that you've been keeping throughout this month-long journey. Was it easier than you expected or more difficult? What was your personal experience with Intermittent Fasting? Casual 'fasters' might want to stick with the skipped meals. More advanced 'fasters' really like the shorter eating windows. Those advanced 'fasters' looking to drop either their weight quickly or reach fitness goals quickly would do well to stay on shorter eating windows and incorporate longer fasts at least once a month.

However your experience went, you deserve to celebrate! Show off your progress by posting "before" and "after" pictures of yourself. Share your journey and help others with theirs, too.

All the Months to Come

There are many more months in your future! Each one of them will have at least 28 new days, where you can make good choices and follow the Keto Diet. Now that you've finished the first 28 days on the Keto Diet with Intermittent Fasting added, how did it go? Only you can answer that question, because your individual experience is so unique. Did you have a good experience? Did it go well overall, with a few rough or rocky patches? Or, was it a struggle?

For those rocky patches, you can take many steps towards making this diet and lifestyle easier on yourself in the future. Many people do well on 8-hour Intermittent Fasting eating windows four or five times a week. You'll have to do a bit of tweaking to see how the fasting/feeding schedule can best fit into your lifestyle. Fasting is not a one-size-fits-all practice. It's based on too many factors!

As for the Keto Diet, I'm more than happy to give you as many tools as possible. In the next chapter, you'll get a complete 7 Day Meal Plan, complete with all of its recipes!

Chapter 7: Look At What's Cookin

Last chapter's definitive twenty eight day guide to starting the Keto Diet together with Intermittent Fasting has given you some idea of how those two work in tandem together. It's like the Keto Diet is driving the car, and then all of a sudden Intermittent Fasting jumps in to help navigate. Now the Keto Diet is accelerated. It's when the two of them come together that you'll really start to see the kinds of results worth posting on social media!

In this chapter, we'll go into the 7 Day Meal Plan that will kickstart your Keto Diet and it also uses Intermittent Fasting, too. This meal plan follows Week One of the previous chapter's guide, which includes three days of skipped meals. Those days have all of the Macros that you need.

This 7 Day Meal Plan is amazing to follow whether you're new to the Keto Diet or have been on it for several months. In the Appendix is a grocery list that contains all the ingredients you'll need for the complete 7 days. It's a good idea to shop for everything you need before starting, so that you can just focus on eating and incorporating the fasting as well.

Following the meal plan chart, you'll see all of the recipes to follow.

You get 22 recipes in total. They cover breakfast, lunch, dinner, and an extra, like a snack, dessert, or smoothie. It's perfectly fine to make substitutions or switch out days. However, you should recalculate your Macros if you're doing that to make sure you're getting the proper percentages. This is a diet about numbers, so meeting your Macros is so important!

Each recipe lists the calories and Macros, plus totals them up. The meal plan is based on an approximate Macro ratio of 70% to 80% fat, 10% to 20% protein, and 5% to 10% carbohydrates. Your Macro ratio will vary, so adjust as you see fit!

Your 7 Day Meal Plan

	7 Day Meal Plan				
Day	Breakfast	Lunch	Dinner	Snack/Dessert	Calories/Macros
1	Avocado Smoothie 587 cal 58 g fat 6 g protein 4 g carbs	Keto Chicken Salad 430 cal 30 g fat 32 g protein 8 g carbs	Crockpot Keto Chili 387 cal 24.6 g fat 33.5 g protein 7 g carbs	Seed Crackers (5) 350 cal 25 g fat 15 g protein 15 g carbs	Calories: 1754 Fat: 146.5 g Protein: 86.5 g Net Carbs: 34 g
2	Skip Breakfast Today (or choose another meal and recalculate Macros)	Leftover Chili 387 cal 24.6 g fat 33.5 protein 8 g carbs	Mahi Mahi with Beurre Blanc 360 cal 30 g fat 20 g protein 1 g carbs	Chocolate Fat Bombs (4) 488 cal 52 g fat 4 g protein 4 g carbs	Calories: 1235 Fat: 106.6 g Protein: 57.5 g Net Carbs: 13 g
3	Skip Breakfast Today (or choose another meal and recalculate Macros)	Italian Chopped Salad 469 cal 44 g fat 14 g protein 4 g carbs	Steak Sheet Pan Dinner 508 cal 34 g fat 37 g protein 6 g carbs	Vanilla Smoothie 669 cal 70.8 g fat 5.5 g protein 4 g carbs	Calories: 1646 Fat: 148.8 g Protein: 56.5 g Net Carbs: 14 g

4	Skip Breakfast Today (or choose another meal and recalculate Macros)	Steak Salad with Cilantro Lime Dressing 663 cal 44 g fat 37 g protein 7 g carbs	Thai Chicken Coconut Red Curry 310 cal 26 g fat 14 g protein 7 g carbs	Chocolate Fat Bombs (4) 488 cal 52 g fat 4 g protein 4 g carbs	Calories: 1461 Fat: 122 g Protein: 55 g Net Carbs: 18 g
5	Spinach, Feta, and Tomato Omelet 287 cal 22 g fat 16 g protein 5 g carbs	Broccoli Cheddar Soup 285 cal 24 g fat 12 g protein 2 g carbs	Keto Meatballs with Mozzarella 622 cal 49 g fat 39 g protein 4 g carbs	Raspberry Chocolate Fudge (3) 222 cal 24.3 g fat 1.8 g protein 2.7 g carbs	Calories: 1416 Fat: 119.3 g Protein: 68.8 g Net Carbs: 13.7 g
6	2 Eggs (any style) and 2 strips of Bacon with Bulletproof Coffee 585 cal 56.5 g fat 21 g protein 3 g carbs	Kale Salad 322 cal 30.9 g fat 2.9 g protein 9 g carbs	Indian Butter Chicken with Roasted Cauliflower 592 cal 52 g fat 24 g protein 6 g carbs	Pink Power Smoothie 310 cal 29.9 g fat 3.8 g protein 9 g carbs	Calories: 1809 Fat: 169.3 g Protein: 51.7 g Net Carbs: 27 g
7	Mexican Breakfast Scramble 452 cal 35 g fat 23 g protein 7.5 g carbs	Leftover Broccoli Cheddar Soup 285 cal 24 g fat 12 g protein 2 g carbs	Keto Pizza 479 cal 39 g fat 25 g protein 7.8 g carbs	Raspberry Chocolate Fudge (2) 148 cal 16.2 g fat 1.2 g protein 1.8 g carbs	Calories: 1364 Fat: 114.2 g Protein: 61.2 g Net Carbs: 19.1 g

We hope you can't wait to get started and that you have a great week of cooking, eating, and enjoying meeting your Macros. The Intermittent Fasting days are built in, but you'll meet all of your numbers in other meals.

The following recipes correspond to the seven days above. For these recipes, you don't need anything special in the kitchen, but the following equipment would help:

- A high-speed blender for smoothies
- A 12" skillet
- A crock pot or slow cooker
- A soup pot
- A food processor
- A mini muffin pan for Fat Bombs
- Parchment paper for baking

All the ingredients are listed by food category in the Appendix, so after you've shopped for those items, then you're ready to begin!

Day One

These are excellent recipes to get you started on the Keto Diet! The Avocado Smoothie takes minutes to prepare, the Keto Chicken Salad is packed with both good fats and protein, and the Keto Crockpot Chili can be simmering in the crock pot all day. That way, when you get home, you can just scoop up a big bowl and enjoy with your special Keto Seed Crackers.

Avocado Smoothie

Absolutely packed with good fats from the avocado, this light green and yummy smoothie is the perfect Keto start to your day. It's also low carb enough to help you reach your Fat Macro at any time of day and would make a wonderful post-workout treat. This is best if done in a Vitamix blender, but you can certainly use a regular blender, too. Just make sure it can crush the ice.

Serving: 1

Serving Size: whole recipe

Prep Time: 5 minutes

Cook Time: 0 minutes

Ingredients

> 1/3 cup unsweetened almond milk
>
> 1/3 cup heavy whipping cream
>
> 1/8 teaspoon Stevia (to taste)
>
> 1 avocado
>
> 6 ice cubes

Instructions

In this order, add the almond milk, heavy whipping cream, and Stevia to your blender.

Slice the ripe avocado in half. Take out the pit and remove all the flesh from the skin.

Drop it in the blender. Add in 6 ice cubes.

Blend on the "smoothie" setting of a Vitamix or similar setting on a different blender. Smoothie should be about yogurt consistency.

Pour into a smoothie cup and enjoy!

Nutrition: 587 calories, 58 g fat, 6 g protein, 4 g net carbs

Keto Chicken Salad

This salad is such a hearty meal, that it could even be a dinner option! It's loaded with delicious chicken, asparagus, avocado, and mozzarella. You can substitute out different veggies for the asparagus if you like. Try zucchini, cauliflower, or broccoli.

Servings: 4

Serving Size: ¼ recipe

Prep Time: 10 minutes

Cook Time: 8 minutes

Ingredients for Salad:

     1 boneless chicken breast

     1 Tablespoon olive oil

     1 avocado

     100g mozzarella balls

     1 tomato

     ½ red onion

     5 asparagus spears

     4 cups fresh spinach

     Salt and pepper to taste

Ingredients for Dressing:

     2 Tablespoons olive oil

     1 ½ Tablespoons red wine vinegar

     1 teaspoon Dijon mustard

     1 clove garlic

     Salt and pepper

Instructions

Prep your salad by slicing the red onion, dicing the tomato, dicing the avocado, and cutting the asparagus spears into 1" pieces.

Mince the garlic clove. Heat your 12" skillet on medium heat.

Slice the chicken breast in half lengthwise and sprinkle each side with salt and pepper to taste.

Add 1 Tablespoon of olive oil to skillet and pan-fry chicken pieces on each side for about 3 minutes until golden brown.

Add the asparagus and cook until softened. When chicken is cooked, take out and slice.

In the bottom of your salad bowl, add the dressing ingredients and mix. Then add the rest of the salad ingredients to the bowl – spinach, tomato, onion, mozzarella, the chicken, and the asparagus.

Toss to coat with the dressing and enjoy.

Nutrition: 430 calories, 30 g fat, 32 g protein, 8 g net carbs

Crockpot Keto Chili

This chili will make your house smell good as it cooks in the crockpot all day. You can also make it in an Instant Pot, which takes about 40 minutes. It also makes amazing leftovers, because the flavors continue to marinate in the fridge overnight.

Servings: 6

Serving Size: 1 cup

Prep Time: 15 minutes

Cook Time: 6-8 hours

Ingredients

    1 lb ground beef

    1 lb ground sausage, any flavor

    1 green bell pepper, chopped

    1 yellow onion, chopped

    1 14.5 oz can diced tomatoes

    1 6 oz can tomato paste

    1 Tablespoon chili powder

    ½ Tablespoon ground cumin

    3-4 garlic cloves, minced

    Salt and pepper to taste

    1/3 cup water

    Garnish: shredded cheddar, sour cream, green onions

Instructions

Heat 12" skillet on medium heat.

Add both the ground beef and sausage. Brown until no longer pink.

Add the meat and the drippings to the crockpot. Then add the rest of the ingredients – bell pepper, onion, diced tomatoes, tomato paste, all the spices, and the water. Mix to combine.

Put the lid on the crockpot, turn to low, and cook for 6-8 hours.

Scoop into bowls and top with shredded cheddar, sour cream, and finely chopped green onions.

Nutrition: 387 calories, 24.6 g fat, 33.5 g protein, 7 g net carbs

Seed Crackers

Make up a batch of these crackers to pair with your chili, soups, and salads. Just one has only 3 grams of carbs, so you can have several at one time. These are very filling and can be a great snack when you're craving something crunchy.

Servings: 22

Serving Size: 1 cracker

Prep Time: 15 minutes

Cook Time: 1 hour

Ingredients

½ cup chia seeds

½ cup sunflower seeds

½ cup pumpkin seeds

½ cup sesame seeds

1 cup water

1 garlic clove grated

¼ teaspoon sea salt

Instructions

Preheat oven to 300 degrees F.

Line a cookie sheet with parchment paper.

Add the chia, sunflower, pumpkin, and sesame seeds to a bowl. Then add the water, garlic, and sea salt. Stir with a spatula to combine. Let sit so chia seeds can absorb water. After several minutes, stir again.

Spread the cracker dough onto the cookie sheet in two smaller rectangles. Each should measure 12" x 7" and be less than ¼" thick. Sprinkle more salt on top.

Bake for 35 minutes. Flip each cracker rectangle over and bake the other side for about 25 – 35 minutes, until golden around the edges.

Let cool for at least 10 minutes before breaking into 22 evenly sized crackers.

Store in an airtight bag for up to 2 weeks.

Nutrition (each): 70 calories, 5 g fat, 3 g protein, 3 g net carbs

Day Two

You'll skip breakfast today, so a bowl of leftover Crockpot Keto Chili with all the toppings will be sure to satisfy your hunger pangs. Since you're trying to get all of your Macros into two meals instead of three, you can have a bit of a larger serving or pair it with a Seed Cracker or two. For dinner is a delicious Mahi Mahi with Beurre Blanc, and you can have Chocolate Fat Bombs as snacks or a dessert.

Mahi Mahi with Beurre Blanc

A classic French butter sauce with delicious fresh herbs dresses a light and yummy fish. This dish is both easy and elegant. You can serve it with a low carb veggie like asparagus, zucchini, broccoli, or cauliflower. If you do, don't forget to add those Macros to the rest of your day.

Serving: 6

Serving Size: 1 piece of fish

Prep Time: 5 minutes

Cook Time: 10 minutes

Ingredients

   3 strips bacon

   6 Mahi Mahi fillets, 3 oz each

Salt and pepper to taste

¼ cup olive oil

¼ cup white wine (Pinot Blanc has the fewest carbs)

¼ cup heavy cream

1 stick butter, sliced thinly into little pats

Juice from 1 lemon

1 Tablespoon chopped fresh dill

2 Tablespoons chopped fresh parsley

Instructions

Cook the bacon in a skillet. Reserve the fat.

Heat the olive oil in a clean skillet on medium-high heat.

Season both sides of mahi mahi fillets with plenty of salt and pepper. Sear the fish fillets for 3 minutes on one side until half cooked, then flip and sear the other side until fish is cooked. Remove fish from skillet, but keep heat on.

Add white wine to skillet with oil and reduce until it's a syrup texture. Then add the heavy cream and the reserved bacon fat. Turn off the heat. Whisk in the thin butter pats until melted into the sauce. Then add lemon juice, dill, parsley, cooked bacon, and a bit more salt and pepper.

Put fish on dinner plates and pour sauce over to serve.

Nutrition: 360 calories, 30 g fat, 20 g protein, 1 g net carbs

Chocolate Fat Bombs

Fat Bombs are one of the great Keto Diet foods! You can make 20 of these yummy Chocolate Fat Bombs and each one packs a punch that can help you meet your Fat Macro on fasting days. Plus, they're chocolate! Giving up sugary treats is difficult, so these Chocolate Fat Bombs will satisfy that sweet tooth.

Serving: 20

Serving Size: 1 Fat Bomb

Prep Time: 10 minutes

Cook Time: 10 minutes

Ingredients

    2 cups dry salted macadamia nuts

    2 Tablespoons Coconut oil

    2 Tablespoons MCT oil

    1 teaspoon vanilla extract

    ¼ cup cocoa powder

    1/8 teaspoons Stevia

Instructions

Process the macadamia nuts in a blender or food processor until very finely chopped.

Melt the coconut oil either in the microwave or in a saucepan. When warmed, add it to the nuts, then add the MCT oil and vanilla. Puree until very smooth. Then add the cocoa powder and Stevia and puree again until smooth.

Pour into lined mini muffin tin cups. Freeze until hardened, and store in the fridge or freezer.

    Nutrition: 122 calories, 13 g fat, 1 g protein, 1 g net carbs

Day Three

Another day of Intermittent Fasting by skipping breakfast. For lunch, a hearty Italian Chopped Salad gives you plenty of good fats. You'll love the Keto Steak Sheet Pan dinner, and for a snack or dessert to help you get your Macros is a yummy Vanilla Smoothie.

Italian Chopped Salad

This chopped salad is so easy to throw together, and super versatile! Add in your favorite marinated meats and veg to make this your own! This salad will keep in the fridge for up to 5 days, so make a big batch and have it on hand for snacking or fast lunch options.

Serving: 2

Serving Size: half recipe

Prep Time: 15 minutes

Cook Time: 0 minutes

Ingredients

    12 Romaine leaves, chopped

    2 oz prosciutto, sliced into ribbons

    2 oz salami, chopped

    ¼ cup artichoke hearts, chopped

    ¼ cup green olives

    1 jalapeno, sliced

    1 Tablespoon olive oil

    1 Tablespoon lemon juice or white wine vinegar

    1 Tablespoon Italian herbs

Instructions

In a large bowl, whisk together the olive oil, lemon juice and herbs.

Toss in the rest of the ingredients, making sure everything is well mixed.

Season with salt and pepper. Serve immediately, or store in an airtight container in the fridge for up to 5 days.

    Nutrition: 469 calories, 44 g fat, 14 g protein, 4 g net carbs

Steak Sheet Pan Dinner

Just one large cookie sheet or baking tray is all it takes for this amazing Steak Sheet Pan Dinner. You'll need to buy some ghee, which is high fat clarified Indian butter. This steak dinner has a unique broiling method for cooking the meat. You'll have dinner on the table in just about half an hour. Very quick!

Servings: 4

Serving Size: 1 piece of steak with veggies

Prep Time: 5 minutes

Cook Time: 25 minutes

Ingredients

> 4 pieces of steak cut to 1" thick each
>
> 1 cup button mushrooms, chopped
>
> 1 cup green beans cut to 1" pieces
>
> ¼ cup ghee, melted
>
> 2 garlic cloves, minced
>
> Salt and pepper to taste

Instructions

Preheat the oven to 425 degrees F.

Add foil to your cookie sheet.

Spread the mushrooms and green beans over the pan. Stir the garlic into the melted ghee to combine, then drizzle half of that over the veggies. Sprinkle with salt and pepper and toss to combine.

Roast for 12 minutes. Take the veggies out of the oven and preheat the broiler. Move the veggies aside and nestle the steaks on the sheet pan.

Drizzle with the rest of the ghee / garlic. Season well with salt and pepper.

Broil the steaks about 4-6 inches from the heat for 5 minutes per side or until done to your liking. Take out and serve with the veggies.

> Nutrition: 508 calories, 34 g fat, 37 g protein, 6 g net carbs

Vanilla Smoothie

This creamy vanilla shake is the perfect thing to have as a snack or even a yummy dessert before bedtime. It's a simple recipe that only takes 5 minutes of prep time and gives you an amazing high fat boost of energy. Both the coconut oil and the coconut milk boost the fat content right up!

Serving: 1

Serving Size: whole recipe

Prep Time: 5 minutes

Cook Time: 0 minutes

Ingredients

>   1 cup coconut milk
>
>   1 Tablespoon coconut oil
>
>   ½ Tablespoon vanilla extract
>
>   1 teaspoon Stevia

Instructions

Combine all ingredients in a blender until smooth. Serve immediately.

>   Nutrition: 669 calories, 70.8 g fat, 5.5 g protein, 4 g net carbs

Day Four

It's the last day of the week where you'll be skipping breakfast and making sure you get enough Macros the rest of the day. A Steak Salad takes advantage of leftover steak from last night, and your dinner is a delicious Thai Chicken Coconut Red Curry. Snack on at least four Chocolate Fat Bombs from Day Two as a delicious way to meet your numbers!

Steak Salad

You can have the Steak Sheet Pan Dinner for leftovers as a lunch option. Or, you can turn it into this healthy Steak Salad that gives you bright flavors with its Cilantro Lime Dressing. That recipe is below. This is a quick lunch because the meat is already cooked. All you need to do is prep the veggies and make the dressing.

Servings: 2

Serving Size: Half recipe

Prep Time: 10 minutes

Cook Time: 15 minutes

Ingredients:

    1 leftover steak from Steak Sheet Pan Dinner

    ¼ red onion, sliced

    ½ tomato, diced

    1 avocado, diced

    1 serving Cilantro Lime Dressing (recipe below)

Instructions:

Slice the steak into strips.

Transfer to a bowl with the rest of the ingredients, and toss well to combine.

Sprinkle with salt to season and serve immediately.

Nutrition: 663 calories, 44 g fat, 37 g protein, 7 g net carbs

Cilantro Lime Dressing

This zingy dressing is perfect for the above Steak Salad, but will work on any Southwest inspired salad creations! Cilantro and lime add a nice zingy twist. The avocado oil is an unusual item, but we've included it here to boost that good fat content.

Servings: 4

Serving Size: ¼ cup

Prep Time: 10 minutes

Cook Time: 0 minutes

Ingredients:

    ½ cup avocado oil

    4 limes, juice and zest

    2 cups fresh cilantro, chopped

1 jalapeno, chopped

Instructions:

In a blender or food processor, combine all ingredients until smooth. Store in an airtight container in the fridge for up to a week.

Nutrition: 60 calories, 3.9 g fat, 1 g protein, 4 g net carbs

Thai Chicken Coconut Red Curry

This is such a fragrant and easy dish. It's adaptable, so you can make substitutions depending on what you have. You can use shrimp, beef, or pork instead of the chicken. Try yellow or green curry paste instead of the red. Use any combination of fresh Keto vegetables you prefer.

Serving: 4

Serving Size: ¼ recipe

Prep Time: 10 minutes

Cook Time: 20 minutes

Ingredients

    1 Tablespoon olive oil

    2 Tablespoons red curry paste (or yellow or green)

    13.5 ounce can of full fat coconut milk

    ½ cup chicken broth

    1/8 teaspoon Stevia

    1 Tablespoon fish sauce

    1 1b boneless skinless chicken cut into 1" pieces

    3 cups assorted bite-size cut fresh vegetables (green peppers, broccoli,

    cauliflower, onion, bok choy, tomatoes, zucchini, etc.)

    1 Tablespoon thinly sliced fresh basil (optional)

    Squeeze of fresh lime

Instructions

Put your large skillet or wok on medium heat. Add the olive oil and heat it.

When warm, add the curry paste and stir fry with a wooden spoon for 1 ½ - 2 minutes until fragrant.

Pour in entire can of coconut milk and the chicken broth. Raise the temperature to medium-high. Bring to a simmer.

Then stir in the Stevia (no more than 1/8 teaspoon or to taste) and the fish sauce until well blended.

Add the meat and all of the vegetables and stir to coat everything in the curry.

Simmer uncovered for 5-7 minutes until the chicken is cooked through.

Remove from heat. Stir in the basil and a squeeze of fresh lime. Could also add sliced spring onion and a sprinkle of fresh finely chopped cilantro.

Nutrition: 310 calories, 26 g fat, 14 g protein, 7 g net carbs

Day Five

Back to eating breakfast today, so you'll start with a hearty Spinach, Feta, and Tomato Greek-style omelet. That will fill you up until you have your Broccoli Cheddar Soup. A hearty Italian dinner of Meatballs with Mozzarella and a Raspberry Chocolate Fudge dessert finishes a great day of Keto eating!

Spinach, Feta, and Tomato Omelet

The Greek flavors in this omelet go really well together. The spinach is packed with essential minerals to help your body recover from three days of Intermittent Fasting. Cubed feta cheese and eggs increase both good fats and protein, while the sun-dried tomatoes are packed in oil for even more fat.

Serving: 1

Serving Size: whole recipe

Prep Time: 5 minutes

Cook Time: 8 minutes

Ingredients

 2 large eggs

 ½ Tablespoon salted butter

 ½ cup fresh spinach

 2 Tablespoons oil-packed sundried tomatoes

 2 Tablespoons crumbled Feta

 Salt and black pepper

Instructions

Chop the fresh spinach and sun-dried tomatoes into small pieces.

Crack both eggs into a bowl and add salt and black pepper to taste.

Whisk until yolks are combined. Warm a 10" or 12" skillet on medium heat. Add the butter and melt it. Then pour in the eggs to spread throughout pan and cook until just set, which is about 2 to 3 minutes.

Sprinkle one side with the spinach, tomatoes, and Feta. Flip the other side over the fillings.

Transfer to plate and serve.

 Nutrition: 276 calories, 22 g fat, 16 g protein, 5 g net carbs

Broccoli Cheddar Soup

Here is a Keto twist on a classic that eliminates all the carbohydrates. This has a thinner consistency without any thickeners like potato or cornstarch. That makes it a perfect light lunch after your filling omelet breakfast. You can pair this with one of the Seed Crackers, too.

Servings: 4

Serving Size: ¾ cup

Prep Time: 5 minutes

Cook Time: 20 minutes

Ingredients

 2 Tablespoons butter

2 Tablespoons diced onion

½ teaspoon minced garlic

2 cups chicken broth

1 cup fresh broccoli, chopped into 1" pieces

1 Tablespoon full-fat cream cheese

¼ cup heavy whipping cream

1 cup shredded cheddar

Handful of cooked, crumbled bacon

Instructions

Set large soup pot on medium heat. Add butter, then add onion and garlic.

Saute until onions are softened and translucent, about 5 minutes. Then add the broccoli and pour in the chicken broth.

Cook broccoli until tender. Season soup with salt and pepper.

Heat cream cheese in a bowl in the microwave for 30 seconds until soft.

Stir both heavy cream and cream cheese into soup.

Bring to a boil. Turn off the heat. Add cheddar cheese and stir throughout soup.

Ladle into bowls and garnish with bacon.

Nutrition: 285 calories, 24 g fat, 12 g protein, 2 g net carbs

Keto Meatballs with Mozzarella

We're continuing our Mediterranean theme for today with this delicious dinner that packs all the flavors of Italy – without the pasta! But if you've been craving Italian, this is the perfect dish to have. It's warm, comforting, and flavorful. The Keto Diet never tasted so good!

Servings: 4

Serving Size: 6 meatballs

Prep Time: 10 minutes

Cook Time: 45 minutes

Ingredients

> 1 lb ground beef
>
> 2 oz shredded parmesan cheese
>
> 1 egg
>
> ½ Tablespoon basil
>
> ½ teaspoon onion powder
>
> 1 teaspoon garlic powder
>
> 1 teaspoon salt
>
> ½ teaspoon black pepper
>
> 3 Tablespoons olive oil
>
> 14 oz can whole tomatoes
>
> 2 Tablespoons fresh parsley, finely chopped
>
> 5 oz fresh mozzarella

Instructions

Take out a large bowl. Add the beef, parmesan, eggs, salt, pepper, onion powder, and garlic powder. Blend thoroughly.

Form into small meatballs about 1.5" in diameter. Heat a large skillet on medium. Add the olive oil. Saute the meatballs until golden brown on all sides.

Reduce the heat to medium-low. Pour in the tomatoes and simmer for 15 minutes, stirring occasionally. Season with salt and pepper to taste. Add the parsley and stir.

Top with fresh shredded or whole mozzarella, torn into bite-sized pieces.

> Nutrition: 622 calories, 49 g fat, 39 g protein, 4 g net carbs

Raspberry Chocolate Fudge

This rich, chocolaty fudge is the perfect thing to hit the spot when you're craving something sweet. Raspberries are a rare treat in a low carbohydrate diet, and they pair so well with the chocolate. Best of all, it's virtually carb and protein free and high fat, which keeps you in ketosis. Fudge is decadent!

Servings: 16

Serving Size: 1 piece

Prep Time: 2 minutes

Cook Time: 10 Minutes

Ingredients

½ cup cocoa powder

2 Tablespoons unsweetened dark chocolate, shaved

2 Tablespoons Stevia

½ cup coconut oil

¼ cup raspberries, mashed lightly

¼ cup almond milk

Instructions

Mix all ingredients together until well combined.

Prepare a 10" baking dish with parchment paper or plastic wrap, and carefully spoon the fudge mixture into the center.

Using a spatula, spread the mixture evenly into the baking dish, and cover with plastic wrap.

Refrigerate for an hour, and cut into 16 equal pieces. Store wrapped in the fridge for up to one month.

Nutrition: 74 calories, 8.1g fat, 0.6g protein, 0.9g net carbs

Day Six

An old-fashioned bacon and eggs breakfast gets a Keto twist with Bulletproof Coffee. Then you'll enjoy a mineral rich Kale Salad that gives your body plenty of good nutrition and flavor. Dinner is an Indian Butter Chicken with Roasted Cauliflower that will wow you with its spices. A Pink Power Smoothie is a great snack for a mid-afternoon pick-me-up.

Bulletproof Coffee

This amazing Keto Diet approved beverage takes regular black coffee and increases its good fats. Pair it with a breakfast of 2 eggs (any style you like) and 2 strips of bacon for a fat-packed start to any day. You can certainly try this version of coffee with other breakfast options, too. Just include the Macros.

Serving: 1

Serving Size: whole recipe

Prep Time: 5 minutes

Cook Time: 0 minutes

Ingredients

    1 cup black coffee

    1 Tablespoon grass-fed unsalted butter

    1 Tablespoon MCT oil

    ½ Tablespoon heavy cream

    ½ teaspoon vanilla extract

Instructions

Mix everything together by hand or in a blender. Serve warm or cold! You can substitute almond extract for the vanilla or leave it out.

    Nutrition: 255 calories, 28.5 g fat, 0 g protein, 1 g net carbs

Kale Salad

This low carb salad is just the thing to ensure you're getting the vitamins and minerals you need, while still watching your Macros! It's super crunchy, so it will keep in the fridge with the dressing for about a day without going soggy. This salad is great on its own or you could top it with proteins like chicken, pork, or steak.

Servings: 1

Serving Size: about 1 ½ cups

Prep Time: 10 minutes

Cook Time: 0 minutes

Ingredients:

> 1 cup kale, chopped
>
> ¼ red onion, sliced thinly
>
> 2 Tablespoons olive oil
>
> ½ Tablespoon Dijon mustard
>
> ½ Tablespoon mayonnaise
>
> 1 teaspoon thyme
>
> 1 teaspoon salt
>
> ½ teaspoon Stevia

Instructions:

In a large bowl, whisk together the olive oil, Dijon, mayonnaise, thyme, salt and Stevia to make a dressing. Toss in the rest of the ingredients, and mix well. Serve immediately, or keep in an airtight container in the fridge for up to two days.

Nutrition: 322 calories, 30.9 g fat, 2.9 g protein, 9 g net carbs

Indian Butter Chicken with Roasted Cauliflower

If you live in a cold climate, there is nothing more warming or comforting than Indian food! You can find the garam masala at Asian stores or online. This recipe is packed with chicken, butter, and spices. It's delicious. Use ghee to increase your fat intake. In place of naan or rice, the cauliflower gives you that same crunchy texture that pairs so well with Indian food.

Servings: 6

Serving Size: 1/6 recipe

Prep Time: 30 minutes

Cook Time: 30 minutes

Ingredients

> 1 2/3 lbs boneless chicken thighs
>
> 1 tomato, cored
>
> 1 yellow onion
>
> 2 Tablespoons ginger
>
> 2 garlic cloves, peeled
>
> 1 Tablespoon tomato paste
>
> 1 Tablespoon garam masala seasoning
>
> ½ Tablespoon ground coriander (cilantro)
>
> ½ Tablespoon chili powder
>
> 1 teaspoon salt
>
> ¾ cup heavy cream
>
> 3 oz butter or Indian ghee

For Cauliflower:

> 1 lb cauliflower, chopped into bite size pieces
>
> ½ teaspoon turmeric
>
> ½ tablespoon coriander seed
>
> ½ teaspoon salt
>
> ¼ teaspoon black pepper
>
> 2 oz melted butter

Instructions

In a blender or food processor, blend the tomato, onion, ginger, garlic, tomato paste, and the spices – garam masala, coriander, chili powder, and salt. Blend until smooth.

Add the heavy cream and stir in. Pour into a bowl and add the cut up chicken until well coated. Cover with plastic wrap and marinate in the fridge for at least 20 minutes. You could marinate for several hours to infuse the flavor.

When ready to cook, heat up a large frying pan over medium high heat with 1 ounce of the butter. Add the chicken to the pan and fry on each side for several minutes.

Then pour the rest of the marinade over the chicken, together with the other 2 ounces of butter. Turn heat down to medium and let simmer for 15 minutes until chicken is fully cooked.

For the cauliflower, preheat your oven to 400F. Spread the chopped cauliflower over a foil cookie sheet or baking tray.

Sprinkle the seasonings and butter over. Bake for 15 minutes.

Serve the butter chicken over the cauliflower and garnish with fresh cilantro and plain unsweetened yogurt.

Nutrition: 592 calories, 52 g fat, 24 g protein, 6 g net carbs

Pink Power Smoothie

This smoothie is full of good fat, and it also has a great flavor and color! Keep any leftovers in an airtight container in the fridge for up to 24 hours so you can enjoy a quick pick me up! The pink color comes from its raspberries, and you'll taste the tangy zing from the lemon zest, too.

Serving: 2

Serving Size: half recipe

Prep Time: 5 minutes

Cook Time: 0 minutes

Ingredients

     1/2 cup raspberries

     1/2 Tablespoon lemon zest

     1 cup coconut milk

     1 Tablespoon flaxseeds

Instructions

Start by pouring the coconut milk into the blender to avoid the ingredients sticking at the bottom. Add in the rest of the ingredients.

Turn the blender on, starting at a low speed and increase as needed. Add extra water if you desire your smoothie more on the liquid side.

Once it looks even, pour into a cup and serve immediately.

Pour any leftover smoothie into an airtight container and enjoy within 24 hours.

Nutrition: 310 calories, 29.9 g fat, 3.8 g protein, 9 g net carbs

Day Seven

Day Seven starts with a flavorful Mexican Breakfast Scramble. You'll have some leftover Broccoli Cheddar Soup for a light lunch, which leaves you plenty of Carb Macros for Keto Pizza! There are also Raspberry Chocolate Fudge pieces for a sweet dessert.

Mexican Breakfast Scramble

Let's go south of the border to enjoy the bright flavors of Mexico in this hearty breakfast scramble. It only takes 20 minutes and is very filling and hearty. This would also make a great option for dinner, too. It's a meal in one pan.

Servings: 2

Serving Size: ½ recipe

Prep Time: 5 minutes

Cook Time: 15 minutes

Ingredients

      1 Tablespoon butter

      ½ small yellow onion, diced

      ½ cup green bell pepper, chopped

      1 cup zucchini, chopped

      ½ cup fresh tomato, chopped

      6 oz chorizo, thinly sliced

      2 cups fresh spinach, chopped

      2 large eggs

      ½ cup diced avocado

Salt and pepper

Fresh cilantro

Instructions

Heat 12" skillet on medium high heat.

Add the butter and swirl to coat. Then add the onion and cook for about a minute. Add the green peppers and stir together. After 3 minutes, add the zucchini and tomatoes.

Cook an additional 3-4 minutes to soften, stirring occasionally. Then add the chorizo and mix in. Cook for about 5 minutes.

Then add the fresh spinach and cook another 2-3 minutes to wilt.

Turn on the oven broiler to high and move oven rack to top. Create a well in the center of the scramble mixture.

Crack in the eggs. Season with salt and pepper, then stick in the oven under the broiler for about 3-5 minutes.

The yolks should be slightly runny. Top with diced avocado and cilantro.

Nutrition: 452 calories, 35 g fat, 23 g protein, 7.5 g net carbs

Keto Pizza

Yes, you can have pizza on the Keto Diet! It wouldn't be that much fun if you couldn't at least have pizza once a week, right? This amazing recipe is a basic one you can certainly dress up with other Keto friendly ingredients. What about broccoli, cauliflower, zucchini, mushrooms, spinach, or bacon?

Serving: 1

Serving Size: whole pizza

Prep Time: 5 minutes

Cook Time: 15 minutes

Ingredients for Crust:

1/3 cup shredded full fat mozzarella

¼ cup almond flour

1/8 teaspoon garlic powder

Pinch of salt

1 large egg yolk

Toppings:

1.5 Tablespoons pizza sauce

¼ cup shredded mozzarella cheese

5 slices pepperoni

¼ teaspoon Italian herbs

Instructions

Put the oven rack on the top position, and preheat the oven to 425 degrees F.

Add the mozzarella, almond flour, garlic powder, and salt to a microwave-safe bowl. Microwave for 25 seconds. Then knead the dough in your hands for a few seconds.

Add the egg yolk when the dough is still warm. Knead until combined and roll into a ball.

Form a disk and place the round disk on a parchment-lined cookie sheet. Press the dough into a 5-6" diameter circle and ¼" thick.

Use a fork to poke holes around the top of the crust.

Bake on the top rack for 8-10 minutes, until golden brown.

Take the crust out of the oven and flip it over. Then spread the pizza sauce on top. Sprinkle with half the cheese. Add the pepperoni slices and the rest of the cheese. Top with the Italian herbs and bake for another 3-4 minutes to melt the cheese.

Nutrition: 479 calories, 39 g fat, 25 g protein, 7.8 g net carbs

Chapter 8: Creating Your Own Meal Plan

Last chapter gave you one of the most helpful tools in this book: a meal plan.

Meal plans require some thought, focus, and Macro calculations up front, but they are extraordinarily useful in helping you stick to your Keto Diet. Meal plans can also help you keep track of your Intermittent Fasting days, too. That way, you'll see all of your calories, fats, proteins, and carbohydrates at a glance.

What else can a meal plan do?

- Take the guesswork out of food decision-making. It can be stressful, especially when on a diet like the Ketogenic one, to come up with meal ideas on the spot. You're more likely to reach for an old favorite meal you used to like, which probably has too many carbs.
- Provide an at-a-glance map of your Keto Diet journey. Just like a real map guides ships, the Keto Diet meal plan will guide you as you sail past all of the tempting sugar and carbohydrate options. It's about sticking to the plan.
- Help you incorporate shopping and cooking times into your diet, too. Eating Keto isn't just about the eating; it's also about purchasing Keto friendly foods and then putting them together into meals each day. That's why the diet is more of a lifestyle.
- Give you meals to look forward to. It's easier being on any diet when there are foods in a meal plan you really love. Put your favorite Keto breakfasts, lunches, dinners, snacks, and desserts in your meal plan.
- Establish an eating routine you like. We all love Taco Tuesdays, pizza on Fridays, lazy Sunday morning brunches, and other routine meals each week. A Keto meal plan gives you these options that also have great Macros.
- Encourage you to try new recipes. A meal plan helps you bust an eating rut, which then could lead to deprivation and falling off your Macros. Perhaps once a week or once every ten days, you could include a new recipe you've never tried. It keeps things interesting!

Now that you've read about the benefits of creating a meal plan, how exactly do you go about it?

How to Create Your Own Meal Plan

A meal plan starts with your own personal weekly schedule. There's a blank meal plan template below. It has spaces for you to write down your daily activities, which include work, family obligations, the gym, events, hobbies, personal time, and everything else you do. That gives you a baseline schedule, where you'll work your Keto Diet meal plan around it. There is no one-size-fits-all meal plan template, because we all have busy lives and plans change a lot, too.

So, the first step is to answer the following questions:

What is your weekly work schedule?

What are your family members' schedules like?

Any weekly obligations you have? Going to the gym or church?

Include all other weekly activities and personal time

Put your answers to those questions into the blank meal plan template. There's enough space for you to write three different activities and the times they are during the day.

It really makes it much easier to then plan your Keto Diet and Intermittent Fasting times around them.

Keto Diet Foods You Can Eat

With every passing month, there are plenty of new Keto Dieters who share their amazing recipes online for you to try out for yourself. As you plan your meals, you'll also need to keep eating plenty of the Keto Diet approved foods. Below, we'll give you the 10 most popular foods in each food group that you should already be familiar with as part of the diet.

Produce:

1. Avocado
2. Lemons
3. Onions
4. Bell Peppers
5. Button Mushrooms
6. Fresh Spinach
7. Kale
8. Broccoli
9. Cauliflower
10. Fresh Garlic
11.

Meat & Seafood:

1. Steak (Flank and Skirt)
2. Ground Beef
3. Bacon
4. Shrimp
5. Cod Fillets
6. Boneless Chicken Breasts / Thighs
7. Pork Chops
8. Salami
9. Prosciutto
10. Lamb
11.

Eggs & Dairy:

1. Eggs
2. High Quality Grass-Fed Butter
3. Heavy Cream
4. Cheddar Cheese
5. Mozzarella Cheese
6. Parmesan Cheese
7. Cream Cheese
8. Sour Cream
9. Goat Cheese
10. Plain Greek Yogurt

Herbs & Spices:

1. Salt
2. Pepper
3. Fresh Herbs (parsley, cilantro, dill, etc.)
4. Dried Italian Herbs
5. Cinnamon
6. Thyme
7. Chili Powder
8. Onion Powder
9. Ginger
10. Paprika

Oils & Condiments:

1. Olive oil
2. Coconut oil
3. Sesame Oil
4. Flavored oils
5. Mayonnaise
6. Dijon Mustard
7. Fish Sauce
8. Hot Sauce
9. Lemon Juice
10. Soy Sauce

Nuts & Seeds:

1. Macadamia nuts
2. Pecans
3. Walnuts
4. Almonds
5. Nut Butters
6. Pumpkin Seeds
7. Sunflower Seeds
8. Sesame Seeds
9. Ground Flax Seeds
10. Chia Seeds

Baking & Broths:

1. Almond Flour
2. Coconut Flour
3. Cocoa Powder
4. Baking Powder
5. Vanilla Extract
6. Sugar-Free Dark Chocolate
7. Stevia
8. Full Fat Coconut Milk
9. Unsweetened Almond Milk
10. Chicken Broth

Other:

1. MCT Oil
2. Green Olives
3. Black Coffee
4. Black or Green Teas
5. Wine
6. Dill Pickles
7. Canned Tomatoes
8. Cocoa Butter
9. Curry Pastes (red, green, yellow)
10. Psyllium Husk Powder

Those are the most essential eighty ingredients! There's plenty here to get you started. I definitely encourage you to get creative in the kitchen. You can combine these ingredients in any number of ways.

There are certain types of foods that we love to eat for our meals. This will help you put together your meal plan, by thinking of foods in terms of categories.

Breakfast

At breakfast, the most typical options for a Keto Diet include high fat-packed smoothies, egg dishes, meat dishes, and breakfast bowls that combine multiple ingredients. Smoothies get their high fat content from either an avocado or coconut milk base. Egg dish options include baked eggs, scrambled eggs, frittatas, and omelets. Meat options have bacon, sausage, or even steak. Breakfast bowls are popular, and you can search for those recipes online.

Lunch

Many of us take last night's dinner to work the next day as a lunch option! That's perfectly fine and helps you not only stick to your Macros, but clean out the fridge, too. Other lunch options include the full range of Keto Diet friendly soups and salads. Soups start with either a chicken or beef broth base, and then you add ingredients. Salads start with a Keto base of hearty greens like Romaine lettuce, fresh spinach, and kale, then feature a protein and more veggies and cheese. Top them with extras like seeds and nuts. You'll definitely like making your own dressings, too. They have an oil base and then you add ingredients.

Dinner

Keto dinners feature one high fat and hearty protein choice like chicken, beef, pork, lamb, or fish. That's usually served alongside a cooked vegetable like broccoli, cauliflower, zucchini, asparagus, mushrooms, or even tomatoes. Sauces are featured, usually having a high fat content from butter or cream. Many dinners have been turned into Keto friendly versions, like Keto burgers and fries, Keto pizzas, and Keto casseroles. Just look for those types of meals online. Chances are, someone has turned your favorite entrée into a Keto version!

Snacks / Desserts / Beverages

Keto snacks help you stick to your high fat Macros. That's why the Fat Bombs are so popular! You can find dozens of flavor combinations of those online and in Keto cookbooks, both sweet and savory versions. Other Keto snacks include veggies with almond butter dip, seeds, nuts, olives, and cheese. You can make your own crackers, like the ones in this book. Keto desserts pack a lot of flavor and tiny amounts of sugar into nice morsels that usually feature treats like chocolate, peanut butter, vanilla, and raspberries or strawberries. Besides smoothies, Keto friendly beverages include regular coffee, bulletproof coffee, black or green teas, a glass of wine, and water with lemon.

So, that is the range of recipes that you can make, from your morning smoothie to your Keto chocolate dessert. When you create your own meal plan, you can include both dishes that you love to eat and those that you would like to try.

Seek out recipes online. After you've found them, you can save them in PDF form to a folder on your desktop marked "Keto Recipes." Then you can organize them and put them into your meal plan, or organize them into other folders like "Recipe Ideas for September."

Many people like to put together actual recipe folders. That could work for you, too! Just print out your recipes and tuck them into a binder or folder until it's that day to make them.

Does it matter which day you begin your meal plan? It does not!

Some people like to do them on a Sunday or Monday, because that's the start to the week. But if you can only plan a few days at a time due to a busy or hectic schedule, that's totally fine! We really just want you to have a delicious time eating this diet!

Calculating Your Own Macros

So, you've got your foods that you can eat and the recipes for all of your meals. How do you calculate Macros for a meal? You've got to keep track of your fats, proteins, and carbohydrates to meet both your weight loss and health goals.

The most important thing when calculating Macros is to determine the portion size of the food that you're eating. It's easy to underestimate how many calories or Macro grams are in foods. The average portion size in a restaurant is at least twice as big as it needs to be. Check your portion sizes, especially for meats, soups, and salads.

Many recipes online tell you what the Macros are in their dishes. Look in the "Nutrition Facts" portion of the recipe to find the fats, proteins, and carbohydrates. They'll be listed in grams. Then, you can just add those numbers to your blank meal template.

If the recipe doesn't have the Macros listed, then you'll have to calculate them yourself. Some smartphone apps already do this, but you can do this by hand, too.

Start by finding the most prominent item in the recipe. It could be eggs in an egg dish, meat in a meat dish, or an avocado in a vegetarian dish. Look up the Macros for that item. That's your base number of fats, proteins, and carbohydrates in this recipe. Then look up the Macros for another prominent item in the recipe. Add those Macros together. You can find the Macros for pretty much every food that is on the Keto Diet online.

After researching and then adding the Macros for the top four or five items in the recipe, that should give you a pretty good idea of the count in grams. You can also contact the person who created the recipe to post their "Nutrition Facts" for that recipe. On the Keto Diet, those nutritional labels are your best friend!

As you become more experienced with the Keto Diet, you'll quickly estimate the Macros in a particular dish. You'll also be able to make substitutions in recipes and still calculate Macros properly and accurately.

Creating a Grocery List

After you've made your meal plan, it's time to make up a grocery list. Divide it into sections, like the one in the Appendix. It has Produce, Meat & Seafood, Eggs & Dairy, Herbs & Spices, Nuts, Seeds & Baking, and

Other. Then, just go through your recipes on your meal plan and add the ingredients to the list. You'll also want to check your fridge, pantry, and freezer at the same time to make sure you're not purchasing duplicates of ingredients.

Instead of dividing your grocery list up into food category sections, you could divide it up by the aisle of your favorite supermarket. Grocery stores sometimes put odd ingredients in the same aisle, so it could be more helpful for you to do that, instead.

You might also want to make a special grocery list for specialty items that you can only find at one particular store or online.

With a meal plan, recipes, and a grocery list, you're all set to make your Keto Diet work for you!

Vary Up Your Diet

Diets get a bad rap because their restrictiveness can become boring, repetitive, and too routine. That's when you want to give it up forever! Well, I sincerely hope you don't. The Keto Diet has given me and countless others amazing benefits. I want you to have all the success you desire!

So, to keep the Keto Diet fun and exciting, it's important you add variety to your diet. The best way to do that? Change up your flavors! Each cuisine around the planet has their own unique flavor profiles. Step out of your geographical region and have fun exploring all the amazing flavors out there. Professional cooks work with flavor combinations, which are certain ingredients that just go together. You can use these flavor profiles to create meat marinades, build your own salads, experiment with soup recipes, or create other types of recipes.

Give these cuisines a try:

Southern / Barbecue Flavor Profile:

- butter, Creole seasoning, garlic powder, onion powder, paprika, chili powder, sugar-free barbecue sauce, bacon, collard greens, mustard greens, turnip greens, tomatoes, jalapenos, cabbage

Italian Flavor Profile:

- olive oil, garlic, pesto, tomatoes, onions, olives, basil, oregano, mozzarella, Parmesan-Reggiano, Asiago, Provolone, lemons, dry red wine, zucchini, broccoli, eggplant

Mexican Flavor Profile:

- olive oil or chili oil, garlic, tomato, onion, cilantro, ground cumin, chili powder, lime juice, Monterey jack cheese, pepper Jack cheese, sour cream, salsa, jalapenos, hot chilis

Greek Flavor Profile:

- olive oil, olives, Greek yogurt, dill, tzatziki (yogurt / dill / garlic dip), cucumbers, zucchini, eggplant, summer squash, tomatoes, lemon juice

French Flavor Profile:

- butter, cream, tomatoes, onions, shallots, garlic, mushrooms, herbs de Provence (tarragon, parsley, lavender, thyme, rosemary), Brie, Gruyere, dry red and white wines

Indian Flavor Profile:

- ghee (Indian clarified butter), tomatoes, onions, curry powder, ground cumin, chili powder, garam masala, turmeric, coriander, coconut milk

Thai Flavor Profile:

- garlic, scallions, ginger, lemongrass, onions, tomatoes, red Thai chili, Thai basil, cilantro, curry powder, coconut milk, fish sauce, sriracha, red curry paste, green curry paste, yellow curry paste

You can come up with your own 'flavor profiles,' as well, centered around the foods that you most enjoy eating and cooking. Take a basic protein like chicken, and you can add the above ingredients to it to make an interesting dish. With the above Keto Diet friendly flavor combinations, you'll be on your way to making this your favorite diet ever.

Besides flavors, the second most popular way to change up your Keto Diet when creating your own meal plan is to pay attention to texture! A lot of the times, our food cravings are not just about flavor, but about texture. Reaching for salty carb foods like chips and pretzels also give you that satisfying crunch. Sweet desserts are not just loaded with sugar, they're also full of creamy textures.

So, on your meal plan, take into account these popular food textures:

Crunchy:

- Celery sticks
- Cucumber slices
- Green bell pepper slices
- Almonds
- Walnuts

- Pecans
- Macadamia Nuts
- Seeds
- Keto Seed Crackers (see recipe in previous chapter)

Creamy:

- Butter
- Heavy Cream
- Cream Cheese
- Cottage Cheese
- Soft or Hard Cheeses
- Yogurt and Yogurt-based dips

- Coconut milk
- Unsweetened Almond Milk
- Almond Nut Butter
- Smoothies
- Cream-based Soups

You can certainly combine these textures, too! Many Keto Diet recipes for Fat Bombs have both creamy and crunchy elements. Keto salads and soups do, too.

When you add variety to your diet, it makes it that much more successful! You'll not just be focused on the end goal of losing weight or dramatically improve your health, but will enjoy the foods themselves each and every day. When you change from just going through the motions to actually enjoying the Keto Diet and everything it offers?

That's when you've found the perfect diet for you!

Eating Out

While you're Intermittently Fasting on the Keto Diet, chances are during your feeding times that you'll want to go out and eat as well! If you like to eat at certain restaurants on a weekly or monthly basis, that should also be included in your meal plan. It's best to think about this before heading out, rather than at the table with a restaurant menu and the waitstaff looking at you, wanting you to order!

There are many wonderful restaurants to try, and you are encouraged to try them. However, it is the rare restaurant that posts their Macros. So, it'll be up to you to make sure you're staying diligent on your diet. Write down the name of the foods that you ate in your meal plan and follow the above tips to estimate the Macros.

What are some other tips that will help you as a Keto Dieter on a meal plan at a restaurant?

- Remember how hefty those portion sizes are! It's not going to be in your best interest to chomp down your entire meal, even if it is made up of good fats and healthy proteins. Eat just half, and take the rest home for another meal.
- Ask the restaurant for any gluten-free options. That will help eliminate carbs.
- Go for the same types of Keto dishes in a restaurant that you can make at home – steak with vegetables, Keto soups and salads, Thai curries, and egg dishes. That way, there's less chance of carbs or other unwanted ingredients sneaking past you.
- Instead of a single entrée, try putting together two or three Keto appetizers to make a meal. This is especially useful when dining in a restaurant that has lots of carb options.
- Enjoy your meal with a partner who's also on the Keto Diet. That way, both of you can have fun sticking to your meal plans together!

More and more restaurants are offering carb free options and providing more Keto friendly ingredients to you. So, hopefully, you'll be able to find something you like when you go out to eat!

Meal Planning on a Budget

While some Keto ingredients like MCT oil, avocado oil, psyllium husk powder, and Stevia might be more expensive because they're harder to find, most of your Ketogenic food list can be found at your local grocery store. As long as you can bypass the bakery and head right to the cheese and meat counters, you'll do just fine!

Many of us do have a monthly food budget. So, it's great to not just follow a successful meal plan, but to have it work within your budgetary constraints. You can definitely do this!

Here are our top tips for meal planning and dieting the Keto way on a budget:

1. Keep a Well-Stocked Pantry

Pantry staples make up the bulk of your diet, whether you're going Keto or not. So, keep a well-stocked pantry full of these Keto foods like the coconut oil, coconut milk, chicken broth, olive oil, almond flour, baking ingredients, and a full herbs and spice cabinet. Try to buy these items in bulk and store them in airtight containers. That way, your weekly grocery list will be about restocking perishable foods like produce, meats, and dairy. It helps your budget.

2. Plan, Shop, and Eat Seasonally

You might want to change your meal plan to go with the seasons. Seasonal foods go on sale, simply because they're more plentiful. Spring foods are ham, asparagus, lemons, and eggs. Summer foods are the produce, fruits, and fresh herbs. Fall foods are earthy foods like onions, mushrooms, arugula, and red wine. Winter foods are the cold-weather veggies like broccoli and cauliflower, together with heartier or game meats. You'll save money, too.

3. Always Shop with a List

This is especially important when you're on the Keto Diet! You want to stick to the grocery list that you've made based on your meal plan. That way, you'll stick to meeting your Macros, prevent impulse buying, and save money, too.

Your Blank Meal Plan Template

Below is a great blank meal plan template! You can certainly print this out and have a new one for each week. Or, you can recreate the template in a spreadsheet program on your computer, customize it, and print it out to post where you can see it each week.

My Meal Plan

Day	Breakfast	Lunch	Dinner	Snack/Dessert	Calories/Macros
1	Food cal g fat g protein g carbs Activity: Time: Activity: Time: Notes:	Food cal g fat g protein g carbs Activity: Time: Activity: Time: Notes:	Food cal g fat g protein g carbs Activity: Time: Activity: Time: Notes:	Food cal g fat g protein g carbs Activity: Time: Activity: Time: Notes:	Calories: Fat: g Protein: g Net Carbs: g
2	Food cal g fat g protein g carbs Activity: Time: Activity: Time: Notes:	Food cal g fat g protein g carbs Activity: Time: Activity: Time: Notes:	Food cal g fat g protein g carbs Activity: Time: Activity: Time: Notes:	Food cal g fat g protein g carbs Activity: Time: Activity: Time: Notes:	Calories: Fat: g Protein: g Net Carbs: g

3	Food cal g fat g protein g carbs Activity: Time: Activity: Time: Notes:	Food cal g fat g protein g carbs Activity: Time: Activity: Time: Notes:	Food cal g fat g protein g carbs Activity: Time: Activity: Time: Notes:	Food cal g fat g protein g carbs Activity: Time: Activity: Time: Notes:	Calories: Fat: g Protein: g Net Carbs: g
4	Food cal g fat g protein g carbs Activity: Time: Activity: Time: Notes:	Food cal g fat g protein g carbs Activity: Time: Activity: Time: Notes:	Food cal g fat g protein g carbs Activity: Time: Activity: Time: Notes:	Food cal g fat g protein g carbs Activity: Time: Activity: Time: Notes:	Calories: Fat: g Protein: g Net Carbs: g

5	Food cal g fat g protein g carbs Activity: Time: Activity: Time: Notes:	Food cal g fat g protein g carbs Activity: Time: Activity: Time: Notes:	Food cal g fat g protein g carbs Activity: Time: Activity: Time: Notes:	Food cal g fat g protein g carbs Activity: Time: Activity: Time: Notes:	Calories: Fat: g Protein: g Net Carbs: g
6	Food cal g fat g protein g carbs Activity: Time: Activity: Time: Notes:	Food cal g fat g protein g carbs Activity: Time: Activity: Time: Notes:	Food cal g fat g protein g carbs Activity: Time: Activity: Time: Notes:	Food cal g fat g protein g carbs Activity: Time: Activity: Time: Notes:	Calories: Fat: g Protein: g Net Carbs: g

7	Food cal g fat g protein g carbs Activity: Time: Activity: Time: Notes:	Food cal g fat g protein g carbs Activity: Time: Activity: Time: Notes:	Food cal g fat g protein g carbs Activity: Time: Activity: Time: Notes:	Food cal g fat g protein g carbs Activity: Time: Activity: Time: Notes:	Calories: Fat: g Protein: g Net Carbs: g

Intermittent Fasting on Your New Meal Plan

Notice on the above meal plan that your Intermittent Fasting times weren't included?

That's because I do want you to follow the twenty-eight day structured Intermittent Fasting guide back in Chapter 6. That Fasting guide is very dependent on how your initial Intermittent Fasting experience goes for you. So, if you want to include fasting, you're encouraged to follow Chapter 6 very closely and stick to the 7-Day Meal Plan in Chapter 7.

Since Intermittent Fasting has so many benefits, it's tempting to try and jump right into it! I mean, you've got pretty much every tool that you need to succeed:

1. Your 7 Day Meal Plan
2. The Recipes to Go With the 7 Day Meal Plan
3. The Grocery List in the Appendix for the 7 Day Meal Plan
4. Your 28 Day Structured Guide to Intermittent Fasting
5. A Blank Meal Plan Template

Yes, for those of you who would love to jump right in and start the challenge, go for it!

You're encouraged to go at your own pace. But of course, if you want to create meal plans with your Intermittent Fasting times put in, then please do so. That will be really helpful if you're diligently following the Structured Guide, too.

Meal Planning Ahead for Keto Success!

Ask any Keto Dieter what one of their secrets to success was, and they'll gladly tell you: it was finding a foolproof plan and sticking to it. Meal plans do take a couple of hours per week to put together. But it's enjoyable time spent browsing recipes, because that's very fun to do! You get to see really nice color photos of the meals you'll love to make. Many Keto Dieters have videos on YouTube, so you can walk through the recipes step by step.

The time that you put into meal planning will pay you back in so many rewards: pounds lost, greater energy, improved health, and all the benefits that you can't see. Those are the ones happening at the cellular level in your body. You'll only see what's happening on the outside.

So, print out the above template or make your own, and get started this week with your first practice meal plan. It doesn't have to be perfect or set in stone. It just needs to be your first step towards not just trying to make this Keto Diet work for you. But assuring its success!

Conclusion

You remember reading about my personal Ketogenic Diet story, along with my personal experience of Intermittent Fasting. That was back in the very first chapter, because I wanted you to get to know me more than just these words on a page.

All of the Keto Diet and Intermittent Fasting information in this book comes not just from personal experience, but from science. I've studied nutrition science and why exactly those Macros (fats / proteins / carbohydrates) interact with our bodies the way that they do. It's pretty fascinating stuff, even if you aren't a science geek like me. I personally was shocked that both fats and carbohydrates are made up of similar atoms, just in a different order. But that makes sense, if you think about it. We need those atoms as fuel for our bodies. We'll take in fuel any way we can get it. Our brain, heart, lungs, stomach, liver, intestines, muscles, and bones require incredible amounts of those atoms to survive.

We each have a human body that's run on fuel. Are you going to get your fuel from carbohydrates and continue to go through blood sugar cycles that also cause you to gain weight?

Or, are you going to make the commitment to be in the ketosis metabolic state? Like a happy marriage, it's a commitment that gives you back far more than it takes! It'll give you a slimmer, trimmer body. It will give you better health. It will give you so much more energy, because you won't feel sluggish or stuck in a carb coma cycle. It will give you back the person that you have always dreamed you could be. When you continue to eat a moderate or high carbohydrate diet, you're not just enjoying sugar, you are keeping yourself further and further away from the kind of body that you want. The kind of body that prompted you to pick up this book.

But, when you go into a ketosis metabolic state? That is when real results happen. Many Keto Dieters are shocked when the pounds start to quickly drop off. But that is what you should expect when you switch metabolic states. You are struggling to burn the existing weight, not burn the fuel from what you just ate at breakfast this morning. Ketosis is the state which burns your existing weight.

That number on the scale just keeps getting lighter and lighter.

Numbers Are Your Friend

You have probably noticed one huge recurring theme that has run throughout this entire book:

The power of numbers.

On the Keto Diet, numbers are your biggest friends and closest allies. It's the numbers that will help you reach your goals. It's the numbers that will help you find the perfect Intermittent Fasting schedule for you. It's the numbers that will help you lose weight and gain all that incredible energy that you have been wanting.

When you are feeling tired or unmotivated to continue, then just go back to the numbers. They are your friends on this Keto Diet!

What numbers do I mean?

1. Your Macros. Find the perfect percentages for you, and follow those percentages. Calculate your specific Fat, Protein, and Carbohydrate daily counts.
2. Your Calories. Calories have a unique relationship to your Macros. If you're struggling, count your calories and make sure you're not eating more than you burn.
3. Your Ketone Counts. You find these by measuring with a Ketone Breath or Blood Monitor.
4. Your Fasting Hours / Feeding Hours. This is your personal Intermittent Fasting Cycle. It could be a six hour, seven hour, eight hour, or ten hour eating window. No matter what amount of time it is, stay consistent.

Think of all these numbers as the firm foundation for your Keto Diet experience. Once you have put this foundation in place, then you are ready to start adding in the fun stuff that will really make this diet the best you have ever been on. That fun stuff includes the recipes, the different flavors, and the new dishes to try.

Fast Forward to Your Future

This isn't the only book you will read about the Keto Diet and Intermittent Fasting. You will keep expanding your knowledge about this diet, and I really encourage you to do that. It is important to be informed about what goes in your body. To eat mindlessly is no better than starving.

So, I encourage you to enjoy your Keto Diet journey. Enjoy what you're eating, enjoy what you're cooking, and enjoy taking the daily steps towards meeting your goals. We all start out with the best intentions, with such high hopes for the future. Dropping 15 pounds in 30 days sounds amazing!

But if every single one of those thirty days feels like torture, you'll stop after just five days. You want to not only enjoy your future body, but you want to enjoy each day towards getting that future body too, right? Otherwise, you'll quit – and rightfully so!

The Keto Diet does restrict certain foods, but that doesn't mean it can't also be the best diet of your life. By following all the tips and tricks in this book, you'll make the Keto Diet the only one that you will want to be on.

That's because it not only gives you the body you want in the future, it gives you the foods that you'll enjoy eating every step of the way!

Now if you have taken one , or two or three pieces of great advice and found them to be of good value, please please

Do pop over to amazon and leave a review and share your thoughts with the rest of the folks who might be looking out for the same information as you have.

Thank you so so much!

Appendix

Here is a grocery list for you! It contains all the ingredients to make every single one of the twenty-two recipes in the 7 Day Meal Plan back in Chapter 7.

7 Day Meal Plan Grocery List:

Produce & Fresh Herbs:

13 cloves garlic

3 lemons

4 limes

5 asparagus

5 avocados

4 yellow onions

2 red onions

1/4 lb. green beans

2 green bell peppers

1 zucchini

6 tomatoes

2 jalapenos

1 fresh head of broccoli

1 fresh head of cauliflower

1 package button mushrooms

1 package fresh spinach

1 bunch spring onion

1 bunch Romaine lettuce

1 bunch kale

1 bunch fresh cilantro

1 bunch fresh dill

1 bunch fresh parsley

1 package fresh raspberries

Meat & Seafood:

7 strips bacon

1 boneless chicken breast

1 2/3 lbs boneless chicken thighs

2 lbs ground beef

1 lb ground sausage

6 3 oz. Mahi Mahi fillets

2 oz prosciutto

2 oz salami

4 steaks

6 oz chorizo

1 package fresh pepperoni

Eggs & Dairy:

1 carton of dozen large eggs

3 sticks butter

1 large container heavy whipping cream

100g mozzarella balls

5 oz fresh mozzarella

1 package shredded mozzarella

1 package shredded cheddar cheese

2 oz shredded parmesan

1 container sour cream

1 container unsweetened almond milk

1 container Feta cheese

1 tub full-fat cream cheese

1 jar Indian ghee

Nuts, Seeds, and Baking:

almond flour

1 container cocoa powder

Stevia

2 large containers coconut oil

vanilla extract

macadamia nuts

chia seeds

sunflower seeds

pumpkin seeds

sesame seeds

flaxseeds

Herbs, Spices, and Condiments:

salt and pepper

sea salt

chili powder

ground cumin

turmeric

coriander seed

Italian herbs

dried basil

dried thyme

chili powder

onion powder

garlic powder

garam masala

ginger

1 bottle fish sauce

red wine vinegar

1 container Dijon mustard

1 container mayonnaise

1 jar Thai red curry paste

1 large container olive oil

1 bottle avocado oil

Other:

MCT oil

3 cans full fat coconut milk

1 container chicken broth

1 jar oil-packed sun-dried tomatoes

1 jar artichoke hearts

1 jar green olives

1 14 oz can whole tomatoes

1 14.5 oz can diced tomatoes

1 6 oz can tomato paste

1 small container pizza sauce

1 bottle white wine

black coffee

Intermittent Fasting For Women 101

The Essentials For Proven Weight Loss Results

Will Ramos & Gin Fung

Intermittent Fasting For Women 101

Chapter 1:
Introduction

I want to admit something to you, dear reader, right up front.

When I first heard that fasting could be an amazing, natural, and healthy way to lose weight and have a healthy lifestyle, I shuddered. All I could picture was the times I myself had been ravenously hungry ('hangry', right?). It wasn't exactly appealing.

But when I realized that it wasn't about starving myself for hours and hours on end and it was more about using fasting times to lose weight, I became intrigued.

I became even more intrigued when the weight started to drop off.

That started me on an incredible journey. It's a journey that I will share with you in multiple ways throughout this entire book.

It's not a physical journey. I didn't start in New York and ended up in California. No, not at all. I started in an unhealthy, overweight body and then I kept trying the fasting times each day. I made that journey to the destination where I am today:

My extra weight is gone. I look great. Do you know how it feels to stand in front of a mirror and say to yourself, "I look great"? If you had asked me to do that two years ago, I would have cried because I was so unhappy.

Not any longer.

Girls Only Wanted!

This book was written for women, by a woman! You won't receive advice that is better suited for men. You know why? Well, they have a completely different body than you do! A male physicality just isn't the same as a female physicality. I'm not just talking the obvious differences here.

Our women's bodies were designed to create and grow beautiful babies, and that means massive differences in our basic physiology. Our cells function differently, our organs function differently, and our entire metabolism processes nutrients differently. We're not male, and so that means big changes from male dieting and fasting advice.

You've probably seen this yourself in the real world. You try to set the same weight loss goals as a boyfriend or husband, only to watch them effortlessly lose weight just by cutting out cheeseburgers! Meanwhile, your stubborn weight doesn't budge. You're cutting out one hundred calories per day, and you're spending your thirty minutes three times a week at the gym. But nothing is happening! What's up with that? It's completely frustrating and demoralizing.

Well, in this book, I'm going to walk you through the exact female only biological processes that are going on in your cells. I want to give you real scientific answers as to why it's more difficult for you to lose weight. We'll delve right down into the cellular level and examine what's going on every time you reach for the next bite.

Forget the male Intermittent Fasting and dieting advice. This book is for women only, and I'll peel back the curtain to show you the reality of what's going on in your body.

Once you have those scientific answers, then we will work together to craft a fasting and feeding schedule that takes advantage of your body! We will work with what we've got and stop trying to make you into something you're not. Bypass that advice and choose this book instead. It's Really All...

About Eating

This book is about Intermittent Fasting for women – but we're also going to spend the vast majority of this book talking about food, too! That's because in between your fasting cycles, you've gotta eat, girl.

But as soon as I mention food, dozens of questions pop up in your mind:

~What am I supposed to be eating to help me lose weight?

~What foods burn fat the fastest?

~What are the most delicious foods to help me lose weight?

~What are the 'no no' foods I can't eat?

~What am I allowed to eat while fasting? Or is it just water?

~How many calories should I eat each day?

~What kinds of calories should I be eating?

~How can I fit my meals into my busy life?

~What's the relationship between Intermittent Fasting and food?

~How many meals should I be eating?

~When should I be eating my meals?

~How big are the portion sizes that I'm allowed?

~Is it okay to be vegetarian or vegan and still do this Intermittent Fasting?

~What if I get hungry?

~Is it okay to try it for just a few days out of each week?

~How do I keep my blood sugar levels up?

~How do I know if I'm burning fat and this is working?

Yep, it really is a lot about eating. You are going to find every single answer to these questions – and more – inside this book. I have covered this food topic in-depth, especially in Chapter 4. That's because eating is such a huge part of any diet plan. Even when Intermittently Fasting, you have got to eat the right foods.

I'll also talk about exactly what you can eat during your fasting times. Yes, you can have some calories, but they have to be the right calories at the right times. We'll go into that, too!

Follow Me Step by Step

So, Intermittent Fasting is about abstaining from eating in order to lose weight and burn fat.

Okay.

But, where do you start?

You need some massive help – and this book will lay it all out for you in easy, practical steps. There are no abstract theories or vague advice present here. I live in the real world, and so do you!

You are a busy woman. You have a full work load of at least forty hours a week, you have your family with your husband and kids, you have to grocery shop, you are probably helping out with chores around the house, and many of you have added responsibilities like taking care of elderly parents, being involved with local organizations, and trying to squeeze in a little time to yourself. Not to mention fun times with friends and going out!

How in the world are you supposed to Intermittently Fast, eat the right way, and have this busy life all at the same time?

I had those exact same questions, too. Which is why when I embarked on my own Intermittent Fasting journey, I made sure to track every single little thing I was doing. In the beginning, I made plenty of mistakes, I didn't feel as good on a daily basis as I did later, and I goofed up a lot. I was also held back by my lack of knowledge about what exactly was going on in my body. I had no idea what I was doing!

But you will!

Just follow this book step by step, and you will get my results, but in a lot faster, more efficient, less time-wasting, and more informed way. That is such a relief, isn't it? Knowledge really is power. Once you have the correct knowledge about Intermittent Fasting and eating, you can rocket right to the top and achieve those weight loss goals that have been so elusive in the past.

A Brief Introduction ...

Hello, and thanks for reading about Intermittent Fasting. My name is Will Ramos, but I'm not the main author of this book! I'm just here to introduce the amazingly talented, beautiful, and successful Gin Fung. She's your Intermittent Fasting success story.

But before I do, I wanted to share my own diet, weight loss, fitness, and health story with you. Yes, I'm a man! But that does not mean I don't know the frustrations of struggling to have the body you want.

There are so many hidden carbohydrates (including all kinds of sugars) lurking in the foods you eat, that even someone who appears healthy on the outside can suffer from unexpected and severe health problems on the inside.

That's exactly what happened to me. I was a hale and healthy male athlete in my teens! I was playing sports, getting outside a lot, didn't carry any extra weight, and my BMI was totally normal. If you saw me, you'd have no idea that I was secretly unhealthy. I sure didn't know.

So, imagine my total surprise when I was suddenly diagnosed with diabetes.

Wait, what?

Yeah, whatever stereotypes you think about the average diabetes sufferer, that surely wasn't me. But suddenly, it was. I now had a disease that radically changed my relationship with food. I'd always exercised frequently, that I just didn't think it was necessary or important to care about what was on the plate. I just burned all those calories, anyway.

But diabetes has nothing to do with calories, being thin, exercising, or sports. That was eye-opening. I was thrown for a loop and struggled with my life into my early adulthood, trying everything I could think of to lessen my symptoms and get my diabetes under control. It took longer than I want to admit (especially to you!) to finally realize there was this incredible link between diet and health. Hey, I was a teenager okay?

Yet, once I recognized this link, my whole outlook changed immediately. I started with the Atkins Diet, which was popular at the time, then shortly thereafter started exploring the Keto Diet. This was around the early 2000s. The Ketogenic Diet sounded weird and extreme to me, with its ridiculously high fat contents and ridiculously low carb contents, but hey – I was already experimenting, so why not?

Well, needless to say, that Keto Diet experiment turned into a full tilt obsession as soon as my diabetes numbers started looking healthier. The more I ate this diet, the better my numbers got. Each doctor visit I was improving. I read everything I could get my hands on, including all about the nutrition, the science, the practical application, the recipes, and the meal plans. I absorbed this knowledge even better than a sponge, because my own health was at stake!

My experiments and personal field tested knowledge paid off. You might not believe me, but it's the truth:

The diabetes is gone. A long gone memory by this point.

And, I've been on the Ketogenic Diet for fourteen years.

I changed the metabolic process in my own body, I'm in ketosis 100% of the time, and I've never been healthier. On the inside and the outside this time. That was my story, and I am happy to say that it could be yours too. But wait! I see your furrowed brows. Isn't this about intermittent fasting for women, by a woman? Indeed!

So, let me introduce the real author of this book. She is the awesome superwoman hero who has put her heart and soul into this book, just so she can share it with you!

Learning From Gin's Story

Thank you, Will! Yes, my name is Gin Fung. I'm definitely a woman. Nice to meet you! I tried Intermittent Fasting for the first time five years ago, with little success. I thought it was okay, but it certainly didn't live up to the hype that several of my close girlfriends kept trying to convince me was the latest thing! I'm a skeptical person by nature. I did do the Intermittent Fasting for just a month, but I did not plan for it, I didn't commit to it, and I was mostly half-heartedly doing it just to lose a few pounds.

Needless to say, I didn't do well at all! Of course, then I thought to myself, "Oh, this whole Intermittent Fasting thing doesn't work. You just starve yourself and you're supposed to lose weight. But it didn't for me, so it doesn't work."

That was my take away from it. Until, about eight months later, I went on a dieting retreat. And, what do you know? A main portion of the retreat incorporated Intermittent Fasting. After just a week of doing it – and doing it right this time – I was shocked at the changes. I felt more energy, my basic body energy was stabilized, I felt slimmer, my clothes fit looser, and I just didn't feel as heavy, sluggish, or bloated.

Inspired, I came home and this time, I did it right! I planned for my eating windows in between fasting times, I ate the foods I was supposed to, I had my meals at the same time each day, I tracked my results ... and the weight loss was actually pretty effortless after that. Yes, I said effortless! I was so focused on the eating aspect that I didn't really feel hungry or deprived during the fasting times. It helps that my life is busy – as is yours, too!

The longer I was on Intermittent Fasting, the more results I experienced. As my energy increased and my weight loss started to escalate as the weeks went by, I embarked on a little personal research project to discover the exact scientific reasons as to why Intermittent Fasting worked so well in my body. I ran into a couple of snags here and there, which have to do with the female only body while fasting. But I went back to the science, read more about what my cells were doing, and then I was able to overcome those snafus to move forward and keep losing weight!

You can keep reading about the scientific evidence that I discovered and wrote about in Chapter 3. You will be as fascinated as I was to discover just exactly what is going on inside you when you either fast or feast. It's pretty eye-opening.

Not to mention life-changing. You won't want to go back to previous ways of dieting or eating, because you will realize that those diets are not in tune with how your body actually works. So, they are doomed to fail! Intermittent Fasting will not doom you to fail. It will launch you towards success.

So, yeah! It's been four years since I've been using Intermittent Fasting to not just lose weight, but to maintain both the healthy weight I am right now and to keep my energy levels nice and high. I have not just high energy levels, but they're stable and do not spike or crash throughout the day.

I discovered many unexpected bonuses that went along with the Intermittent Fasting, too. My weekly meal planning is second nature, plus I have a lot of fun finding and trying new recipes for my eating window times. Grocery shopping is a breeze because I know exactly what foods to buy, and I easily bypass the foods I know will disrupt my current healthy metabolism. I am not a hardcore gym user, but I do get out jogging for about thirty minutes three times a week. That keeps my body healthy and slim. I also train with kettlebells to build up my strength. It helps when carrying things! I sleep better, too. I fall asleep easier, I deeply rest all night long, and I wake up feeling refreshed. My stress levels are down, and I'm able to manage my natural cheerful outlook throughout my life, too. I even feel better during my period, without the sore and heavy chest, sluggish tiredness, brain fog, and irritability I used to experience. Just saying farewell to those symptoms alone is worth it!

I'll talk even more about the benefits of Intermittent Fasting, which you can read all about in Chapter 9 on getting the most out of your diet.

So, are you with me? Would you like to get started on a healthy, doable, totally practical, scientifically based, and enjoyable way to get lean? It's just for women, and it works for women. You'll feel great about the way you look!

What's Included in This Book?

There is a wealth of information in this book that covers all aspects of Intermittent Fasting. You will find all kinds of tips, tricks, dos, don'ts, benefits, troubleshooting tips, and more in here. This is just a sampling of what you will read:

~That One Thing you Need to Know about Intermittent Fasting. It might Change Your Life!

~How Intermittent Fasting stimulates changes in a women's body and how you can use that!

~The different types of Intermittent Fasting and the tips to know which is for you

~Your motivation or motivations to stay on Intermittent Fasting and no its not just willpower!

~The How-To and Not-To when fasting

~Dealing with speed bumps while fasting and how to turn them into Positives!

~What we can learn from a Bear and how this is crucial to weight loss process

~The One Main thing you need to note when coming out of longer fasts

~A complete and detailed 30 day Intermittent Fasting challenge

~What to eat, when to eat, and how to eat during your 30 Day Challenge

~Incorporating the Keto Diet into Intermittent Fasting

~Getting the most out of your Intermittent Fasting journey

~... and so much more!

There is plenty to learn in this book! You can skip to the chapters that best suit your needs right now, or you can follow my recommendation and read the whole thing straight through from this page to the last. That gives you the most complete picture of Intermittent Fasting, it answer all of your questions in a logical and timely way, and the natural progression of information was laid out here just for you to best understand it. By the time you get to Chapter 8 and the Intermittent Fasting 30 Day Challenge, you'll be inspired to try it. You'll also succeed!

A Fasting Foundation

The next chapter gives you the basics of Intermittent Fasting: its history, what it is, the three types, and the ways you can customize it to fit your lifestyle. Learning these basics gives you the firmest and most solid foundation for succeeding on Intermittent Fasting. As you already know from previous dieting plans in the past, the basics are always more important than they at first appear! Oh, and if you're having trouble with Intermittent Fasting, it also helps to go back to the basics and work on those.

Fast forward towards Intermittent Fasting success!

Chapter 2:
What is Intermittent Fasting?

Cool, so you want to add Intermittent Fasting to your life and not just shed those pesky pounds, but gain many other rewards along the way!

You definitely can.

In this chapter, we will start with the basics of Intermittent Fasting – what it is, its benefits, its history, and the three types. We'll also examine some of the silly myths around fasting. I want to get you excited to start upon this journey!

So ... What is Intermittent Fasting?

It is exactly what it sounds like!

When you do something intermittently, that means you are not doing it continuously, but in smaller amounts. To fast is to abstain from all foods that have calories for a certain period of time.

When you add those two words together, you get Intermittent Fasting!

This is a scheduled way of combining both extended fasting times and eating times into a continuous routine. It is a way to unlock the exciting features and benefits of Intermittent Fasting, which gives you incredible rewards like:

~A slimmer, trimmer body

~Amazing energy

~Better health

~Having your cells cleaned and revitalized

~Effortless weight loss

~No exercise required!

That is what Intermittent Fasting is designed to do.

But, why has this become a new way of losing weight? What makes it so powerful, and why is it an ideal process for your body to drop the pounds?

Those answers come from how your body actually works and has worked for centuries!

Intermittent Fasting for Human Survival

While in modern times, there is a grocery store or restaurant on every corner ... that was definitely not the case throughout most of human history.

Picture this:

It is thirty thousand years ago, in Europe. It's at the height of summer, but winter is only a few months away. You are expending a lot of calories just doing your daily living. But you're also eating as much as you can while the plants are in season and the animals are plentiful. You eat and eat, basically gorging yourself and eating way more calories than you normally need to survive.

We'll talk more in the next chapter about the science behind food storage in your cells. But thousands of years ago, that's exactly what was happening. Your body stored every tiny extra bit of nutrients in your fat cells. That was their purpose then, and it is still their purpose! You were meant to store extra fuel.

After a few months, the plants died, the animals became scarce, and winter came. Now your body was prepared to face the months and months of vastly reduced food supply. You had spent your summer days storing the food that you needed.

Winter was historically a months' long fasting period. Your body was prepared for it, and your ancestors survived those long, cold winters. You're here!

But your body was built to withstand prolonged fasting times with few calories to sustain you. You were forced to live off of the stored fuel. Consequently, your body switched metabolic states and went into what's called ketosis. Ketosis helped your body use fat as a primary fuel source, not glucose.

Our ancestors survived because their bodies could switch metabolic states so easily, adapt to pretty hardcore fasting, use their stored fuel efficiently, and prevent themselves from starving to death.

Nowadays, though, we live in seriously the most abundant and food plentiful time in human history. Our ancestors would be staggered at the amount of food available to us, the variety, and the constant freshness! They had to make do with whatever they could hunt or gather.

So, that is the history of fasting. It is built into the DNA of each of your cells. Your body was economically designed to conserve and store as much food as humanly possible. It is very efficient and has helped the human race persist and thrive as much as we have for thousands of years.

However, it certainly does not help modern humans like you and me who want to lose that conserved and stored energy! We want to shed that stored fuel, and we want to do it quickly.

The best way to do that?

Turn back the clock on your body. We are going to pretend like it is thirty thousand years ago. We want your body to go into a prolonged fasting mode, so that your existing stored fuel is used. The less stored fuel on your body, the less you weigh. Intermittent Fasting will help you meet those weight loss goals.

That's really all there is to it!

Your Two Fasting Goals

You have two basic goals with Intermittent Fasting:

~Burn even more fat than you would if you weren't fasting

~Boost your energy levels

These are not just goals; they're also benefits! In Chapter 3, you will read more about the specific fat burning benefits, and why fasting kicks your metabolism into high gear. You will also read about the science behind why you get so much energy, too.

When we proceed to the preparations before the 30 Day Challenge, you'll be thinking about the weight loss goals to set. It's great to set a small amount of weight to lose, but don't be surprised if your weight loss far surpasses that! Intermittent Fasting is specifically designed to burn fat. Many women have reported astonishing results. You will, too!

Imagine what you would be able to do if you did have plenty of extra energy. Right now, you're probably feeling sluggish from blood spike and crash cycles. Not to mention that your life is pretty busy. You have a full to-do list each day. How can you expect to get it all done?

That is when the power of Intermittent Fasting comes into play. This is an extremely energy boosting way of eating. It lifts up your energy levels to new heights, and helps you accomplish everything you need to do each day – and then some! Wouldn't it be great to feel younger, refreshed, vitalized, and having a natural positive outlook each day? Well, when you decide to both fast the correct way and eat the correct way on Intermittent Fasting schedules, that's really when great stuff happens.

Are You Fasting or Feeding?

Intermittent Fasting is not just about abstaining from food. You are actually going to both eat and not eat on a continuous looping cycle. There are two parts to this cycle:

~Fasting times

~Feeding times (also known as eating windows)

You are either in one or the other.

You actually already implement a fasting cycle every day of your life! Did you know that? It's when you are sleeping in between dinner and breakfast. The word "breakfast" literally comes from the phrase "break a fast." Yes, sleeping definitely counts as fasting.

Most of us follow a pretty regular weekly feeding schedule of eating breakfast in the morning, lunch around noon, and dinner in the evening. You fast at night when you sleep. You feed and fast, feed and fast, continuously throughout the weeks and months.

With Intermittent Fasting, we are going to take that same schedule, but just apply more rigidity and structure to it. So, instead of being free to eat whenever you want while you're awake, now you'll have a set period of time when you are supposed to be eating. Also, instead of just fasting when you're asleep, you will also set aside certain hours during the day to fast while you are awake.

Creating your own feeding schedule means that you will set up what are called eating windows. You will be consuming all of that day's calories within the window of time.

Your Intermittent Fasting schedule is now entirely dependent on the clock! Are you feeding or fasting? Depending on the time of day and your Intermittent Fasting schedule, you will know.

The 3 Types of Intermittent Fasting

There are three main types of Intermittent Fasting schedules. Let's take a look at them from easiest to the most challenging.

1. Skipping Meals

You have probably skipped breakfast many times before, especially if you were trying to get to class or work on time. You just did not know you were Intermittently Fasting at the same time. Skipping meals to extend a fast is definitely the easiest way to continue the benefits of fasting. You could either skip breakfast to extend your fast from the night before, or you could skip dinner to start your nightly fasting time earlier. When you skip meals, you reduce your eating window. You want to make sure you're hitting your calorie count goals before your next fast starts.

2. Fast a Lot, Eat a Little

This is the second most common type of Intermittent Fasting. You stick to a schedule that includes a long period of time fasting followed by a shorter eating window. These eating windows average between six and eight hours per day. Then, you spend the rest of the time fasting. The most common types of this fasting schedule include:

~8 hour eating window / 16 hour fasting

~7 hour eating window / 17 hour fasting

~6 hour eating window / 18 hour fasting

I'll talk a lot more about this version of Intermittent Fasting, because it is the most common and also helps produce amazing results!

3. Multi-Day Fasting

Once you get the hang of Intermittent Fasting and really want to take it to the next level, then you can try fasting for between 24 and up to 36 hours. This is a more complicated, complex version of fasting. You will need to prepare for it, and you will also need to have special mineral rich foods to eat once you come out of the fast, too. In the 30 Day Challenge, I have included two 24-hour long fasts. Those who do the multi-day fasting are especially pleased with the results. I highly recommend becoming proficient enough at fasting that you are able to go for longer periods of time. Don't worry – I'll walk you through all the tips and tricks you need to do it.

In this book I will go into much greater detail about these three types of fasting, how to do them properly, and exactly how to incorporate them into your lifestyle. For now, just be aware of them and start thinking about which type would best fit your schedule. If you are too busy these days with work, family, and other obligations, you might want to just skip meals. For other women, a shorter eating window of six or seven hours is totally doable.

There is no 'right' or 'wrong' way to do Intermittent Fasting. This is a highly customizable form of losing weight. It is custom tailored to you!

Is Fasting Harmful?

Well, since you fast every single night of your life, fasting is definitely not harmful! It is not unhealthy, either. In fact, fasting is a perfectly normal and natural process that gives your body time to rest in between your eating windows.

What about starvation mode? That is when your brain and vital organs start shutting down because they are completely deprived of any food source. No glucose is being consumed and no glucose is stored, either.

Starvation is serious, but Intermittent Fasting never gets that drastic. We are not suggesting you abstain from food for longer than five days at a time! All we are doing is fasting for up to about 36 hours at a time. Those short fasting windows don't produce any starvation adverse effects. Your liver will be using the stored fat in your cells as the ketones for fuel, in place of glucose.

Another misconception about fasting is that it shrinks or depletes your muscle tissue. Yes, it is true that some stored glucose and fat are deposited in some of your muscle cells. But during the fasting times, your body will use those stored fatty acids and not touch your muscle tissue at all! Only during extreme starvation does that happen.

In essence, the short time periods of Intermittent Fasting prevent many of the really bad problems associated with severe fasting and starvation.

So, not to worry! Fasting for up to three days is not harmful. It's all about using up your stored fat and melting that weight right off!

This Will Work for You

Yes, Intermittent Fasting really will work for you. You have the same DNA and the same cells in your body that your ancestors did, and they will act the same way when you fast intermittently!

So, what are you waiting for? Now that you've gotten the basics of fasting, let's go deep into your cells and see what exactly is going on when you're fasting.

Chapter 3:
The Science Behind Intermittent Fasting

I'm pretty geeky, because I love reading about the science behind nutrition. But that's because these are facts! I'd rather have the scientific evidence behind why I do something. I want it to work, and I want it backed up by real claims! It's easy for yet another diet guru to come down the pike and start spouting all kinds of ideas about this diet or that diet.

I prefer to bypass the nonsense and go right to the science.

And, do you know what the science behind Intermittent Fasting and weight loss tells me?

That your body is a fuel-processing machine. It really is! Every single process that goes on in your digestive system is all about receiving fuel, extracting the nutrients, separating those nutrients, getting the right nutrients to the right organs, and then eliminating the waste.

In this chapter, we will talk all about glucose, which is your body's primary fuel source!

Fueling for Fasts

The top three nutrients that you eat in your foods each day:

~Glucose from carbohydrates and sugary foods

~Proteins and amino acids from protein foods like meat and dairy

~Fatty acids from the good fats like olive oil

Glucose is probably the most important sugar of all, because it is such an important energy source. It's also the simplest sugar, being just a monosaccharide. Glucose is made by plants when they photosynthesize, so that's its primary source in your diet. Glucose is absolutely key when it comes to your normal body functioning. It is transformed into glycogen in your body.

We measure this fuel as calories, not glucose consumption – even though that is exactly what's going on. Glucose also comes from several other types of sugars.

When we talk about carbs, we're talking about the three distinct atoms of carbon, hydrogen, and oxygen. The word "carbohydrate" contains these three words. "Carbo" for "carbon," "hydr" for "hydrogen," and "ate" for "oxygen." By themselves, these are three very harmless elements and are the building blocks of life.

But when combined into carbohydrate molecules, these three atoms become a group of sugars, starches, and cellulose (plant sugars) called saccharides. Your body can process four chemical groups of saccharides: the monosaccharides, disaccharides, oligosaccharides, and polysaccharides. It is the fourth group, the polysaccharides, that are processed by the body and then stored as energy in your cells.

Sugars are even less complex carbohydrates than the saccharides. They come in many other forms besides glucose, including:

Sucrose (table sugar)

This is the regular sweet white or brown sugar you can purchase in stores that's also found in so many food items, especially baked goods. Table sugar comes from the stems of the sugarcane plant and the roots of the sugar beet. It also contains cellulose plant sugars.

Fructose (fruit sugar)

This is what gives fruits like strawberries, cherries, bananas, and apples their characteristic sweetness. It is also present in some natural sweeteners like honey and agave. Fructose is a monosaccharide sugar. It can also bond to glucose and form sucrose. Fructose is easily made into syrups, like the high fructose corn syrup that's so prevalent in foods these days.

Cellulose (plant sugar)

Cellulose is a polysaccharide sugar that's found in plant cell walls and certain vegetable fibers. Some of your favorite vegetables have really high amounts of cellulose. That includes potatoes, carrots, and corn. Humans can't digest cellulose, so it's usually broken down into its smaller glucose molecules and – you guessed it – stored in your cells for future energy.

Lactose (milk sugar)

People who are lactose intolerant can't digest milk sugars, which are disaccharides made up of galactose and glucose. Cows' milk is really high in lactose. Dairy cheeses have smaller amounts of lactose.

Too Much Fuel = Stored Fat

"Fat" is just a short term nickname for the fatty acids that are present in fats. Fatty acids are long chains of molecules with different chemical components that are various combinations of three atoms: carbon, hydrogen, and oxygen.

Too much of a good thing really is too much, in this case.

Did you know that all three types of fuel – glycogen, proteins, and fatty acids – can be stored as excess in your cells?

Which cells are they stored in? Those cells are called adipocyte cells, which are made of adipose tissue. That adipose tissue's entire specialty in life is to store that excess fuel or excess energy. Think of adipocyte cells as little tiny storage centers all over your body.

Carbohydrates provide fuel, contribute towards stabilizing your blood sugar, and are also frequently found in many fibrous foods like seeds, nuts, legumes, and vegetables.

It is when you eat too many carbohydrates, but especially glucose (which is found in regular sugar, fructose and cellulose), that things start to go haywire. Your health will start to take a turn for the worst, and you'll also notice the weight gain, too.

After you eat good fats, your cells break them down into both glycerol and those fatty acids. This process is called lipolysis. Both the glycerol and those fatty acids are released into your blood and travel through your bloodstream to your liver.

That's where those same fatty acids can then be either broken down directly and used for that day's energy, or they can enter into a new multiple step process called gluconeogenesis, which turns those fatty acids into glucose. Amino acids are combined with the fatty acids to manufacture glucose. Then the glucose is used the same way as other carbohydrates are processed, which is explained below.

What about extra fats? Are those used as energy, like glycogen, or are they stored, like excess protein and carbohydrates?

The answer is yes: those fats are stored. They are stored as triglycerides in fat cells called adipocytes. Those cells can expand, but they do have a limit. In addition, that stored fat can also be stored in your muscles to provide extra energy for when you need it. When you're doing moderate intensity exercising, your muscles open up those stored fat cells and use that energy to meet your fuel needs.

After you eat your protein serving, it is digested in the stomach and absorbed by the intestines. Then it goes directly to your liver, where the nitrogen and the amino acids are broken down and separated. Your amino acids are sent to your muscles for fuel. There are nine essential amino acids in protein, and if all of those are present, then your body uses them all up happily. However, any excess protein that's not used by your body is then turned into either glucose (sugar) or fatty acids and sent to your cells for energy and storage purposes.

That's right. If you eat too much protein, it is stored and causes you to gain weight!

Excess Fuel Storage = Excess Pounds to Lose

Now that you've learned exactly how your body processes each nutrient (carbohydrates, fats, and proteins), let's put the whole scenario together in a real-life example.

This is exactly what's happening in your body every day of your life!

Let's say that you eat a balanced dinner with chicken, potatoes, green peas, and an orange. The chicken is made primarily up of proteins and the good fats. The potatoes are carbohydrates, mostly starches, cellulose (plant sugar), and glucose. Both the green peas and the orange are made up of fructose (fruit sugar), cellulose (plant sugar), and glucose.

Then let's say that after you ate this dinner, you watched a half-hour show on TV, and then took your dog out for a fifteen-minute walk around the block. Well, in that time frame, you are going to use a certain portion of that fuel that you just ate at dinner. You will use the proteins and amino acids and fats from the chicken. You will also use the sugars from the orange, potatoes, and peas, which all have been processed into glycogen.

But you won't use all of that fuel. The rest is stored in that adipose tissue present in your adipocyte cells. There are two storage processes: glycogenesis and lipogenesis.

~Glycogenesis is when excess glucose is converted into glycogen and stored in your liver and muscles. Your body stores up to 2000 calories of this! If you fast for up to 24 hours with no incoming glucose, then your body will use this glycogen storage first.

~Lipogenesis is when there's enough glycogen in your muscles and liver, so the glucose is converted into fat and stored in those adipocyte cells. Your fat stores are pretty unlimited, unfortunately. This is the kind of storage we're trying to shed!

That extra fuel is stored for as long as it needs to be, until your body requires it during a time of calorie and nutritional deficiency. Historically, this would have been winter! Today though, our modern American culture doesn't have a starvation period.

Still, your body just keeps on storing those excess nutrients. Too much fuel of all three kinds (proteins, fats, and carbohydrates) makes you gain weight.

That is the real picture of what's going on inside your body.

You ate plenty of the right types of fuel. It was just too much of it!

So, now you want to shed your extra fuel storage. It would be so much easier if we could just reach inside those adipocyte cells and extract that storage. That process would be similar to decluttering your basement. You want to get rid of the excess fuel storage that you've been carrying around for months or even years.

Intermittent Fasting is the most natural way to declutter all of this extra fuel storage that you want to shed from your body.

Fasting Burns Fuel Storage

While we can't just mentally tell our adipocyte cells to start decluttering, Intermittent Fasting is the process that kickstarts your body into doing that!

On a typical day, you eat a lot of those three types of fuel sources – carbohydrates, fats, and proteins. That's plenty of incoming glucose to store as glycogen or convert to fat and store.

But what if you stop eating and start fasting instead? When your body isn't receiving any more incoming fuel sources, what does it do then?

Well, you still need energy to run your brain, organs, skeleton, and muscles. You still need fuel. So, your cells look elsewhere for that fuel source. That's why they go right to those adipocyte cells, into the adipose tissue, and start extracting the stored fuel.

The whole process looks like this:

You Eat Your Daily Calories

|

Fuel is Extracted

|

Some Glucose is Used for Today's Energy

|

Rest is Converted to Fat

|

Fat is Stored in Adipocyte Cells

|

Stored Fat Adds up to Weight Gain

This is what's currently happening, and the whole process happens every day inside your body. It's very gradual, but it adds up to increased weight gain over time.

Unfortunately, the absolutely domineering message in our American food culture is that we are eating the wrong things! Too much fat, too many carbohydrates, too little protein, and on and on it goes.

But, as you've seen in this chapter, it's not so much that we are eating the wrong types of fuel. Your body is extremely well adapted to process carbohydrates, fats, and proteins.

It's that we're eating too much and too often!

The more you eat, the more excess glucose is converted to fat and stored in your adipocyte cells.

It really comes down to this:

Eat Larger, Healthier Meals Less Often

That's a very good mantra to post on your wall, on your fridge, or in your kitchen somewhere. It will help you stay focused on the bigger picture!

You're going to eat larger meals less often than you have been eating your regular three meals a day plus snacks, and you're going to eat healthier ingredients. We will definitely cover which ingredients in the next chapter!

Then on top of this mantra, we're going to add Intermittent Fasting periods to your weekly schedule.

Putting All the Pieces Together

What does your body do after you've eaten all your meals for the day? I'm glad you asked!

After your eating window is done and you're fasting, your body has to seek elsewhere for fuel.

Here is what that process looks like:

You Stop Eating and Fast for 18 Hours

|

No Additional Glucose or Proteins or Fatty Acids Enter the Body

|

Cells Still Need Fuel

|

Cells Extract Stored Fat from Adipocyte Cells

|

Fat is Sent to Liver for Processing

|

Liver Turns Fat into Ketones (called Ketogenesis)

Ketones Used as Fuel

The more consistently you keep up a fasting schedule, the more weight that you lose! That is because your liver is using all that stored fat to make ketones.

What are ketones? Ketones are small organic compounds of fuel made up of carbon and oxygen that are bonded to hydrocarbon groups. That's a fancy scientific way of saying they are an alternate fuel source to fatty acids, proteins, and the glucose from carbohydrates.

When your body is subsisting primarily on ketones for fuel rather than glucose, you are said to be in ketosis. We'll talk more about that in Chapter 10 when discussing the Keto Diet. Many of you will want to get into ketosis and stay there, because you are consistently burning more of that stored fat in your adipocyte cells.

But, you don't have to be on a special diet for your body to use stored fuel. You're just going to eat larger, healthier meals less often.

The Intermittent Fasting will help you take care of the rest!

How Intermittent Fasting Affects Women

So now, you know exactly how your body processes carbohydrates to turn them into glucose and glycogen, fats to turn them into fatty acids, and proteins to turn them into proteins and amino acids.

Yet, there are so many other ways that Intermittent Fasting affects your body. We are not just different than men physically. We are also affected differently when we abstain from eating. Since so much of the female body and our monthly cycle is about preparing for pregnancy and carrying healthy babies, getting the proper nutrients is of the utmost importance. That is why fasting from foods is such a big deal for women. In some ways, we don't have all of the positive benefits that men experience.

So, when you fast, there are certain side effects that you will definitely notice. Let's go through them one by one to explain what they are and what you should expect when you fast.

Your Ovulation Hormones

Intermittent Fasting definitely affects your hormones. Your body is so sensitive to calorie restriction. So, when your calorie intake is low, from fasting for long periods of time, that affects the hypothalamus in your brain. This in turn disrupts the secretion of a hormone called gonadotropin (GnRH). GnRH helps release two reproductive hormones, luteinizing hormone (LH) and follicle stimulating hormone (FSH).

Those two reproductive hormones – LH and FSH – are the ones that communicate with your ovaries to release eggs each month. They trigger the production of both estrogen and progesterone, which are needed to release an egg each month so you can either become pregnant or have your period in your normal 28-day cycle.

But, when those hormones aren't released and there is no communication with your ovaries, that definitely affects your ovulation cycle. No egg is released, because the hormones haven't told it to. Your periods might become irregular, and it can cause problems with fertility, too. This is especially true if you spend a long time on Intermittent Fasting, going up to three to six months at a time or longer. It even causes a reduction in ovary size and irregular reproductive cycles. Some women have reported, and this is in more extreme cases, that it brings on early-onset menopause.

From a historical standpoint, this makes sense! Thousands of years ago when times of food were scarce, the last thing your body wanted to do was bring a baby into the world. It was too high a risk for the infant and the mother, who would probably starve. Your body doesn't know it's the 21st century. So, Intermittent Fasting definitely affects your ovulation cycle.

Your Hunger Hormones

Fasting also affects three hormones that both regulate and react to either hunger or satiety – leptin, insulin, and ghrelin. These hormones' goals are to maintain homeostasis, which keeps everything in balance. That means not too much hunger or too little, as well as not feeling too full or not enough. When you fast and reduce the calories you eat compared to what you're burning, you get hungry.

Both leptin and ghrelin regulate appetite. Leptin is secreted primarily from your fat cells, but also in your stomach – it decreases hunger. Whereas ghrelin is secreted in your stomach lining, and it increases hunger. Both of them are responding to how much you eat!

When you fast, you're reducing those fat cells and secreting a lot of leptin! It decreases your hunger, making you feel less inclined to eat those calories. Oh, cool! You're thinking. I can just fast and won't feel hungry? That's awesome! Well, not so fast. You still have to take in enough calories to eat during the day. We'll talk more about that in the next chapter.

As for ghrelin, that's the 'rumbling in your stomach' hormone, causing you to go to the fridge or poking through cupboards. When your stomach is empty, it makes ghrelin, which travels through your blood up to your brain and triggers that peckish feeling. When studies have been done on ghrelin, scientists have been surprised to discover the levels have stayed stable during longer fasts up to 33 hours. So, eating nothing for a day makes you no more or less hungry! As a bonus, being a woman, your ghrelin hunger hormone decreases much, much faster than a man's when you abstain from eating. So, you will feel less and less hungry the longer you fast.

Your Thyroid

How does Intermittent Fasting affect your thyroid? For women with thyroid conditions, like hypothyroidism, can Intermittent Fasting help you with thyroid issues? Fasting decreases the concentration of the T3 thyroid hormone, while the T4 (thyroxine) levels stay the same. The thyroid stimulating hormone TSH does not increase, either. These changes only occur if you do more serious multi-day fasting, like three days or longer.

So, in effect, when you fast for two days or just Intermittently each day, that has very little scientific bearing on your thyroid function. You're free to continue managing your thyroid condition the same as you would if you weren't fasting.

Your Sleeping Patterns

Another side effect of Intermittent Fasting is that your normal sleeping patterns get disrupted. You'll find you have difficulty getting to sleep, staying asleep, and waking up feeling refreshed. This is especially the case if your shorter eating window is a big change from any previous meal time habits. While this is unfortunate and makes you feel tired, it actually clears up after about a week or so. That's because your circadian rhythm needs some time to adapt, just like when you deal with jet lag by crossing time zones.

Like the hormones, this also has to do with brain function. Your brain needs hours of sleep in order to perform all its processes when you wake back up, like reading, learning, memorizing, coming up with new ideas, remembering, thinking, and everything else. After you get used to Intermittent Fasting, you'll find that it helps to make you feel more calm and grounded throughout the day, with less nervousness, tension, anxiety, and stress.

Remember that your body adapts very well to Intermittent Fasting because this was such a necessary survival mechanism centuries ago.

None of these side effects are guaranteed for every woman who tries Intermittent Fasting! But if you do have them, now you know why. You're advised to keep your fasting to a minimum of every two or three days.

Some women pick up fasting with no problem, have no issue with it, and don't experience any of these symptoms at all. Everybody is different.

Positive Body Changes!

When you incorporate Intermittent Fasting into your life, you are going to see some wonderful and positive body changes!

As you've read in this chapter, there is an amazing wealth of scientific information out there as to how your body processes every nutrient you eat. So, exactly what kinds of foods are you going to be eating in between your times fasting?

I'm so glad you asked, since I love to talk about food. Who doesn't, right? That is exactly what we'll discuss in the next chapter.

Chapter 4:
Eating as Part of Intermittent Fasting

As you can see, Intermittent Fasting has so much to do with what you're eating during the day! In this chapter, I want to talk about what exactly you will be eating, your calories, and ways to make eating fun on this diet.

We came up with an amazing mantra in the last chapter about how to eat in between your fasting times.

Eat Larger, Healthier Meals Less Often

Yep, we're going to kick a lot of eating myths right to the curb. Myths about three meals a day, myths about small portion sizes, myths about eating the wrong things, myths about eating the right things, and myths about calories or calorie counting.

Intermittent Fasting is about four huge eating concepts:

~Eating in a small, specific window of time, within 8 hours or less

~Eating healthy meals that contain proteins, carbohydrates, and fats

~Eating fewer meals, usually two or even one a day instead of three a day plus snacks

~Eating to meet your calorie requirements

We'll go over each one of these in-depth in this chapter, starting with calories!

Calories and Intermittent Fasting

Calories were discovered by Nicolas Clement in 1824 as a unit of heat energy. But nowadays, we think of calories as the basic unit of how food will burn as fuel in your body.

What is your recommended daily calorie intake? In other words, how many calories does your particular body require to maintain that balance your own body is looking for?

To find out how many calories you need to eat, just go to an online calorie calculator. You will fill in your information, including your age, your current weight, and your height. You will also provide your current level of weekly exercise. This is to determine whether you're burning more calories than you currently take in.

You know calories because they're listed on food packages or you can Google them, right? Most of us who've been dieting for some time actually have a pretty firm grasp of how many calories are in fruits, vegetables, meats, dairy, and grains. No biggie there.

For women, the average amount of calories is about 1800 per day. That depends on many factors, but it is a nice round number and a good place to start. That's your base level.

Did you know that you can actually eat more calories and lose more weight just by adding Intermittent Fasting?

Whoa! That's pretty life changing.

Let's take an average 1800 calorie day. You split up your calories throughout the day, eating several hundred for breakfast, several hundred for lunch, some for an afternoon snack, several hundred for dinner, and the rest in the evening. Even though you're proud of yourself for getting in a lower calorie diet, you're running into several problems:

~Lower calorie foods just don't fill you up and satisfy your hunger, so you feel pretty ravenous throughout the day.

~You're not eating a lot of calories, but you are eating frequently.

You're not eating too many calories, but you are eating too often!

On the Intermittent Fasting eating plan, you can eat up to 2000 calories per day in a shorter eating window – and lose weight faster!

Yes, it's absolutely true.

How is that even possible?

It's because of how your body processes the nutrients from your foods. We talked a lot about nutrients back in Chapter 3, and the three main nutrients are fats, proteins, and carbohydrates.

Your body actually prefers if you consume lots of these nutrients in one sitting. We're talking 1000 calories in one meal. In our modern era, it's almost unheard of to try and eat so much in one meal unless you're trying to gain weight. But you split up all of those 2000 calories into just two meals a day, at 1000 calories each, and get rid of all snacking in between. You eat those two meals within a 6-hour window. Then, you fast the rest of the time. You'd actually feel incredibly full longer, you'd meet all of your calorie requirements, and you'd lose more weight because you ate enough fuel and nutrients to not just sustain yourself during the fast, but increase the rate at which that fat from your adipose cells are burned.

Pretty incredible, huh?

It's still a good idea to get your base calories for your body type and fitness level, just to give yourself a baseline number. But you can safely stick to a 2000 calorie diet on the Intermittent Fasting plan – and still drop those pounds.

Losing weight is NOT just about cutting calories! That is the standard conventional wisdom, but we have much more scientific evidence to back up our claims and provide you with all the information you need.

Cutting calories is also NOT the only possible way to lose weight. If that were true, then every single person who ever ate fewer calories would automatically start dropping the pounds. That would be a magical weight loss fantasy indeed! But that's not what is happening.

Thankfully, more and more women are waking up to the fact that simply cutting your calories doesn't work for weight loss. This is one of the many reasons why Intermittent Fasting and the Keto Diet have suddenly jumped in popularity.

You are free to eat up to 2000 calories a day, and still lose weight.

Hallelujah!

Okay, So What Should I Be Eating?

Well, just because you can eat 2000 calories per day doesn't mean those calories should come from junk. We want to eat healthy! Intermittent Fasting is all about eating windows, which I'll talk about below. But before we get there, let's talk about exactly what kinds of foods you should be eating. Remember that you can eat up to 2000 calories, so we're not dealing with restrictive diets.

We're dealing with healthy, balanced diets. Diets that contain healthy amounts of those three awesome nutrients we were talking about earlier:

~Carbohydrates (starches and sugars)

~Proteins

~Fats

So, a healthy diet would include healthy amounts of each of those three nutrients. While you have a lot of leeway here, the percentages that I have personally used in the past are:

~Carbohydrates – 40% of daily total calories

~Proteins – 30% of daily total calories

~Fats – 30% of daily total fats

This means that on a 2000 calorie diet, you'd be eating 800 calories of healthy carbohydrates, 600 calories of healthy proteins, and 600 calories of healthy fats each day.

You have a lot of flexibility here – an entire grocery store's worth, actually!

There are a number of diets out there to choose from, like Atkins, the Paleo Diet, or the Ketogenic Diet, which is discussed in depth in Chapter 10. You could even go vegetarian or vegan if you like! Again, Intermittent Fasting is more about when you're eating your calories, not so much exactly what those calories should be.

However, common sense tells us that calories from fried foods aren't the same as calories from organic chicken. Eating 2000 calories in larger meals is not a carte blanche excuse to just go crazy. Healthy is key.

There are good and bad carbohydrates, good and bad proteins, and good and bad fats. You want to stay away from the bad kinds and choose the good kinds.

Speaking of grocery stores, let's go shopping and take a look at each of the food groups to see which foods fall under the healthy category.

Vegetables

The produce section has some wonderful options to get in your healthy carbohydrates. You can't go wrong with leafy greens like Romaine lettuce, fresh baby spinach, and kale. They make a great base to salads. You can also eat onions, tomatoes (although they're a fruit), broccoli, cabbage, cauliflower, celery, cucumbers, green peas, fresh green beans, bell peppers, beets, Brussel sprouts, carrots, squash, zucchini, eggplant, and asparagus. Starchier veggies like potatoes, sweet potatoes / yams, and turnips have higher carbohydrate counts if you're watching those numbers.

Fruits

Many diets, especially the Keto Diet, advocate a very low carbohydrate gram count that doesn't include hardly any fruits. But fruits are high carbohydrate foods with lots of natural fructose, which can convert to glucose and provide great energy for your body. Excellent healthy fruits include apples, oranges, bananas, berries, grapes, pineapple, lemons, limes, and melons. Avocados are popular, too.

Eggs & Dairy

Dairy foods provide proteins, some lactose (milk sugar), and good fats, too. Try to get dairy products either organic or grass-fed, since those are the healthiest and provide you with the best protein sources. Milk, cream, real butter, cottage cheese, cream cheese, plain unsweetened yogurt, goat cheese, and other types of cheeses will give you yummy calories. Whole large eggs are a versatile food that also have plenty of good fats and proteins.

Meat & Fish

It's perfectly fine to get all of your calories from non-meat sources on a vegetarian diet with Intermittent Fasting. But you can also get your proteins from sources like chicken, turkey, beef, ham, high quality bacon, lamb, fish, and seafood like clams, shrimp, scallops, crab, and lobster. Buy good quality meat and fish. They'll provide plenty of proteins and the good kinds of fats to meet your calorie requirements.

Carbs & Grains

The carbohydrate category is one of the more controversial, because those carbohydrates from flours, sugars, and starches convert right to glucose in your body. On the Keto Diet, your carbohydrate count is 25 grams or less. But if you're following an Intermittent Fasting plan with more carbs, then you can increase the count. Don't go overboard in this category, though! You want some good fats and proteins, too. Examples of great carbs that have plenty of fiber and give you long-lasting energy include oats, barley, quinoa, lentils, beans (kidney, cannellini, navy, black beans), brown rice, wild rice, chickpeas, and bran. As for breads, you can get whole wheat, rye, pumpernickel, or sprouted grain. Try to keep your corn, white rice, and white flour consumption to a very small percentage of your carbohydrate intake.

Herbs & Spices

Herbs and spices have their own very low carbohydrate counts because of the plant sugars. They add their own unique and amazing flavors to the above food groups. You can change up cuisines and eat different kinds of dishes. You can find fresh herbs and garlic in the produce section, but you should also stock plenty of dried herbs and spices, too. One fun thing about cooking is getting to try a new herb or spice you're not familiar with. Herbs and spices pack a punch with flavor that excites your taste buds and turn healthy ingredients from blah to blasting.

More Healthy Foods

There are hundreds of other healthy ingredients that you can add to your cupboards, fridge, and freezer. You can try the different types of nuts and seeds. There are many healthy condiments like olive oil, balsamic vinegar, soy sauce, Dijon mustard, low sugar barbecue sauce, full fat mayonnaise, and hot sauce. Black coffee and teas can be mixed with cream. Some Intermittent Fasters stock baking ingredients. It's up to you whether you'd like to have sugars. Remember that they convert to glucose and become stored in your cells.

Treats

Yes, you can have some treats on this diet! Dark chocolate is yummy, and so is a glass of wine. Many ice cream brands are pretty healthy, so look for ones that are just milk, cream, sugar, and natural ingredients. Even pizzas and French fries have healthy versions. Whatever your personal indulgence is, keep note of it. You don't have to write it off completely. Just have a tiny portion of it with as few artificial ingredients as possible, factor in the calories, and only have it occasionally, like once a week. This is not a meal plan about deprivation.

Any Off-Limit Foods?

While it's more important when you eat in between your fasting times, there are certain foods you shouldn't be eating on this diet. That is because they're just plain unhealthy! They are made in a laboratory, so that makes them stuffed with artificial sweeteners, colors, flavors, and preservatives. These chemicals are the bad kinds of carbohydrates, fats, and proteins. They're not all natural straight from the ground or the animal.

Avoid:

~Boxed pastries and baked goods

~Boxed meal kits

~Margarine in any form

~Frozen boxed lunches or dinners

~Canned soups

~Frozen breakfast foods

~Canned meals (Chef Boyardee, etc.)

~Frozen pizza

~Kids' lunch packaged meals

~Grocery store packaged foods

~Pre-packaged sauce mixes

~Dried soup mixes

~Potato chips

~Cheesy crunchy snacks

~Bagged microwave popcorn

~Cheese crackers

~Any packaged salty or cheese snack food

~High sugar coffee drinks from Starbucks or other coffee shops

~Soda, even if it says zero calories

~Energy drinks

~Sports drinks

~Alcohol, unless it's the occasional glass of wine

Most of these are pretty self-explanatory as to why they are on the naughty list. They're packed with nasty ingredients like high fructose corn syrup, trans fats, and manufactured items like partially hydrogenated oil, aspartame, xylitol, and dextrose. Not to mention the ridiculously high amounts of sodium, caffeine, and sugars.

Yuck!

Honestly, anything packed with seventy ingredients you can't pronounce is not good for your wonderful body. Stick to an eating plan that works for you, incorporates at least 90% good, healthy ingredients, and provides you with those amazing carbs, proteins, and good fats.

Your Eating Windows

The Intermittent Fasting plan focuses more on WHEN you eat! We're going to squeeze all of your 2000 calories into a shorter period of time than the average day. Most of us begin eating in the morning, and we don't pay attention to the clock. We might have our last bite or two very late at night.

That's not going to work with Intermittent Fasting. Your diet is not just dependent upon what you put in the grocery cart.

It's about the clock, too.

So, the maximum amount of time you should be eating for weight loss is a 9 hour daily window. A minimum time is about 5 hours, but that's only if you are doing one meal a day (OMAD), which I will discuss in more detail below.

You get a lot of flexibility with choosing how long your eating window is.

Eating Window Examples:

~Eating window of 9 hours, fast for 15 hours, repeat

~Eating window of 8 hours, fast for 16 hours, repeat

~Eating window of 7 hours, fast for 17 hours, repeat

~Eating window of 6 hours, fast for 18 hours, repeat

~Eating window of 5 hours, fast for 19 hours, repeat

You can see that your eating windows and fasting times keep repeating, over and over, on that cycle.

Which one is best for you? I personally have found the shorter eating windows of 6 or 7 hours to be the most effective for weight loss. I am just not hungry in the morning, so my eating window starts at noon and stops at 7:00 pm each day. I eat all of my 2000 calories within that time frame. I eat 30% of my calories at lunch at 12:00 pm noon, and then have a 70% calorie dinner at 5:30 pm. I like to eat a lot at dinner! Once that clock hits 7:00 pm, I stop for the day.

That is how an eating window works.

The 8 Hour Eating Window and the Hunger Hormone

Remember back in Chapter 3 I mentioned the hunger hormone, called ghrelin?

Well, it turns out this hunger hormone lives on its own natural 8 hour eating window every single day of your life.

Ghrelin levels are pretty low even after you wake up, those levels peak at noon, and then those levels steadily decrease throughout the day, corresponding with a smaller peak around 8:00 pm at night. Sound familiar? You are definitely your hungriest at lunch time, throughout the afternoon, and at dinner. Millions of people skip breakfast not necessarily because we're trying to, but because those ghrelin levels are low. We're simply not hungry!

These ghrelin levels also give you the most perfect 8 hour eating window between 12:00 pm and 8:00 pm. Pretty neat, huh? It's like you were biologically designed to have this 8 hour eating window. Your ghrelin hunger hormone levels certainly support it. This is an eating window that works with your body, rather than against it.

The only rule of thumb when it comes to finding the best eating window of time, is that your last meal should occur about two to three hours before bedtime. Eating windows of time last around six hours, which gives you eighteen hours of fasting. So, for example, if you go to bed at 11:00 at night, your six-hour feeding window could be between 3:00 pm and 9:00 pm. That's the latest it could be. This is a perfectly fine Intermittent Fasting eating schedule.

Here are some possible examples:

~Have a full time nine to five job? Try an eating window between 7:00 am and 1:00 pm. Take in most of your calories at breakfast and then the rest at a noon lunch time.

~Work a late shift? Schedule your feeding window between 9:00 am and 3:00 pm, in the middle of the day before your shift starts.

~An early riser? Then your eating window can be between 5:00 am and 11:00 am. You'd take in all of your calories in the morning.

~What about the night owl? Your eating window is shifted to later in the day, starting at 3:00 pm and ending at 11:00 pm. If you have a very late bed time of 1:00 in the morning, this would be a great time for you.

Spend some time looking at your weekly schedule to find the best times that work for you.

Splitting Up Your Calories in the Eating Window

The percentages of calories that you're consuming at each of your meals in your eating window is really important. Consistency is key on the Intermittent Fasting plan, so whatever calorie percentage template you use, please keep repeating it for each of your eating windows.

You get several options here of how many meals you'd like to have. I started out with three meals per day within a 9 hour eating window. That was because I wasn't sure if I would be ravenous with having to fast for the other 15 hours. I also was still locked into the mindset of 'three meals a day is normal.' In fact, I was more used to eating six meals a day, because I ate smaller portion sizes and just grazed all day! That is not a meal plan for weight loss – that's a meal plan for weight gain!

So, on the Intermittent Fasting eating plan, you can cut back from three meals a day to just two or even try one meal a day (OMAD).

Sample Templates: 8 Hour Eating Window with Three Meals a Day

This is an excellent beginning sample template for starting out with Intermittent Fasting and getting used to the whole process. It's also perfect for women who are in college taking classes, women who work full time, and women who would like smaller portions rather than eating two larger meals per day. For the times, you can definitely move your eating window to be earlier in the day or later in the day.

Your schedule could look like this:

~Meal 1 is between 12:00 pm and 2:00 pm, when you eat 30% of your calories.

~Meal 2 is between 3:00 pm and 5:00 pm and that is when you eat another 30% of your calories.

~Meal 3 is between 6:00 pm and finishes before 8:00 pm, when you consume 40% of your calories.

This template is really balanced.

You could still follow this template with the exact same number of meals, but only the calorie percentages are switched.

~Meal 1 is between 12:00 pm and 2:00 pm, when you eat 30% of your calories.

~Meal 2 is between 3:00 pm and 5:00 pm and that is when you eat another 20% of your calories.

~Meal 3 is between 6:00 pm and finishes before 8:00 pm, when you consume 50% of your calories.

For busy moms with families when dinner is the biggest meal of the day, this template would be ideal. You would have a large dinner with your family in the evening.

Do you work a later shift or have more time earlier in the day to get in most of your calories? If you are a breakfast lover within your 8 hour eating window, then check out the following meal plan template:

~Meal 1 is between 6:00 am and 8:00 am, when you eat 60% of your calories.

~Meal 2 is between 10:00 am and 11:00 am and that is when you eat another 15% of your calories.

~Meal 3 is between 12:00 pm and finishes before 2:00 pm, when you consume 25% of your calories.

Notice that I also moved the eating window up to starting at 6:00 am instead of 12:00 pm? That is the power of eating windows. You can start them at any time you want. The important thing is to stop all food consumption at the end of the eating window and fast until the eating window starts again tomorrow. You can have water, but that's it. No other calories!

All of these meal percentages were for 8 hours. You can certainly shorten the time frame down to 7 hours and use the same percentages.

Sample Templates: 8 Hour Eating Window with Two Meals a Day

Now that you've gotten an idea of what exactly Intermittent Fasting looks like on a three meal a day plan, we are going to stick with the same eating window time of 8 hours. But this time, we will reduce your meals from three to two. This also changes the calorie percentage. You will consume more calories per sitting. Many of us skip breakfast, so eating just two meals a day comes naturally! I've eaten two meals a day for years, and I feel so much fuller and so much better. Think back to 30,000 years ago. Our ancestors could probably only eat once or twice a day, because the rest of the time was needed for actually hunting the food! It is very natural to eat just two meals a day.

For an 8 hour eating window, your schedule could look like this:

~Meal 1 is between 12:00 pm and 2:00 pm, when you eat 30% of your calories.

~Meal 2 is between 6:00 pm and finishes before 8:00 pm, when you consume 70% of your calories.

I call this the Dinner Lover template! If you love to have a sit down supper with your family in the evening, then you would try this template. Keep in mind that a two meal a day plan does not provide any calories for snacking in between meals. You are consuming all of your calories within two meals, and in two meals only.

What about if you need to or want to eat the vast majority of your calories earlier in the day? You could definitely do that in your 8 hour eating window.

~Meal 1 is between 12:00 pm and 2:00 pm, when you eat 70% of your calories.

~Meal 2 is between 6:00 pm and finishes before 8:00 pm, when you consume 30% of your calories.

Don't forget that you could move your eating window earlier, to consume that 70% of your calories starting at six in the morning if that fits in your schedule. If you do that, you would plan your second meal so that it stops at 2:00 pm.

Sample Template: 6 Hour Eating Window with Two Meals a Day

The longer you fast, the more weight you will lose. So, many women love to increase their fasting times, shortening their eating windows to 6 hours instead of the usual 8. You will gain more and more benefits from fasting from longer periods of time. In a 6 hour eating window, you really only have enough time to enjoy two large meals. You can split up the calorie percentages to have it be either top heavy (most of your calories in the beginning) or bottom heavy (most of your calories at the end).

Check out this sample 6 hour eating window with two meals:

~Meal 1 is between 12:00 pm and 2:00 pm, when you eat 70% of your calories.

~Meal 2 is between 4:00 pm and finishes before 6:00 pm, when you consume 30% of your calories.

This is the top heavy version, where you have a huge lunch. Would you rather have a huge dinner? That is great, too! You could reverse the calorie percentage for your 6 hours:

~Meal 1 is between 12:00 pm and 2:00 pm, when you eat 30% of your calories.

~Meal 2 is between 4:00 pm and finishes before 6:00 pm, when you consume 70% of your calories.

As with the 8 hour eating windows above, you can move this eating window to be earlier in the day or later in the day. Just make sure that you are finishing your meals before the end of the 6 hour eating window and that you are having your last bite at least two hours before bed time.

One Meal a Day Intermittent Fasting - OMAD

Now, we get to the pinnacle of the amazingness of Intermittent Fasting, and that is consuming just one meal a day (OMAD for short). Yes, that is right – you would eat all 2000 calories in a single sitting. But that also means it is your only meal that day, and you are not to eat any other calories and have no other foods until you break your fast tomorrow to eat your 2000 calories again. So, it is more difficult than simply reducing meals or playing around with calorie percentages like in the above sample template meal plans.

However, there are some awesome perks to eating OMAD:

~You can eat your OMAD whenever you want – have fun picking the time that works best for you

~Forget planning multiple meals – now you can just find about 1 hour each day in which to eat. That's it!

~You only have to cook once a day, for just one huge meal

~You will feel like an Olympic athlete consuming that many calories in a single sitting

~You will greatly simplify your grocery shopping and meal planning

~After you have eaten your OMAD, you don't have to think about food the rest of the day

With OMAD, the ratio is 23:1. So, you are fasting for about twenty-three hours and only eating for one hour. Eating just once a day is extraordinarily beneficial for women who have very busy lives, who travel frequently, who are stay at home moms, who have a full college course load, who are high performance athletes, and for any woman who would love to just eat all their calories in one huge sitting. It's like having your own personal banquet each day!

There are some tips to eating OMAD, because of how your body processes those key nutrients. If you are doing OMAD specifically for weight loss purposes, you would want to try and reduce your carbohydrate count down to about 15% of your daily calories or less. That is because the less glucose you consume, the fewer grams turn into glycogen and the more fat is used as fuel from your adipose cells. You might also want to try the full Keto Diet, with is extremely low carb counts that kick your body into ketosis much faster and use up that stored fat for ketones. Read about the Keto Diet in Chapter 10.

The other tip to eating OMAD is to ease into it slowly. This is not an eating plan about deprivation. 2000 calories is a lot to consume in one sitting! But the other twenty three hours of fasting is a long time. So, go easy on yourself. You are used to eating multiple meals a day, so there is an issue about changing your mindset, too.

The third tip? Keep that huge meal stuffed full of good, healthy nutrients. When eating just once a day, you could be tempted to just binge on one type of food. But you want to be sure you're getting enough variety. This is not an eating plan that will work if it becomes boring! Change up your flavors with each of your single meals. You will deeply enjoy eating and fall in love with this meal plan.

Difficult fasts don't equal better results if you're feeling deprived. You don't get bonus points for starvation or deprivation. You just feel deprived.

So, find an eating window and a meal plan that works for you!

Eating by the Calendar and the Clock

Your eating window is as unique to your lifestyle as you are! That's because it starts with your weekly calendar and how you can find the best time each day in which to eat your meals. In the 30 Day Challenge chapter, you will actually get to sample multiple types of Intermittent Fasting schedules. It's more about when you eat, as long as what you eat is healthy.

Chapter 5:
Dos and Don'ts for Intermittent Fasting

How are you doing so far? Lots of nutrition information, meal planning information, eating window information, and calorie information! It's a lot to take in. But just like starting a new class in school, those are the basics to Intermittent Fasting. They are a solid foundation that will help support your entire weight loss and health journey!

But, as you spend each day alternating between your eating windows and your times for Intermittent Fasting, you will also run into some obstacles here and there. That's why I've set up an entire list of 'Dos' and 'Don'ts' to help guide you in this chapter.

These are just a bunch of really helpful tips, and they provide the true keys to success when you decide to embark on this Intermittent Fasting lifestyle. How do you know what will bring you the results you need? How do you know what pitfalls to avoid, including many mistakes that I made! Here's your first don't: don't skip this chapter! Learn from me and do it the right way.

DO: Ease Into Your Intermittent Fasting

Breathe with me. Just breathe. In ... and out. Good!

It's easy to get overwhelmed when you start a new dieting plan.

Intermittent Fasting is not a race! I know you want to lose the weight quickly and have that goal number on the scale.

But please don't let impatience or eagerness cause you to bite off more than you can chew. Intermittent Fasting is going to give you the maximum success if you not only ease into it, but take your time to plan everything out. It's not just a diet; it's an entire lifestyle change. And it's only a lifestyle change that will benefit you if it's not rushed, if it really works the best with your schedule, and if you decide to put in the committed effort to make it work for you.

Patience is not just a virtue – it's also the key to losing lots of weight with Intermittent Fasting! Plan for your eating windows, prepare yourself for the hours of fasting, and spend as much time as you need finding the perfect eating window of time and the perfect meal plan schedule for you. Only then will you see the weight drop off ... and you'll be a happier woman on each step of the journey, too.

DO: Stay Hydrated While Fasting

While you are abstaining from all calorie consumption during fasting, you want to make sure you stay well hydrated. In one of the below tips, I mention to keep a food diary. As part of your food diary, track how much water you are drinking as well. It's good to get in your eight glasses per day. Many of us don't realize that we're not drinking as much water as we should!

Water has so many other benefits, too. Your body is mostly made up of water, so every single cell needs it for optimum functions. To flavor plain water while you're Intermittently fasting, try adding a squeeze of lemon or a few berries to infuse a fruity flavor.

DO: Rest As Much As You Can

When was the last time you woke up refreshed from an amazing night's rest? It is one of the best feelings to be well rested. While you're Intermittent Fasting, your body is working hard to repair cells, help you lose weight, digest the healthy foods you've been eating, and perform all of its different functions – and it's best when your body is able to do these at night, while you are asleep.

So, get as much rest as you can while on the Intermittent Fasting plan. Sometimes making sure to sleep enough is even harder than going to the gym! But your mental alertness levels, your mood, your overall health, and your best weight will all be improved by a proper night's rest. How much sleep you need is completely individual! I need at least eight hours, while my husband seems to function well on only six or seven. Every person is different. Just make sure you're getting the optimum amount of rest for you.

As a bonus, the more you sleep, the faster those hours of fasting go by!

DO: Listen to Your Hunger Signals

In the previous couple of chapters, I mentioned the ghrelin hunger hormone a few times. Some women have a more difficult time fasting because this hormone has not adjusted to your fasting schedule yet. Give it time to ease into your shorter eating windows. If you have to start with a longer eating window, like ten hours, that is perfectly fine. Pay attention to your own ghrelin levels and when your hunger is the most ravenous.

It's a good idea to plan your eating windows around those peak hunger hormone times. This is all about working with your body's natural processes. Pay attention to your inner hunger signals. That is when you can eat your largest meal, with the highest calorie percentage. Then you can custom tailor your meal plan around that largest meal.

What about when you're hungry during times of fasting? You don't have to suffer through on sheer willpower. Within your first month or two of fasting, especially while you are in the 'testing the schedule' phase, you are allowed to have a very tiny amount of calories to see you through. This is especially helpful at night, if you're trying to fall asleep on an empty stomach. You can have a very small amount of nuts, one slice of cheese, half of a banana, half a glass of milk, or one other reduced serving of a food. This is not meant to satisfy your hunger, but to ease it. Only see these calories as a crutch.

As you spend more and more weeks Intermittent Fasting, the fasting will get easier. It also helps to eat plenty of protein, fiber-rich carbohydrates, and good, healthy fats to keep your tummy satiated between meals and eating windows.

DO: Meal Plan

Yes, yes, and more yes! You read about the sample meal plan templates in the previous chapter, so hopefully by now you're thinking about which one will fit best into your lifestyle.

Once you've decided on your first eating window meal plan template that works for your schedule, then start to calculate your individual calorie count requirements. From there, you can search online or in cookbooks for healthy recipes. Build healthy meals from the suggested ingredients list in Chapter 4. Then plan out your meals each week in your day planner or calendar.

Meal planning can be a pain. I mean, it's one more thing to do in my busy week! Meal planning takes a bit of time up front, but it saves you enormous amounts of time throughout the rest of your week. Since Intermittent Fasting is all about the clock, meal planning becomes that much more pertinent. It should be an essential part of your week. I'll talk more about Intermittent Fasting preparations in Chapter 7. It's so important!

DO: Keep a Food Diary

This is also really important. Every woman's eating and fasting journey is going to be unique, so there's no way you can compare mine to yours. I can give you plenty of tips, but I can't walk the road for you! A food diary not only keeps you accountable, but it also provides the most helpful and useful road map for the daily changes in your body.

Use a food diary to track:

~Your daily eating windows

~Your daily fasting times

~Your calorie percentages for each meal

~What you eat each day and the calorie counts

~How many glasses of water you drink each day

~How you feel each day

~What you weigh each week

~What ingredients to shop for

~And more!

While I am old school and like to keep my food diary in a paper planner, you can certainly find an app for your smartphone that works just as well. Make it personalized to your lifestyle, and you'll not only use it more, but it will be that much more helpful to you in the long run.

I've kept food diaries for years. It's amazing to look back and see not just how many pounds I've lost, but the daily steps it took to lose those pounds. Every weight loss journey takes weeks and months of time. A food diary helps you see all that time at a glance.

DON'T: Force Yourself to Fast

Fasting is not the same as starving or food deprivation. Far from it! Fasting is more similar to a resting period between meals. You are helping your body's digestive processes work better by fasting. You are not starving your body of nutrients or kicking your cells into more harmful things, like diabetic ketoacidosis, muscle deprivation, organ failure, bone weakening, or anything else. Those are serious conditions.

But have no fear. So, don't force yourself to fast, either. You don't have to fast to be healthy and lose weight. It's just one of the most natural ways to do so! If you are having difficulty with a particular fasting schedule or eating window, you can either cut back and only fast a few days a week instead of each day, or change your eating windows. To force your body to fast would only add more problems in the long run, so it's definitely not worth it!

On the other hand, if you enjoy fasting and you love both your eating window and your schedule, then by all means keep on doing what you're doing! If it isn't broke, don't fix it. Continue on the same path, use your food diary to monitor how you feel, and enjoy watching those pounds gradually and pretty effortlessly drop away. You'll also look and feel a whole lot better, too.

DON'T: Wing It

Yes, it's true. This is not an eating plan where you just wing it and hope for the best! It requires a lot of planning, consistency, and the ability to stick to the confines of the Intermittent Fasting schedule. That is why above I made the strong suggestion of meal planning. This is a diet where you are also watching the clock, so it's that important to make sure you're following a consistent routine. You need to be accountable to yourself.

So, once you have nailed down your ideal eating window / fasting schedule ratio, then please stick with it. Watch the clock, eat your meals on time, finish eating before the end of your eating window, plan for your one, two, or three meals per day, and just wash, rinse, repeat until you reach your weight loss goals.

This is definitely the kind of eating plan that works best with a consistent weekly schedule, but you can definitely do it if your life is crazy, too! That type of lifestyle just takes more planning.

If you are also following the Ketogenic Diet, which I'll chat about in Chapter 10, you shouldn't wing it with your Macros, either! Also, that is not a cheat day diet, where you can just jump off the wagon. It could knock you out of ketosis. So, when you're combining both the Keto Diet and Intermittent Fasting, you want to put in your due diligence to stick with it.

DON'T: Go This Alone

Even if you're doing Intermittent Fasting with a male partner or friend, his experience might not give you an accurate picture of this type of eating plan. So, find other women who are doing Intermittent Fasting! There are thousands of helpful gals out there who've had success, who've also gone through what you're going through, and they want to help you! Your feelings about how you live in your body each day are important. No one will understand that better than a fellow woman going through the same thing. She can also help hold you accountable to sticking to this!

So, in that light, don't try to go it alone with this Intermittent Fasting. Join an online forum or a dieting group in the real world. Talk about what you're going through. You might want to share your food diary, share your thoughts, and share your journey every step of the way. A blog could be a helpful place to just air your thoughts and experience with this. Any kind of outlet that helps you sort through your relationships between eating, fasting, and feelings is going to be so incredibly beneficial. You'll not just feel better when you finally achieve your weight loss goals. You will also have a better day to day experience!

DON'T: Be Afraid to Tweak Your Fasting Schedule

Life happens! It's okay to tweak and change your Intermittent Fasting schedule. If you become pregnant, are planning a huge life event like a wedding, have to take care of elderly parents, change jobs, move locations, suffer an emergency situation, or other big circumstances, that can certainly throw a wrench into your fasting schedule. There are just some times when being on an eating plan is too much work and one more thing to throw into an already overloaded schedule.

That's perfectly fine. Just give yourself the space and time to tweak your fasting schedule. You can move your eating window up by a few hours, go back to three meals instead of two (or drop down to two meals instead of three), or other changes. Just keep listening to your body, paying attention to your hunger hormones, and you'll still gain the benefits of fasting.

This has happened to me. I was on a two meal a day 6 hour fasting schedule, when I had an emergency situation happen in my husband's family. Our whole life seemed to stop and was put on hold for a month. My fasting schedule suddenly didn't work anymore, since our lives were so topsy turvy. I went down to OMAD and ate it in the morning, so I could attend and help out for the rest of the day without worrying about getting myself lunch or dinner. I could just be there in the hospital. After everything had smoothed over and I'd gone back to normal, I spent a few days tweaking my fasting schedule and increasing back to the 6 hour eating window.

So, if something happens to you, just know that your fasting schedule is not set in stone. It's there for you to customize depending on how your life is going.

Do the Intermittent Fasting Your Way

Every woman's life is different. We all have our own lives with our families, friends, work, home, hobbies, and other things that fill up our time. Intermittent Fasting is the most flexible eating plan you'll ever be on, so take advantage of it and make it work for you. These tips in this chapter prevent most of the issues with Intermittent Fasting for women and are helpful signposts along the way as you navigate through your own dieting journey.

Oh, and one last do for you: show off your progress! Take those awesome 'before' and 'after' pictures that are so fun to see and share on social media. Take a picture of yourself each month and watch those pounds come off.

You'll have so much success just by using Intermittent Fasting!

Chapter 6:
Being a Mom on Intermittent Fasting

Hi there fellow moms!

Now, this is a chapter you won't see in a lot of Intermittent Fasting books, especially those written by men.

But for me to not include my husband and children on my Intermittent Fasting journey would be so incredibly difficult, that I wouldn't be able to do it! I'd be doomed from the start. In fact, a huge part of my own personal success has happened because I took my family into account, too.

So, this is a book that is for the mothers who want to lose weight. If you don't have children, you can certainly get a lot of great tips from this chapter, too. I'm a mom who has committed to this lifestyle and not only changed my body for myself, but changed it in a better way that benefits my entire family. I feel better, and a happy mom equals a happier home life. That's for sure!

The moms who commit to this and make a change for both yourselves and your children are super happy. You can read many success stories online.

You want to be happier for your sons and daughters, too. They mean the absolute world to you, and it's the easiest thing in the world to put them first. First, meaning above yourself.

But what about your own health? You want to live for your kids. You want to change the future of what you see for yourself. You've probably already tried different things to lose the weight, but the failures have piled up.

How about doing something different this time? You will feel better trying Intermittent Fasting than any other kind of dieting or eating or fitness plan. Let's pick a diet you can sustain for the rest of your life. That also means starting slow with workouts, too.

So, whether you're trying to lose weight after giving birth, want to get back to your former size before children, or just want to have more energy, vitality, and a better overall outlook with your husband and kids, I'm here to help you succeed on Intermittent Fasting!

Balance vs. Busy Life

If every woman who's heard the term "work-life balance" was paid a dollar, we'd all be millionaires! It seems that no matter how hard we try, we can't be super moms and have it all for longer than a few months before becoming exhausted and burning out. You have to look out for your kids, help out around the house, feed those hungry mouths, have your own full-time job (or multiple jobs), and somehow have enough time to follow an eating plan, let alone have success on it?

No wonder so many of us have been stuck in 'yo-yo' dieting purgatory for years.

Intermittent Fasting has so many extraordinary benefits for even the busiest lifestyle. In fact, the busier my life gets, the easier it becomes for me to fast and lose weight. Yep, you read that right:

The busier your life gets, the easier Intermittent Fasting becomes.

What kind of magical statement is that? I'm not surprised you're skeptical.

The reason Intermittent Fasting is the ultimate eating plan for your busy lifestyle is because you customize it to work around all that hectic craziness.

As you read in Chapter 4, there are a bunch of sample meal plan templates for you to choose from. Each of them will work beautifully if you just follow them every day. Each of them is a path towards losing weight.

The only thing you have to do is pick one of those templates and stick to it. You can also definitely tweak and customize your schedule if life throws you a curveball. I talked more about that in the last chapter.

Doing Intermittent Fasting is actually easier than if you weren't fasting! Do you have a certain busy time of day where it's just impossible to prep and cook a meal? Then add that time of day to your fasting period, and set up your eating windows around it.

For me, this is the morning. I need to wake my kids up, get them ready for school, and make sure they have a packed lunch. I already meal planned to make sure that their breakfasts are ready to go, but it's just too much to also try and eat something for myself at the same time. They finish breakfast quickly and get out the door. I break my fast with my first meal of the day two hours after they leave, which is plenty of time to prep and cook that meal. I've grown used to this schedule, so I'm not even hungry in the morning until that meal time comes around.

Pretty simple. It also takes all the guesswork out of trying to balance your life.

Life is full of ups and downs, but even more so when you have kids. Embrace the ups and downs. Add Intermittent Fasting and your eating windows to your life. They will help you work with your crazy schedule – and before you know it, the weight will start to drop off.

Planning Mom Equals Happy Mom

As a mom, do you know what really helps both my sanity and my weight loss?

Having a plan. Specifically, my meal plan each week. I actually plan out two meal plans into one large meal plan: my own Intermittent Fasting meal plan, and my kids' meals. I don't cook entirely separate meals from my kids, but I make sure that they have their own healthy things that they're eating. I include what they want each week as part of their meal plan, too.

When I'm done meal planning for my kids, I post their meals on the fridge each week, so that they can see it. Do I still get asked what's for dinner? Yep, sometimes! My kids can forget. But I pretty much always have the answer right there on my fridge.

In addition to just writing down what we're having for meals in my family, I also include grocery shopping lists. That makes it super easy to shop for exactly what I need for those meals!

I'm a mom who plans, and boy, am I a happy mom because of it!

So, for my fellow moms out there, I urge you to plan out not just your own Intermittent Fasting meals, but those for your children as well.

Meal planning is definitely one weekly task of mine that I actually look forward to! That is because it saves so much time in the long run. I know that the hour or two that it takes to sit down with your kids on a weekend afternoon to plan out the meals and shopping lists for ingredients is time that will not just be saved, but will also pay me back in pounds of weight loss.

Remember that:

A Meal Plan Saves Time and Pays You Back in Weight Loss!

The same goes for you, too!

Eating for You, Eating for Kids!

What kinds of recipes are going to go on your meal plans for the adults and the kids in the house?

Children like to eat simpler, blander meals than adults do. Their taste buds are more sensitive, and they like to eat things that have lots of sugars, salts, and creamy or crunchy textures. They will gladly reach for the junk food! Kid fave food choices include ice cream, pizza, burgers and fries, hot dogs, popcorn, potato chips, chicken tenders with dipping sauce, macaroni and cheese, spaghetti with meatballs, and candy. While you can find some healthy versions of these foods, they are definitely not going to help you with your weight loss goals. It's time for more greens and more proteins!

When you're putting together your meal plan, don't forget to slowly but steadily shift away from unhealthy recipes and choose healthier ones instead. Also, try to include common ingredients in both meal plans that will appeal to both kid and adult palates.

What kinds of foods are great for both kids and you?

~All those wonderful healthy vegetables listed back in Chapter 4. You can roast vegetables, put them into soups, add them to a wrap, stir-fry them, make salads, or puree them to serve with a main entrée course of meat or fish.

~Fruits are also delicious for both kids and adults. Apples, bananas, oranges, berries, and sliced melon are usual favorites.

~Fill your kids' bellies with a good amount of proteins for growing muscles, healthy brain function, and energy. You'll both enjoy chicken, turkey, ham, pork, beef, fish, and different kinds of seafood.

~Kids love cheese, and moms do, too! Look for yummy full fat cheeses and other healthy dairy products.

~Kids can really enjoy fiber rich carbohydrates, like whole grain bread, oatmeal, canned beans, barley, and other options.

~Both you and your kids can include nuts and seeds in your diets.

Search online for more kid friendly and all natural breakfast, lunch, and dinner options. As with the adult options, stay away from packaged foods and anything stuffed with chemicals, artificial flavors, colors, and especially sweeteners. Kids' smaller bodies are especially susceptible to spikes in blood sugar, which you will definitely see as they go crazy from a sugar rush!

I don't know about your kids, but mine love eating the same ten or fifteen meal choices over and over. They don't seem to get bored! I introduce new foods to them every couple of weeks, just for a bit of variety. It also seems like, since they have a lot of input into their own meal plans, that they understand the whole process of grocery shopping, cooking, and eating a lot more. They are interested in it, and they actually help me out quite a bit.

These are wonderful life lessons to help teach your kids. Your weight loss and health journey is a part of their lives, too. Maybe they will grow up understanding the essential links between diets, fitness, health, and weight loss. That is a valuable thing to learn!

Exercising and Intermittent Fasting as a Mom

When you're a busy mom with a packed schedule, exercising seems a like a whole lot of extra work that you just wouldn't be able to fit in. Unless you involve your kids with you, it takes time away from them, too. Who is going to watch them while you work out at the gym?

It is also both natural and normal to be intimidated, scared, or otherwise averse to going to the gym.

I know I was.

I had plenty of really good reasons why I wasn't getting any exercise, but most of them had to do with fear. I was afraid of going to the gym and looking like an idiot, sweating profusely in front of others. Maybe that is a silly fear, but it kept me from exercising – and it kept me from losing the weight I wanted to.

So, I just started out with Intermittent Fasting, eating windows, and choosing healthier ingredients. I put exercising on the back burner. After a month, I'd gotten used to fasting, I was much more comfortable with my eating windows, I'd already lost ten pounds, and I finally felt like it was time to add exercise to the mix. I wanted to up my weight loss, too!

But I really had no idea where or how to start. My favorite exercise has always been walking. I love to walk everywhere. Would walking be exercise enough to shed pounds while fasting? I had no idea, but it was a question I wanted to answer with a yes!

I began a daily walking routine of just fifteen minutes. That is once around the block of my neighborhood. After a few days, I increased it to thirty minutes by walking twice around the block. I kept up that routine for several weeks, and I was shocked at my results. I mean, all I was doing was walking twice around the block! But that was when the weight really started to drop off. My body also felt better, I felt lighter inside, and my legs felt better, too.

That's when I finally bit the bullet and bought a gym membership. I was very scared the first few times! I just tentatively started on the treadmill and walked for thirty minutes, increasing my incline. But you know what? After that first week, it definitely got easier. The days passed, and I enjoyed the treadmill. It took me about a month to get used to just going to the gym as part of my daily routine. My kids sometimes joined me, too! They loved using the equipment.

Gradually, I went from the treadmill to using other machines at the gym, like the stationary bikes and rowing machines. Then, I started using kettlebells as part of weight training.

Nowadays, I'm a much more confident gym goer! I work out for thirty minutes each day, using a combination of different machines and the kettlebells. I still get a bit trepidatious, but then I remind myself of all the pounds of weight I've lost because I added exercise to my Intermittent Fasting. I also look better than I have in years. I feel stronger, leaner, and fitter.

I hope my story can give you some idea of how you can add exercise to your eating plan, too!

Just start with a simple walking routine. If you can't get to the gym, then you can buy a treadmill. Just fifteen minutes of walking today, to start. Even with kids, you can do this!

Build a Support System

Any kind of diet plan while you're a mom can feel like its own upward hill climb when you're living in a house full of people who aren't doing what you're doing.

So, it's absolutely essential that you have a support system. You need girlfriends and relatives and other Intermittent Fasting women to talk to! You need to be able to rant about a difficult day, vent about the rocky patches, and just share what you're feeling and what you're thinking with like-minded, compassionate souls.

The women who have experienced the most successful weight loss journeys have had support to do it. You can find this support system online or through reaching out to other women in your community. These women will help cheer you on, hold you accountable, and you can support their goals, too.

Don't forget to include yourself in your support system, too. Support your own weight loss goals and fitness goals. Ask for help around the house when you need it. Teach your kids how to be there with you along the way as you get healthier.

The more support you have, the more successful you will be!

Your Body is For You

What's great about Intermittent Fasting, is that I have done so much of the nutrition research for you! If you'd like, you can go back to Chapter 3 and read all about the actual science behind what is going on in your body. And yes, all of that stuff is true even after you have had children! Your body doesn't magically stop processing nutrients the way it did before you got pregnant. So, that's good news! That means this will work.

While you may be inspired to get healthy for your husband or your children, ultimately, they don't live inside your body. They don't know how you feel each day, they are different people with their own trials and tribulations, and they aren't going to take the same journey as you.

Just like any journey, this Intermittent Fasting one begins with the proper preparations. That is what you will read about in the next chapter!

Chapter 7:
Easy Guide to Starting Intermittent Fasting

Let's say you want to go on a two tropical vacation to the Caribbean. You can't wait to have fun in the sun. Would you leave the house without packing for your trip? Of course not! You need your bathing suit, sunscreen, beach towels, clothes, makeup, and other stuff to take with you. I also never go on vacation without at least having a packing list!

Think of this chapter as similar to a travel packing list. We are going to go over absolutely everything you need to know to prepare yourself for Intermittent Fasting. The next chapter is my favorite in the book and has your 30 Day Challenge. But before we get started, it's time to get ready!

Prepping for the Journey

I want you to go through each step of preparing for your Intermittent Fasting 30 Day Challenge. Take as much time as you need, but the whole process shouldn't take longer than a week or so. It's okay to fit this into your busy schedule!

By now, you have read through many aspects of Intermittent Fasting, and you are probably starting to realize this is definitely an eating plan and fasting plan that has as much to do with mental preparations as any other endeavor. You are going to get your mind ready to go as much as anything physical that you'll do. Your mindset should be one of openness, curiosity, excitement, and be flexible enough to handle any and all challenges that come your way.

Got it?

Okay, good. Now, we will move on to a few of your personal numbers that I want you to calculate before we go about finding recipes and meals.

Setting an Eating Window:

If you have not done so already, go back to Chapter 4 and read over the sample meal plan and fasting plan templates. Choose the amount of time that you'd like for your eating window. You will also pick whether you'd like to eat one, two, or three meals per day. Meals usually last about one to two hours. Then calculate when your eating window will begin and when it will end.

Write all of this information below:

My Eating Window Lasts _____ Hours

Eating Window Start Time: _____ am / pm

Eating Window End Time: _____ am / pm

Number of Meals Per Day: _____ meals

Meal #1 Time: _____ am / pm to _____ am / pm

Meal #2 Time: _____ am / pm to _____ am / pm

Meal #3 Time: _____ am / pm to _____ am / pm

Okay, great! Remember that this information is flexible, and you can change it at any point. This will be personalized to you. I like to write my eating window information on the first page of my food diary. That helps me remember it while I am going about my day.

Setting Your Calorie Requirements:

Next, is to figure out your calorie requirements. You can find that in an online calorie calculator. Then, we will divvy up those calories amongst your meals. Refer back to the sample meal plan templates in Chapter 4 to get a better idea of what percentages work best with either one meal, two meals, or three meals. Those percentages should all add up to 100%.

Write all of this information below:

Calories Per Day: _____

Meal #1 is _____ % of my daily calories = _____ calories

Meal #2 is _____ % of my daily calories = _____ calories

Meal #3 is _____ % of my daily calories = _____ calories

Great! Now you know exactly how many calories to consume in each meal. Those calories are going to be a mixture of the healthy food ingredients you read about in Chapter 4 as well.

Setting Goals:

You have your baseline eating window times, your meal plan times, and your calorie counts. Now it's time to set your goals. You get thirty days' worth of Intermittent Fasting days in the next chapter to get through. So, what are your weight loss goals for the next four weeks? I break my weight loss goals down into smaller five pound or ten pound milestones. That way, I don't get overwhelmed by lots of weight to lose. I just focus on losing the next five pounds.

I also want you to think about your exercise goals, too. That is largely about setting up a gym going or home exercise routine of various activities that will help shed the pounds and strengthen your body at the same time.

Fill in your goals in the spaces below:

Overall Weight Loss Goal: _____ pounds

Current Weight: _____ pounds

Goal Weight: _____ pounds

First Weight Loss Milestone: _____ pounds lost in _____ weeks

Second Weight Loss Milestone: _____ pounds lost in _____ weeks

Third Weight Loss Milestone: _____ pounds lost in _____ weeks

Exercise Goal: _____ minutes per day and _____ days per week

Exercise Start Time: _____ am / pm

Exercise End Time: _____ am / pm

Exercise Routine: _____

I include my goals right on the front page of my food diary. They help keep me motivated, and it's amazing to see how far I've come just by using Intermittent Fasting on a regular basis.

With your numbers prepped, ready to go, and written down in an app or food diary or place where you can see them pretty much each day, you know where you start. The journey begins with finding out where you are today – and these numbers tell you that in great detail.

Finding Recipes and Meals

Here is the fun part of any eating plan – finding recipes and meal ideas to go into your meal plan! Whether you are eating one, two, or three meals a day, you have your calorie counts for each of those meals. Now, it's just a matter of finding delicious foods and flavors that will satisfy your nutritional requirements.

There are just certain types of foods that we love to have with our meals each day. If you think of your meals in terms of categories, that makes it easier. Check out my ideas below:

Meal 1: Breakfast

Whether you're eating two or three meals per day, typical breakfast food options are really popular. These are actually my absolute favorite foods. I could eat breakfast for dinner, too! Breakfast foods are also popular with kids, if you're a mom. Here are some breakfast food options you will love to have to help you when you literally break your fast.

~Smoothies, especially ones with an avocado or coconut milk base to give you plenty of good fats to start your day. Stick in a handful of fresh baby spinach or kale to sneak veggies into your diet.

~Egg dishes, like baked eggs, scrambled eggs, frittatas, quiche, and omelets stuffed with veggies and cheeses.

~Meat options include bacon, sausage, or even steak.

~Breakfast bowls are popular, so have fun searching for ones that contain healthy ingredients like vegetables and different herbs or spices.

~For breakfast beverages, you can have milk, low sugar orange juice, low sugar fruit juice like strawberry banana, coffee, or tea. Bulletproof coffee, which has been enhanced with good fats like butter, is a popular and tasty option, too.

Meal 2: Lunch

Most of us eat lunch at work, and you only get an hour at the most. So, I often take last night's dinner as leftovers for lunch! My favorite lunch options are either hearty and filling soups or salads with plenty of toppings. If you are eating just two meals a day and lunch is your biggest meal, you might want to check out the dinner ideas and have supper for lunch instead. Here are other lunch options:

~Home made soups, usually made in the crockpot to make them easier. Popular ones include chicken noodle, beef stew, chunky minestrone, and hearty vegetable. Kids really love soup, too.

~A hearty salad that starts with a base of greens like Romaine lettuce, baby spinach, and chopped kale. Top with more sliced fresh veggies like mushrooms, bell pepper, tomato, red onion, carrots, cucumbers, or celery. Then add pre-cooked chicken, beef, turkey, or ham. I also add a handful of cheese like Feta or shredded cheddar, and a sprinkling of crunchy extras like seeds and nuts. For dressing, I like many different flavors to add variety. Buy all natural salad dressings that have an olive oil or dairy base, limited chemicals, and no added sugars.

~Healthy sandwiches with whole grain bread, mayo or mustard or pesto, and then plenty of cheese, proteins like chicken or ham or bacon, and lots of veggies. Serve alongside pickles or fresh vegetables with hummus to dip.

~Lunch beverages include milk, green or fruit or herbal teas, low sugar fruit juice, or ice water with lemon.

Meal 3: Dinner

Dinners, also known as your last meal or third meal, usually feature the majority of your daily calories. They are built around one major hearty protein choice like chicken, beef, pork, ham, fish, or seafood. This protein is usually served alongside a cooked or roasted vegetable like carrots, onions, potatoes, broccoli, cauliflower, or mushrooms. You can also expand your palate by choosing foods from around the world for dinner. What else could be for dinner?

~Find healthy recipes for your family's favorite ten dinner options.

~Try a new dinner option every two weeks. Pick a country with different flavors and try to incorporate that dish into the menu. Popular options include French food, Thai food, Indian food, Greek food, Spanish food, and Japanese food.

~Substitute brown rice, wild rice, barley, quinoa, or whole wheat for rice, corn, and white flour carbohydrates.

~Dinner beverage options are ice water with lemon, milk, or the occasional glass of wine.

These meal options are just here to give you an idea of the different things you could eat for your one, two, or three meals each day. On a two meal a day plan, you could have breakfast and dinner, with no lunch foods, lunch and dinner with no breakfast foods, or breakfast and lunch with no dinner foods. This eating plan really is customizable to your life!

It's more about when you eat. As long as you choose healthy, natural ingredients like those above, you will do just fine!

Creating Your Weekly Meal Plan

Meal planning is made a lot easier when you have all the meal ideas and recipes from the last step ready to go. I have a folder on my computer that contains all of my recipes for each meal. That makes it a lot easier to just add those to my weekly meal plan and much easier to create grocery lists, too.

I thought I'd share my weekly meal plan template with you. I eat two meals a day. I type this up on the computer, then print it out and put it on the fridge each week for my kids to see it, too. That way, everyone knows what we're eating when!

Date: _____

Meal 1 at 12:00 pm.

      Recipe: _____

      Calories: _____

Meal 2 at 4:00 pm.

      Recipe: _____

      Calories: _____

Kids' Dinner: _____

Feel free to customize this sample daily meal plan template! I have a 6 hour eating window and eat just two meals a day. Are you eating three meals a day instead? Then add the extra lines for the third meal. Are you eating just one meal a day? Then include all the recipes and calories for the foods in that one meal. You can play around with this basic idea to really make your meal plan your own.

I also have kids, so they get their own dinner option. That way, I know what to make for them, if I have to make something separately. Usually, though, I eat what they're eating! I do make healthy versions of foods, so both Mom and the kids are happy and healthy.

The Kitchen Equipment You'll Need

Do you need to purchase anything fancy and special to make delicious Intermittent Fasting meals?

Not unless you really want to! I am able to make all kinds of delicious items using basic kitchen equipment like my 12" cast iron skillet, several saucepans in different sizes, three large cookie sheets with a cooling rack, a high-speed blender for making smoothies, a large crock pot or slow cooker, and a food processor. Instant Pots have recently become popular, so you could get one in a larger family size to cut down the amount of time to make many crock pot dishes.

Whichever recipes you've decided to make that go with your calorie counts and your personal tastes, they can usually be made using the above equipment. It helps to have everything washed, cleaned, and ready to go as part of your overall Intermittent Fasting preparations!

Creating a Grocery List

Meal planning makes creating grocery lists so easy! With your seven days' worth of meals in front of you, you can quickly rifle through the fridge, cupboards, and freezer to see what you need to stock up on.

I created a grocery list template on my computer that has all the food categories of items to restock. I tend to buy a lot of pantry and cupboard items in bulk that have a long shelf life. Then, I spend about an hour each week purchasing the fresher ingredients for that week's meals. After doing this for several weeks, you'll find that grocery shopping is a breeze. You will also discover that you keep purchasing the same items over and over. That is a good thing! It means you're committed to only buying healthier ingredients, and that you're not tempted to put something in your cart that could slow down your weight loss.

Remember Gin's Golden Rule of Grocery Shopping for Weight Loss:

If It Doesn't Go in the Cart, it Can't Go in Your House and it Won't Get Eaten!

Weight loss begins at the grocery store, lovely ladies. Stick to your healthy shopping list, and you will stick to your weight loss goals.

Here are the grocery store categories that correspond to most grocery stores:

Produce & Fresh Herbs:

~In the produce section is where you'll get your fresh vegetables and fruits for the week.

~You can buy fresh garlic and fresh herbs in this section as well.

Meat & Seafood:

~Buy the best quality proteins, fish, and seafoods that you can afford, since they won't have as many harmful ingredients.

~You can purchase meats in bulk, portion it out into plastic bags, and store them in the freezer.

Eggs & Dairy:

~In the cheese section at your store, you can find all the cheeses to add to your grocery cart.

~The milk, eggs, butter, yogurt, and other dairy items are often kept in a different part of the store. I replenish my dairy items all the time, since we eat them so much in my house!

Nuts, Seeds, and Baking:

~I buy nuts and seeds in bulk and store them in airtight containers in my pantry cupboards.

~Shop in the baking aisle for your baking ingredients. I like to bake some home made healthy treats like crackers, granola bars, and healthy cookies.

Herbs, Spices, and Condiments:

~Dried herbs (fresh herbs go in the produce category) and dried spices. I keep a fully stocked herb and spice cabinet. I sometimes visit different ethnic markets to find herbs and spices that are inexpensive, unusual, or distinctive.

~Condiments include oils, vinegars, barbecue sauce, soy sauce, mayo, ketchup, and similar. Check labels, since these are packaged goods and frequently have too many harmful chemicals.

Frozen Section:

~The frozen section has a lot of packaged foods, so read your labels carefully here.

~I buy frozen vegetables, some frozen meats, and occasionally a small tub of healthy frozen yogurt.

Other:

~Coffee, wine, tea, and other items that don't fit into any other categories go in this part of my grocery list.

You can customize this list to fit your own stores. I sometimes create separate grocery lists for buying items online, at different markets, and at different stores.

Cooking Your Meals

Fasting for at least fourteen hours per day gives you some extra time to prep and cook the recipes for the meals on your meal plan. It's sometimes the prep work that takes the most time, so I cut down on that and save time by slicing vegetables and storing them in sealed plastic bags in the fridge. I also like to pre cook favorite foods like chicken breasts, bacon, and beef ahead of time. That way, it's easy to combine those ingredients with others and make dishes.

While you are planning out your meals for your eating windows, you might want to include the cooking times. It's all about preparing yourself for the 30 Day Intermittent Fasting Challenge to come!

Preparing for Fasting

What about your actual fasting times in between meals? What kind of preparations should you put in place for those?

Water and Hydration

Prepare for your fast by drinking plenty of water! You are also allowed to have water, perhaps with some fresh lemon slices, to sip on throughout the fast, too. It might help to stock up on plastic water bottles, a plastic water jug for the fridge, and any other items you will need to remind yourself to keep drinking water.

Having Tiny Snacks

Throughout your first few weeks trying Intermittent Fasting, it helps to have a few small snacks available during those fasting periods. It helps to get your body over the 'hump' of changing your metabolism, adjusting to fasting, and encouraging your cells to seek fat from your adipose cells instead of relying on incoming glucose. These tiny snacks should be no more than 80 calories at the absolute most. By the third week, your body will have grown used to Intermittent Fasting, and you will no longer need to have any calories for those periods of time between your eating windows.

Longer Fasting

What about preparing for longer fasting periods? In the 30 Day Challenge, I include a 24 hour fasting day. For those longer fasts, you would want to eat all of your calories like normal the day before the fast, but abstain from exercising that day, the day of the fast, and the day after as well. You would also want to break your fast with a well balanced and good protein rich meal that has plenty of essential vitamins and nutrients. I'll talk more about that with the longer fasting in the next chapter.

Support System

If you read the chapter about being a mom on Intermittent Fasting, you read about putting a support system in place. This is another preparation to do before you start fasting. If you haven't already, find an Intermittent Fasting community online and reach out to other women who are doing this along with you! They can give you real life examples of what they're going through and answer more specific questions about their journeys. It's very helpful!

Fasting Activities

Before you begin Intermittent Fasting, you might want to think about what kinds of activities you would do during your fasting periods. I was surprised to discover that, since I had cut out a meal, I now had that free time. If you already have a busy lifestyle, this is definitely one of the perks! You would simply be able to fill the new time with more things in your schedule. But it does help to add more activities into your life during your fasting times.

Tracking Your Progress

As part of preparing for Intermittent Fasting, you want to find the ideal tracking method for you that will be a helpful resource for collecting and writing down your own 'data' about this weight loss plan. You want to treat yourself to a nice paper food diary or find a great app for your smartphone that can be a resource to help you.

There are so many parts of Intermittent Fasting to track! Here are just a few ideas you could put into the diary:

~Track your weight loss goals

~Track how you feel and what you're experiencing each day of Intermittent Fasting

~Track what you eat and the calorie counts

~Track the water that you're drinking each day

~Track the exercise routine that you have chosen

~Track any new recipes you find

~Track how a new healthy recipe tasted

~Track grocery shopping

I am in love with tracking! I do like data and numbers. They give me a much clearer picture of what is really going on in my weight loss journey than just my own memories and experiences of it.

Tracking is also a way of honoring your commitment to changing your body for the better. You are putting how you feel in your body first! Your record of this experience is just confirmation of how much strength and courage it takes to not just try something new, but to believe that it will work. That is inspirational!

Tomorrow is When We Begin

Okay, you are now completely prepped and ready to begin the 30 Day Challenge of Intermittent Fasting! You have accomplished a lot, and you haven't even begun your first day of fasting yet!

Let's see what you did:

~You have found your first eating window in which to begin

~You've decided how many meals you'll eat

~You looked up your daily calorie requirements

~You divvied up those calories amongst your meals

~You set your weight loss and exercise goals

~You found recipes and ideas for eating

~You made an amazing meal plan based on those recipes

~You also created grocery lists that have healthy ingredients

~You stocked your kitchen with equipment to make your meals

~You have what you need to see you through your fasts – water bottle, snacks, etc.

~You have a tracking method, either a food diary or an app

That is a lot, but you will need it all throughout the next thirty days.

The final thing to do to before starting tomorrow? Take a selfie! Make sure that you take a picture of yourself as you are now. Are you ready to work towards changing your body and having a whole new you after fasting?

Then let's get started.

Chapter 8:
Intermittent Fasting 30 Day Challenge

Last chapter gave you so many tools to prepare you for this challenge! I hope you have all of them in place, because today is the day to get started.

We have laid the groundwork for a successful first month spent Intermittent Fasting.

This is the nuts and bolts chapter, that shows you exactly what a life of steady Intermittent Fasting looks like. This is a 30 Day Challenge that you can begin at any time, when it is most convenient for you. I encourage you to just read this entire chapter from start to finish before you begin. That will give you an overall view of the whole thing.

Then, you just start on Day One!

Fasting Foundation for Success

I personally designed this 30 Day Challenge for a complete beginning to start on Day One. We're going to split this into three different sections of 10 days each:

~Beginner – 10 days of skipped meals, getting used to Intermittent Fasting, and finding the perfect eating window that works for you.

~Intermediate – 10 days of locking in your eating window, then getting your recommended calories in that eating window.

~Advanced – 10 days of more advanced Intermittent Fasting, including your first 24-hour fast, as well as a 48-hour fast.

What's awesome about these three levels is that after you've completed the 30 Day Challenge, you can certainly go back to the Beginner or Intermediate section – and stay there for months at a time. Intermittent Fasting is meant to be a lifelong eating and fasting plan, so it's safe for you to do that.

As a quick note, just keep in mind that this guide is just one way to incorporate Intermittent Fasting into your life. As always with this way of eating, you are more than welcome to change it and customize it to suit your needs. If you're confident in your ability to start with small eating windows and you'll be fine with that, you're more than welcome to skip ahead to the Intermediate section.

It's not so much where you start – it's the fact that you will start! I also want you to enjoy yourself throughout your time spent Intermittent Fasting. This is an eating plan you can stick with for your whole life! So, it's worth it to take that extra step to enjoy each day of it.

Ready to get started? Let's go to the Beginner section.

Beginner Intermittent Fasting

Day 1

Day 1 of our 30 Day Intermittent Fasting Challenge has begun. Today is when you are going to ease slowly into this and try to eat your first day within a large eating window. If your ultimate goal is to eat within six hours, that is too much change too fast. It could possibly derail your plans and goals in the long run. You are advised to start out with an eating window of ten hours, which would give you a fasting time of fourteen hours. The ratio is 10:14. I also suggest you start out with a three meal a day schedule, instead of two meals. There will be plenty of time to drop back to eating fewer meals. But the slower you begin this, the more time your body will have to adjust.

You can start your 10 hour eating window at any time you like and whichever time works best in your schedule. Let's say you start it at 8:00 in the morning. Counting forward ten hours, that would give you until 6:00 pm at the latest to eat all of your calories for the day. When 6:00 pm rolls around, cease all food until tomorrow except for water.

If you have not already done so, today would also be the ideal time to plan out your meals for the rest of the week, find recipes using healthy ingredients, and go for a grocery shop to stock up your kitchen. For those who already have an exercise routine, it's perfectly fine to continue that today. But if you don't, that's okay, too! We'll include exercise after you've gotten used to the fasting schedule.

At the end of the day, take out your food diary. Track and record your eating window, what you ate today, and your overall experience. You will do this each day, and it's an excellent habit that will help you lose more weight than you've dreamed of!

Day 2

Great, you got through Day 1! How did that go? Hopefully you had a good experience with it. Today is when you are going to repeat your 10 hour eating window / 14 hour fasting routine. Do it at the same time you did the 10 hours yesterday. Then gently break your fast by eating a healthy meal. Continue on your meal plan until the end of your 10 hour eating window, then stop and begin the fasting part of the cycle.

Did you have any difficulty sustaining a 14 hour fast between yesterday and today? Since we're starting with a larger eating window, fourteen hours is a much shorter time to fast. Track and record in your food diary what you ate today and how your first official Intermittent Fasting period went.

Day 3

If Day 2 was fine and you enjoyed it, then repeat your 10 hour eating window / 14 hour fasting time today. As the days go by, it becomes easier and easier to get into the routine of eating and fasting. How are you doing with your calorie counting, cooking, and eating your meals? Eating all of your daily calorie requirements within a 10 hour window is pretty doable. Are you hungry at all during the fasting periods? Many of us are used to snacking or nibbling on something whenever we feel like it. So, to deliberately fast can seem a little odd at first. Keep pursuing it.

Track and record what you ate today and how your fasting is going for you.

Day 4

Another repeat day of the 10 hour eating window / 14 hour fasting period. Follow your meal plan, eat your meals at the correct times, and eat all of your calories within the 10 hour window.

As your body gets used to fasting, your hunger might start to drop off a bit. You'll also notice during the day when you're the hungriest. Remember that your ghrelin hunger hormones are at their highest around noon, and then taper off as you get closer to 8:00 pm at night. As long as you're eating healthy and following your recipes to cook good meals, you're on the right track.

Track and record what you ate today and how your fasting is going. Are you struggling with hunger or other minor health issues like headaches? Or, has your body adapted well to this so far? Write down your answer.

Day 5

Another repeat day of the 10 hour eating window / 14 hour fasting period. Keep following the meal plan, having your meals at appropriate times, eating all your calories before the end of the eating window, and ceasing all calorie consumption after the ten hour window ends.

Throughout the first five days of this challenge is when you have the most flexibility to tweak your eating window times. For example, you might have discovered that starting your eating window early in the day doesn't work, because you're ravenously hungry during your fasting times. So, you can move it to later in the day. You have options.

Track and record what you ate today and how the fasting is going.

Day 6

Now that you've been Intermittent Fasting for five days, you should have locked in a good eating window by this time. That's the time that works best for you, your family, and your schedule, too. You've also started to grow used to watching the clock, eating meals at certain times, and tracking your calories. I personally love the routine-ness of this diet, where I can just eat at the same times each day. You might like it, too!

As for today, we are going to do one final 10 hour eating window / 14 hour fasting time before we start shortening our eating window tomorrow. After today, you really shouldn't play around with moving your eating window earlier or later. Consistency and routine will be the best for weight loss! Track and record what you ate today.

Day 7

Congrats – you got to the end of your first week of 10 hour Intermittent Fasting! That wasn't so bad, was it? Once you get a hang of the routine, it becomes easier to incorporate it into your lifestyle. Are you doing well during the fasting times? Drinking plenty of water? If you needed to supplement one of the 14 hour periods with a tiny snack, that's perfectly fine.

Today is when you will drop your eating times back one hour. That means your eating window has shortened from 10 hours to 9 hours. Adjust your meal times accordingly. You are welcome to still eat the three meals, or to try just two larger meals per day if you're feeling like you've got the hang of this. You will also increase your fasting time from 14 hours to 15 hours. So, if your eating window for six days has ended at 6:00 pm at night, it now ends at 5:00 pm.

Track and record what you ate today and your new eating window of 9 hours.

Day 8

Day 8's meal times and 9-hour eating window is a repeat from yesterday. You fasted for 15 hours between yesterday and today, so you're starting to push your body a little bit more than just fasting for 14 hours. Drink water, get some rest, and just concentrate on eating all of your calories within the 9 hours. It seems like a lot of time, but it goes by quickly! Every woman I know, including myself, is a busy gal.

Day 8 is also an excellent time to readjust your meal plan, find new recipes for the next week, and go shopping for those ingredients to restock your kitchen.

Track and record what you ate today, your new eating window, and your calories.

Day 9

The 9 hour eating window repeats again today. Eat your meals at their adjusted times. You fasted 15 hours between yesterday and today. You have been Intermittent Fasting for over a week now. If you would like to begin an exercise routine while still in this first ten-day beginner part of the challenge, then today would be the perfect time to do it. Don't push yourself too much. Just increase your heart rate doing an exercise for about 15 to 20 minutes.

Track and record what you ate today, your fasting experience, and the exercise you've started doing.

Day 10

Today is the final day of the beginner section of this 30 Day Challenge. You started out with a 10 hour eating window, dropped back to 9 hours, increased your fasting, learned how to time meals and eat them within your windows, and perhaps also tried some exercising, too.

For today, you can continue on your 9 hour eating window / 15 hour fasting times. It's the final day of this schedule, since we're going to drop back one more hour tomorrow. Continue with your light exercise regimen, too.

Today would be a great time to weigh yourself. Have you lost any weight yet? A healthy weight loss schedule is up to two pounds per week. The combination of healthy eating and Intermittent Fasting really does wonders for your body. If you haven't lost any weight, not to fear. Your body is still adjusting.

Track and record your meals, your meal times, your exercise, and your experience during the first 10 days of this challenge!

Intermediate Intermittent Fasting

Day 11

This intermediate section is all about both reducing your eating windows and reducing your meals from three down to two, plus getting used to longer fasts and keeping up an exercise regimen, too. Since your body is adjusting to a fasting schedule, don't overdo it on your workouts. Start out with light exercise for about 20 minutes a day, then gently increase as the days go by.

Today, you're going to drop back from a 9 hour eating window to an 8 hour eating window. You'll still eat your three meals today, but you might need to adjust the times. You can also adjust the calorie percentages, like the different meal plan templates in Chapter 4. Adjust your meal plan as well. How is your new eating window time? It it is working out, great! After fasting for ten days, your body does start to change!

Track and record your new eating window, meal times, what you ate, your exercise, and your fasting experience.

Day 12

The 8 hour eating window / 16 hour fasting time is one of the most popular Intermittent Fasting schedules. It's especially great for women, since you get a lot of calories in a short period of time, but your body doesn't start to operate like it's a time of true scarcity.

Repeat your 8 hour eating window today. You fasted for 16 hours between yesterday and today. Eat your meals at their scheduled times.

Track and record what you ate and any exercise, too.

Day 13

Day 13 is just a repeat of yesterday: eating for 8 hours and fasting for 16 hours. As a general reminder, get plenty of water during fasting periods. You can increase your exercise up to 30 minutes if you want, but not if you are feeling weak or struggling with this eating routine. Allow your body plenty of time to adjust.

Track and record what you eat, how you feel, and any exercise.

Day 14

Congrats – you've reached the end of your second week Intermittent Fasting! You went from a 9-hour eating window to an 8-hour eating window, and are now fasting for 16 hours within each 24-hour cycle. That's extra hours your body spends pulling fuel sources from existing fat cells rather than any incoming nutrients.

It's time to assess the week. How did you do on increasing your Intermittent Fasting? Was it easy to adjust to 8 hours of eating? Have you been tracking everything each day? Weigh yourself today as well – and take a picture. How is your weight loss going?

Today, you will continue on your 8 hour eating window, just like yesterday. Eat your meals at their scheduled time. By now, you are really getting the hang of Intermittent Fasting. Track and record everything, too.

Day 15

Day 15 starts with an even smaller eating window – this one is just 7 hours. That means you'll be fasting for 17 hours within each 24 hour cycle. As you drop one more hour from eating, readjust both your meal plan and your meal times, too. We'll repeat this for several days, so make sure it's a time you're comfortable with. Get plenty of water during fasting periods. You can do your exercise today, too, if you want.

Dropping from 8 hours down to 7 hours started producing much more dramatic weight loss results for me. That result might be typical for you as well. Track and record your new eating window, your new meal times, and how you're doing. As a brief reminder, you have flexibility with your new eating windows, too.

Day 16

Today is a repeat of yesterday, with your 7 hours of eating and 17 hours of fasting. You fasted for the longest period of yet between yesterday and today, so how did that go? Slowly reintroduce your exercising again today, if you gave yourself a day off yesterday.

Track and record what you ate today.

Day 17

Today is the last day of the 7 hour eating window / 17 hour fasting times, so enjoy it! We're going to drop down to just a 6 hour eating window tomorrow. If you want to do anything to prepare for that shorter eating window, then do it today. Those preparations might include changing your meal times, cutting down from three meals to two, or even trying the one meal a day (OMAD) fasting.

Within your 7 hour eating window today, get all of your calories in before the time is up. Track and record everything that you ate, what you experienced, and any other notes.

Day 18

We're going to drop one more hour off of our Intermittent Fasting schedule today and go down to the 6 hour eating window / 18 hour fasting time. Together with the 8 hour eating window, this is the most common schedule for Intermittent Fasters. Those who do like this schedule usually eat just two meals a day, because the 6 hour time frame is so short. If you do that, then you will need to adjust your meal plan, your calorie percentages, and your meal times accordingly. Check out the two meal a day sample templates in Chapter 4 for exactly how to do this.

Is it okay to stick with an 8 hour or 7 hour eating window instead? Absolutely. Only go down to 6 hours if you feel comfortable with it. This eating window produces great results. You're encouraged to at least try it! Especially when you combine it with exercise. The weight starts to come off faster and faster.

So, eat your meals at your new meal times. Then track and record what you ate and when.

Day 19

We're going to stick with the 6 hour eating window / 18 hour fasting schedule today. How did last night's 18 hour fast go? Were you very hungry when you got up today, or has your body adjusted to fasting? Make any tweaks or changes if necessary. It's also okay to take a break from fasting if you're not feeling well.

However, if you are doing well, then I encourage you to also keep up with your exercise program. Don't forget to track and record what you ate at your meal times.

Day 20

So, you got through the second phase of Intermittent Fasting! You started out with an 8 hour eating window, then dropped down to 7, and are now at just 6 hours per day, with 18 hours of straight fasting. That's quite an accomplishment. You've probably also dropped down to just two meals a day and increased your calorie percentages for those meals. All those extra hours are when your body is using fat sources from your cells as energy, rather than relying on new foods that you're eating. Oh, and when you've added an exercise regimen to it, that is a recipe for success.

It's time to assess the past ten days. How have you been doing? Weigh yourself to see if you've lost more weight. You will start to feel big changes in your body.

In the next ten days, we will go into more advanced fasting, including a 24-hour fast and eating just OMAD (one meal a day).

As for today, just continue with your 6 hour eating window / 18 hour fasting. Track and record what you ate today, too.

Advanced Intermittent Fasting

Day 21

You are going to continue with your 6 hour eating window / 18 hour fasting schedule today. Also, you will want to read over the next ten days and prepare your meal plan accordingly for the 24-hour fast on Day 23 and the OMAD (one meal a day) days as well. After you have prepared your meal plan, today would be the ideal time to create your grocery list and shop for the ingredients you'll need.

As for today, just track and record what you ate, when your mealtimes are, and any exercise routine.

Day 22

Today is all about preparing for tomorrow's 24 hour fast. It's imperative that you make sure to eat all of your calories within your 6 hour window today. Also, abstain from exercising today, tomorrow, and on Day 24, to give your muscles a chance to fully rest. Eat your regular 6 hour eating window today, and begin your fast at the normal time.

Day 23

Today is your first 24 hour Intermittent Fasting day! Count 24 hours from the end of yesterday's eating window. Don't eat any calories throughout the entire time of fasting. For example, if your 6-hour eating window ended at 6:00 pm yesterday, you're not to eat anything until 6:00 pm today.

During your fast, you're allowed to have water. Don't exercise other than a very light walk if you want to do so.

When you do break your fast, do so gently. Eat a meal that has a good healthy protein and mineral rich foods like dark greens, avocados, nuts, and olives. Don't worry about eating your entire calorie percentage for the day. Just stop all eating about two hours before bed-time.

Track and record your 24-hour fast experience, including the meal to break your fast.

Day 24

How did yesterday's fast go? Today, you will return to the normal 6 hour eating window at the exact same times you had it on Day 22. Eat your normal calories like you would on any other day, and eat your meals at the same times as Day 22. Hydrate yourself with plenty of water, since that will also help flush out toxins and get your skin glowing. Help your body refuel from the fast by eating healthy today. Don't worry about getting any exercise today. You can if you want to!

Track and record your meals today.

Day 25

Today, you will repeat your regular 6 hour eating window / 18 hour fasting time. Eat the same number of meals at the same times that you were eating on Day 21. Also today, you will add back in the exercise routine that you have been on. Try for 30 minutes to get your heart rate up. You can do any exercise that you want.

Track and record your meals, the times, and your exercise.

Day 26

Tomorrow is when we are going to try OMAD (one meal a day), so today is about preparing for that. Eat your normal 6 hour eating window with the normal meal times, add exercise, track what you eat, and record your experience. You might want to prepare your singular meal recipes for tomorrow ahead of time.

Day 27

Today is a day to try the advanced fasting technique of OMAD. Choose a 60-minute free period of time today, and eat all of your calories within that 60 minute sitting. It's similar to having a large holiday meal! Don't overstuff yourself, but do get all of your calories in at once. Once the 60 minutes are over, that is when your eating window is done. You will fast until tomorrow, with nothing to consume except water.

Track what you ate today, when, and how you like eating one meal a day. It's definitely an interesting concept to try eating all of your calories just once a day.

Day 28

Repeat your one meal a day from yesterday, eating all of your calories within 60 minutes. Have your single meal at the same time you ate the one meal yesterday, to give your body the complete benefits of a 23-hour fasting time. Don't forget to exercise today, too.

Track and record what you ate and when.

Day 29

Today is a third day to try eating just one meal a day. Do you like it, or do you prefer longer eating windows? Consume all of your daily calories in just one meal. That leaves the rest of the day to fill with all of your activities! You can add in your exercise regimen as well today.

Track and record your one meal, when you ate it, what you had, and how you exercised.

Day 30

Wow, congratulations! You have reached the end of the intense 30 Day Intermittent Fasting Challenge. You got through several days of a short 6 hour eating window, the 24 hour fast on Day 23, and a couple of days of just trying the famous OMAD option! It's been quite the month to start from a 10 hour eating window on Day 1 and then get all the way here. So, congrats again on your success.

Time to weigh yourself again! How much weight have you lost? The successful combination of healthy eating, Intermittent Fasting, and regular exercise can really get you the results that you're looking for. Were you able to hit a goal weight loss? Did you stick with the Intermittent Fasting throughout the month? Even if you just decided to stay with the 8-hour eating window, that's still spending 112 hours a week fasting. It makes such a difference.

No matter how your experience went, you should celebrate! Show off your progress by posting those cool "before" and "after" photos of yourself. Look back over your food diary entries you've kept for the past thirty days. You can share those, too. Post your progress. You never know who you'll inspire – maybe even yourself!

What Works Best For You

The 30 Day Challenge is designed to give you a day by day account of how the Intermittent Fasting eating plans and lifestyle actually fit into a real woman's life.

Where do you take it from here?

Well, this 30 Day Challenge also introduced you to three main types of Intermittent Fasting:

~10, 9, 8, 7, or 6 hour eating windows with the appropriate fasting times

~A longer 24-hour fast that could also be extended up to 36 or even 48 hours

~Eating one meal a day within one hour and fasting the rest of the time

Whichever one you choose is that which works best with your lifestyle and your personal weight loss goals! Some women will do great on just shorter eating windows, and others will want to push themselves in order to try new things. Make this diet yours!

Thank you so much for going on this 30 Day Challenge and stretching your mindset about the link between when you're eating and when you're fasting! Are you ready for even more tips to help you? Then read on to the next chapter.

Chapter 9:
Get the Most Out of Your Intermittent Fasting

Going through the 30 Day Challenge in the previous chapter has certainly given you an amazing foundation for incorporating any type of Intermittent Fasting into your life.

Now, you're going to boost up and derive the most amount of benefits from staying on Intermittent Fasting!

Cleaning Up With Autophagy

We're constantly learning new things about how our body's cells work. Since the dieting industry is such an enormous business, scientists study exactly how nutrients impact our body, how our body processes nutrients, and the link between nutrition and fuel.

One scientist studies a revolutionary cellular process that's the scientific proof behind why Intermittent Fasting works. Japanese cell biologist Yoshinori Ohsumi discovered this process, which is called autophagy. His work was such a breakthrough, he won the 2016 Nobel Prize in Physiology or Medicine.

What's autophagy – and what does it have to do with Intermittent Fasting?

Autophagy comes from the Greek words for "self-devouring." Sounds a bit gruesome, but it is a natural process that your cells go through all the time. In essence, autophagy is cellular spring cleaning. Your cell can actually disassemble its own unnecessary or non-functioning components and recycle those components. Autophagy is activated when you fast, because it is a natural response to the lack of incoming sufficient fuel sources: good fats, proteins, carbohydrates, or sugars.

Cells that perform autophagy are actually removing their own harmful and toxic components. Those components are responsible for so many bad things that happen to your body as you age, including:

~Skin damage, like wrinkles and sagging skin

~Failing eyesight and hearing

~Memory problems

~Loss of energy

~Increasing aches and pains

~A more sluggish metabolism

~Continual weight gain or stagnant weight that won't come off

The cellular components causing all of these issues are just like old junky clutter hanging on inside your cells. But when you are on the Keto Diet and Intermittent Fasting at the same time, your cells get the message that it is time to clean out all that stuff. It's removed as waste or toxins and some parts are recycled to make your cells run better, faster, more efficient, and ultimately healthier for you. The result is that you feel better, look better, and actually slow down the aging process!

But that's the power of autophagy!

You can absolutely trigger autophagy by just fasting on a regular diet that includes higher carbohydrates. But ultimately, it's the combination of Intermittent Fasting and the high fat fuel source on the Ketogenic Diet that really causes your cells to internally clean house!

That's right, ladies – Intermittent Fasting can be a key to slowing down the aging process.

That's because the autophagy from Intermittent Fasting leads to amazing changes at the cellular level.

Speed Up Cell Repair and Regeneration

You are made up of trillions of cells that are continuously going through their life cycles. As time goes on and you age, it's harder to replace cells, repair cells, and regenerate cells. You see it as aging – the loss of energy, being more susceptible to illness, getting creaky joints and arthritis, failing eyesight, hearing loss, and a host of other symptoms.

But you can definitely help turn back the clock by Intermittently Fasting! Especially when combined with a low carb, high (good) fat diet, those processes definitely increase your stem cell production, and stem cells can magically morph into any cell your body needs.

So, those great stem cells can now be used to keep you feeling fit and younger, even down to the cellular level. Just because you can't see it, though, doesn't mean you can't feel it! You definitely will.

Intermittent Fasting Increases HGH

What's HGH (human growth hormone), and why is it a good thing that Intermittent Fasting increases it? Just like other well known hormones such as your estrogen, HGH is a natural substance. It's produced by your pituitary gland and goes straight to your liver for metabolism. HGH is a 'monitoring' hormone that affects many processes in your body, including:

~Muscle and bone growth

~Sugar and fat metabolism

~Body fluids

~Overall body composition

~Cell regeneration and reproduction

~Slowing down aging

~Recovering from both disease and injury

When you don't have enough HGH, then that increases body fat, a lower lean body mass, and even decreased bone mass. In short, it's a good thing when HGH is increased. If you fast for just a 24 hour period, you can potentially increase your HGH production naturally by 1300%. That's plenty to give you all those above benefits all their own.

The HGH production is also triggered by the state of ketosis in your body, which I'll go into detail in the next chapter.

Give Yourself an Energy Boost-Up

Intermittent Fasting does NOT decrease your energy – it actually increases it!

But this is another myth that seems like it should be true. After all, the less we eat, the less energetic we feel, right? But it doesn't make sense from a historical perspective.

Let's say it's 30,000 years ago, and a human hasn't eaten for a single day. If that person's metabolism decreased after just one day of fasting, then they wouldn't have any energy to go out to hunt or gather more food! After a second day, supposedly that person would be even weaker. If energy continually was lost after fasting, our species would not have survived. We needed energy even after fasting to go out and hunt more food.

So, when you're fasting, your metabolism actually goes up. You're burning more stored fat as fuel, and that increases your metabolism. It also means your personal energy supply doesn't run out. As long as you've got plenty of stored fat for your liver to turn into ketones for fuel, your metabolism and energy levels will be just fine!

The Benefits of Exercise

I've touched a bit on exercising in Chapter 6, when talking about how to start with a simple exercise regimen. If you haven't already done so, go back and read that section. It will give you one of the easiest and simplest step by step routines towards incorporating exercise into your lifestyle and combining it with an Intermittent Fasting eating routine.

You can definitely lose weight just by Intermittent Fasting. Simply follow the 30 Day Challenge in the previous chapter to find your ideal eating window amount of time and then fast the rest of the time.

But how would you like to boost up your weight loss into that kind of magical territory that you see online in Instagram pictures, Facebook posts, and magazine stories? You know, the kinds where you see women have lost forty, fifty, sixty, or even a hundred pounds in less than a year?

You will see the common denominator for those women was that they added exercise to their Intermittent Fasting and healthy eating. It really kickstarts your body into a state of significant weight loss!

Would you like to feel not just leaner, but stronger, too? Then I highly suggest adding some mild weight training to your exercise program. I use light kettlebells to help build up my muscles and burn even more fat from my adipose cells. You actually gain muscle when you fast, which is why it's become very popular with men who want to bulk up! But even us girls can have an amazingly toned and well muscled body from combining weight training with Intermittent Fasting.

On the Fast Track

One last benefit that will really turbocharge your Intermittent Fasting? Combining it with the Keto Diet. This is another piece of the weight loss puzzle that thousands of women have had success with.

So, how do you do that? In the next chapter, we'll definitely go in depth into it!

Chapter 10:
The Keto Diet and Intermittent Fasting

By now, you've probably heard of the Ketogenic Diet, nicknamed the Keto Diet for short. This is a very powerful and some say life-changing eating plan. It has some restrictions, so I only recommend it for those women who have really gotten comfortable with your Intermittent Fasting eating windows, eating healthier, and adding your own exercise regimen.

But once you have, then get ready for some miraculous body transformations. The Keto Diet is a diet of extremes. We're going to take the 'balanced diet' idea and completely throw it out!

The Keto Diet is a very high (good) fat, very low carb eating plan. We're talking over 100 grams of fat and less than 30 grams of carbohydrates per day. But it's these kinds of extremes that will get you massive results.

All About Ketosis

The Keto Diet actually changes your body's metabolic processes from one that mostly runs on glucose and glycogen from carbohydrates to one that primarily runs on ketones that come from those fat cells processed in your liver. When you are using ketones as your number one fuel, you're said to be in ketosis.

Ketosis is not a singular bodily function, but rather a series of processes that activate certain cells to stop doing things they were before and start doing new things.

Take a look at the whole process in action:

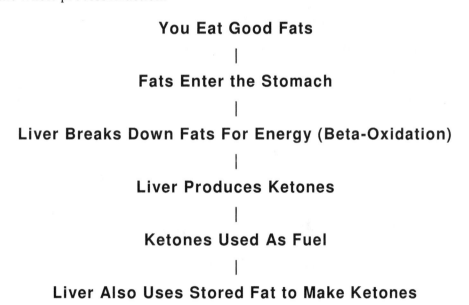

You Eat Good Fats

|

Fats Enter the Stomach

|

Liver Breaks Down Fats For Energy (Beta-Oxidation)

|

Liver Produces Ketones

|

Ketones Used As Fuel

|

Liver Also Uses Stored Fat to Make Ketones

Ketones Used As Fuel

Say, look at that! We're back to using your stored fat as fuel, which is exactly what we want. You want to be in a state of ketosis while you're Intermittently Fasting in order to gain the maximum benefits from both.

How can you tell you're in ketosis? You will need to purchase a special monitor that can test your urine, breath, or blood to be sure. Your reading tells you exactly how many ketones your liver is producing for fuel. These monitors can be purchased online or at a store like Amazon or Walmart.

When you're just starting out on the diet, check for ketosis every day. Once you are in ketosis and you get a feel for that metabolic state in your body, then you can measure your ketones every three or four days. If you eat too many carbohydrate foods, you could knock yourself out of ketosis.

The Keto Macros

Remember how I talked at length about Fats, Proteins, and Carbohydrates back in Chapters 3 and 4? That's because in the Keto Diet world, those three are called Macronutrients. These 'Macros' form the basis for the Keto Diet and are the main thing you track each and every day. On the Keto Diet, calories matter, but not as much as getting the right amount of your Macros.

I suggested back in Chapter 4 that you should eat healthy carbohydrates and grain foods that have a lot of fiber. You can eat up to 30% carbohydrates on some of the meal plan templates.

But your Macros on a Ketogenic Diet are vastly different.

You should be consuming 70% of your daily calories from those good fat sources, 19% of your proteins from natural animal and plant sources, and 5% - 8% of your carbohydrates from healthy sources.

For a woman's Macro requirements, it looks like this:

70% FATS – 19% PROTEINS – 5% CARBOHYDRATES

These are the Macros that you should track, and the proper percentages that you need in order to get into ketosis and stay in that metabolic state.

There are many online Ketogenic Macro calculators, and I encourage you to calculate your exact Macro percentages. They change depending on many factors in your physicality, including your height, weight, current age, and BMI.

As a general guideline when reading about the contents of these Macros on a food label, you should look for these quantities:

167g FATS – 100g PROTEINS – 25g CARBOHYDRATES

That adds up to 292 total grams of food per day. These are the Macros that you should be tracking each day that you're on the Ketogenic Diet.

These are the daily amounts that will kick your body into a ketosis state and start burning massive amounts of stored fat.

Keto Approved Foods

How are you supposed to eat nearly 170 grams of fat per day and yet far less than 30 grams of carbohydrates per day?

By sticking to the Keto Diet approved foods list! Below, I've put together the top 10 most common Ketogenic approved foods. This is an excellent base to get you started on the road towards changing your diet to the Keto one.

Produce:

~Avocados

~Lemons

~Onions

~Green Bell Peppers

~Button Mushrooms

~Romaine Lettuce

~Fresh Spinach

~Kale

~Broccoli

~Cauliflower

Meat & Seafood:

~Steak (Flank and Skirt)

~Ground Beef

~Bacon

~Shrimp

~Cod Fillets

~Boneless Chicken Breasts / Thighs

~Pork Chops

~Salami

~Prosciutto

~Lamb

Eggs & Dairy:

~Eggs

~High Quality Grass-Fed Butter

~Heavy Cream

~Cheddar Cheese

~Mozzarella Cheese

~Parmesan Cheese

~Cream Cheese

~Sour Cream

~Goat Cheese

~Plain Greek Yogurt

Herbs & Spices:

~Salt

~Pepper

~Fresh Garlic Cloves

~Fresh Herbs (parsley, cilantro, dill, etc.)

~Dried Italian Herbs

~Cinnamon

~Thyme

~Chili Powder

~Onion Powder

~Ginger

Oils & Condiments:

~Olive Oil

~Coconut Oil

~Sesame Oil

~Flavored Oils

~Mayonnaise

~Dijon Mustard

~Fish Sauce

~Hot Sauce

~Lemon Juice

~Soy Sauce

Nuts & Seeds:

~Macadamia Nuts

~Pecans

~Walnuts

~Almonds

~Nut Butters

~Pumpkin Seeds

~Sunflower Seeds

~Sesame Seeds

~Ground Flax Seeds

~Chia Seeds

Baking & Broths:

~Almond Flour

~Coconut Flour

~Cocoa Powder

~Baking Powder

~Vanilla Extract

~Sugar-Free Dark Chocolate

~Stevia

~Unsweetened Almond Milk

~Chicken Broth

~Beef Broth

Other:

~MCT Oil

~Green Olives

~Black Coffee

~Black or Green Teas

~Wine

~Dill Pickles

~Canned Tomatoes

~Full Fat Coconut Milk

~Curry Pastes (red, green, yellow)

~Psyllium Husk Powder

Those are the most essential eighty ingredients! There's plenty here to get you started. If you're having trouble meeting such a high fat requirement throughout your eating window, then take a look at the following foods and their high fat percentages:

~Butter – 100% fat

~Olive Oil – 100% fat

~MCT Oil – 100% fat

~Heavy Cream – 95% fat

~Green Olives – 88% fat

~Macadamia Nuts – 88% fat

~Cream Cheese – 88% fat

~Sour Cream – 86% fat

~Coconut Cream – 86% fat

~Walnuts – 84% fat

~Brazil Nuts – 84% fat

~Almond Butter – 79% fat

~Avocado – 77% fat

All of these foods are not only delicious, they can help you meet those fat gram requirements.

Just like in the 30 Day Intermittent Fasting Challenge chapter in this book, you want to be diligent about tracking your Macros each and every day. When you're on the Keto Diet, it's largely about the numbers. Eat as many good fats as you can to hit that high level required, keep your healthy protein intake to a medium level, and slash that carbohydrate number down to one that is very small.

If you have any questions about putting together meals from these ingredients and finding even more ingredients that are Keto approved, I suggest you buy a specific Keto book! That will go into so much more detail.

The Keto Diet and Intermittent Fasting

Why do Intermittent Fasting and the Keto Diet work so well together?

That's because Intermittent Fasting helps your body get into ketosis faster and helps maintain that metabolic state even longer than if you weren't fasting.

What this means, is that you can supercharge the benefits that you get from Intermittent Fasting. You will go into ketosis quickly, and also begin burning the fat from your cells that much sooner.

Going Keto is the ultimate boost up for Intermittent Fasting.

Chapter 11:
Conclusion

Thank you so much for reading all the way down to this chapter! I've had a lot of fun putting this book together for you. I've shared with you my personal story, my own tips and tricks, and I've also shown you that I'm a woman just like you who is looking for the same things as you are:

A healthy, natural, and pretty effortless way

to reach and stay at my goal weight.

When I first stumbled across Intermittent Fasting, I was skeptical and I messed it up. It's only when I really began to take it seriously and find ways to make it work in my real life (house, husband, kids, job, and all!) that I was finally able to reach that goal weight number.

Intermittent Fasting and You

Now it's your turn to take this book with you on your own Intermittent Fasting journey. It won't look like mine, although you'll find my advice so helpful and useful. But your journey will be unique. You may have a different eating window than me. You have a different life than me.

That's why I urge you to take Intermittent Fasting seriously and spend the time to make it your own. See it as a great challenge to incorporate it into your existing life. This isn't an eating plan that's only for celebrities, women in warm climates, women who are really well-off or wealthy, women who do have kids or don't have kids, or any other kind of woman!

This is an eating plan for you. It's so flexible that it fits every woman. Think of it like finding that absolute perfect fitting outfit. It's the perfect color, perfect fabric, perfect fit, it shows off what you want to show off, it conceals what you want to conceal, it's comfortable, and it even has decent pockets! Now that really would be the perfect outfit, right?

Intermittent Fasting is like that. It's great for you, because you make it your own.

A Calendar and a Calculator

If you really want to know the secrets to dieting success, let me point you to two very simple, very inexpensive office tools:

~A calendar

~A calculator

Your Intermittent Fasting lifestyle is intricately connected to your calendar days. It is a schedule as much as it is an eating plan. You schedule your eating windows, you schedule your fasting times, and you schedule in exercising, too.

Eating on the Intermittent Fasting way also requires a calculator to stay within your Macro percentages during your meal times in your eating windows. You are calculating the calories that you eat as well. If you decide to try the Ketogenic Diet in conjunction with Intermittent Fasting, you will be calculating and adding up your Macros each day, too.

So, that's it – just a calendar and a calculator are your primary weight loss tools. That's how I started, and that's an excellent place for you to get started, too.

How to Enjoy Intermittent Fasting

I don't know about you, but if something is not enjoyable for me, I just won't do it. I learned long ago that trying to force myself (different than getting out of my comfort zone) was just completely counter-productive.

Then, I discovered something. It happened while I was trying to get my kids to do chores. I realized that if I made it enjoyable in any way – singing, make it a game, playing – then they happily responded and helped do their chores.

Well, even though I'm a mom and an adult, I'm still just a big kid. I knew I had to make Intermittent Fasting enjoyable for me in some way as well. The same goes for you. When you make this eating plan enjoyable, it stops being about work and starts being more about a great part of your life. You might think I'm a little nuts, but I actually look forward to fasting!

So, how can you enjoy Intermittent Fasting and have a great time doing it? Here are things I've done myself:

~Play around with flavors and recipes in the kitchen. I just love trying new dishes, expanding my palate, and discovering a new spice, fruit, vegetable, herb, or grain I've never tried before. With online choices from Amazon, you can buy all kinds of wonderful ingredients.

~Use your fasting times to do something fun for yourself that doesn't involve food. I only eat twice a day, so I am able to squeeze in some extra time to do stuff I love to do.

~Share your fasting story with friends. I love to text my girlfriends about my latest fasting experience. We cheer each other on. It's a lot of fun.

I just see my eating windows and fasting times as two different facets of the same thing – an eating plan that I can enjoy because it gets me results. Plus, I have fun with it along the way, too.

Future You Will Thank Today You

You can be on the Intermittent Fasting plan for as long as you like.

Think about how you'll feel two months, two years, two decades from now. Today really only is temporary. Think of how quickly the last two months have gone. It just flies by.

There are so many perks to this. I mean, have you ever kept your bigger clothes from season to season because you thought you might need them in the future? What if the future you is the same size for months at a time?

You can use Intermittent Fasting to obtain your goal weight and to stay there for months or even years at a time.

Happy Feelings, Healthy Body

Your happiness is tied to how you feel in your own skin. Your Intermittent Fasting success story is waiting for you to write it. When I started writing this book, I first outlined what I wanted to say, and then I spent many hours writing the words for you to read them. Your weight loss journey will be just like that.

You will spend time reading about Intermittent Fasting, just like you've done in this book, and then you will follow the 30 Day Challenge day by day towards losing the weight. That alone will give you an amazing variety of eating windows and fasting times.

Life is a wild ride, girl! Isn't it? It has its ups, downs, times when you're steadily going forward, and times when it feels like time has stopped and maybe you are even going backward.

You need an eating plan that can keep up with all of these crazy changes. You need to give Intermittent Fasting a try.

You'll feel better, and you'll have a healthier body, too. It's for yourself, for your family, for your friends, and for your own future, too. Fasting is your friend!

So we have reached this point where I hope to say that it is just a temporary good bye. I hope to see you in my other books focused on health, diet and nutrition.

Before you go though, could you do me a favor?

Please let us know what is the 1 or 2 things you picked up that is of value to you in this book and please share it as a review on amazon. This will be super helpful to others and also to let others know what you have learnt!

Thank you so so much !

The Complete Guide To A Fast Keto Diet For Beginners

Ketogenic Diet Recipes And Meal Plans For People On The Go

Suzanne Summers

The Complete Guide
To A Fast Keto Diet For Beginners

Introduction

A Little Bit About Me

As I sit here typing this book I am flooded with memories of my life before the ketogenic diet. I was stuck in a body I wasn't happy with and a way of eating that made me feel anything but good about myself. After years of yo-yo dieting and losing and regaining the same 20 pounds, I knew it was time for a change.

Now, as you are probably aware, there is literally an ocean of diet plans out there to choose from. I had already done a bunch, including fad diets that didn't really work in the long-term. So, how do you know which one to choose?

Well, for starters, you must change your thought process. You see, for so many years I was looking for the perfect diet. Guess what? It doesn't exist. I've learned over the years that diets are temporary fixes that typically cannot be sustained over the long haul. I needed to find a way of eating that I could commit to for the rest of my life.

Thus, began my search. I read books, visited Facebook groups, watched documentaries, and even visited a nutritionist. My mind was flooded with words like, "low-fat", "calorie restriction", and "low-carb". I literally had to take a seat in my office (which is actually a hike on a wooded bike trail) and think about all the information I received.

There was one way of eating (WOE) that I kept coming back to. During my research, I continually saw the word "keto". At the time, I had no clue as to what that even was. After determining that it was some sort of low-carb diet, I chalked keto up to be an Atkins plan.

Boy, was I ever wrong!

After returning from my hike, I went into my actual office, sat down at the computer, and started to research this keto thing a bit more.

Ladies and gentlemen, the scales had been removed from my eyes.

Keto, or rather the ketogenic diet, is not an Atkins Plan at all. Yes, there are similarities, but keto is focused on eating high healthy fats and moderate protein. The Atkins plan is the opposite. However, each WOE focuses on very low-carb.

What caught my eye about the keto WOE is that you got to eat FAT. Have you ever heard of such a thing? Eating fat to lose weight? I had always been taught that fat makes you fat. That is so not true, and I'll cover why as you dive deeper into this book.

I knew, from that point on, that I wanted to give keto a try. You get to eat fatty foods like burgers, bacon, and butter. Who wouldn't want to do that? Plus, you lose weight in the process.

I totally immersed myself in the science behind this WOE and was impressed by what I found. I was glad to know that the ketogenic diet was not a fad diet or trend. This WOE has strong roots and has been around since the 1920s.

Over the course of a year, I stayed true to keto and the results were more than I ever could have imagined. Not only did I lose weight, but I felt better and certain health issues in my life improved.

We've all been in a place where we needed something special in our lives to really take hold of who we are and change us for the better. Keto did that for me. I was sick and tired of being sick and tired. For me, the key to a drastic change was within the foods I was eating. This is the case with most people.

I want you to know that I've been overweight, and I haven't liked who I saw in the mirror, just like you. I know what it feels like to go to the store and leave in tears because the clothes just don't fit right.

I also know what it feels like to be successful in an eating plan.

The days of losing and regaining the same weight are over for me and they can be for you, too. Keto changed my entire world and how I think about food and dieting.

I am not a doctor or a dietician but rather a woman who got tired of yo-yo dieting and wanted a new lease on life. It is my intention that this book will open your eyes to the wonderful world of keto, that has been backed by science, and change your life like it changed mine.

Who This Book Is For

Essentially, this book is for everyone. Keto focuses on zapping the sugar out of your life and there isn't one person on this planet whose health didn't improve from doing that. However, there are some specific folks out there that keto is targeted towards.

Here's a list of questions to ask yourself:

- Do I want to lose weight?
- Do I want to maintain my weight after I have lost it?
- Do I have health issues that need to be reversed?
- Do I desire to eat a healthier diet?
- Do I want to feel energized throughout my entire day?

If you answered "yes" to at least one of these questions this book is probably for you. Keto is designed with all types in mind. It is a WOE that can help anyone, and everyone feel better, look better, and even think better.

What This Book Provides

In addition to a wealth of information, this book gives you easy-to-understand meal plans that are well thought out, tasty, and perfect for your busy lifestyle. I not only include 1 meal plan, but 2. The second plan focuses on simple meals that can be prepped and prepared quickly. So, even if you are a busy mom, a working dad, or a young student at college, you can still create keto meals that are tailored towards your on-the-go lifestyle.

Don't worry. These meal plans come with step-by-step recipes, ingredient lists, and even nutritional information. I've literally done all the legwork for you. All you have to do is turn the pages of this book.

This book also contains a detailed section on how to get started with the ketogenic lifestyle. There is a little something called "ketosis" and I'll give you the tools to help you better understand what that is and how to get your body into it.

What's a weight-loss and healthy eating book without the bones to back it up? Not very good. That's why I've included scientific evidence throughout this entire book, so you know what you're reading is legit and not just a bunch of hogwash. By the time you finish reading you'll have an in-depth understanding of the ketogenic diet and why it works.

Lastly, I provide you with strategies and tips to make keto work for you forever. If you're anything like me, you are tired of diets that don't work. You'll learn how to sustain your new keto lifestyle without getting burnt out in the process.

So, are you ready to get started on your keto journey? Yes? Great! Let's do it!

CHAPTER 1
What Is Keto, Ketogenic?

What is the Ketogenic Diet?

To simply put it, the ketogenic diet (keto) is a high healthy fat, moderate protein, and very low-carb way of eating (WOE). Many folks confuse keto with the Atkin's Plan, and although there are similarities, Atkins focuses on high protein, moderate fat, and low-carb intake. In the big scheme of things, these are major differences.

So, you may be wondering, "Why choose keto"? Well, my friend, there are many reasons as to why the keto WOE might be good for you. For starters, the keto diet is backed by evidential science. There have been over 20 studies showing the efficacy of a high-fat, low-carb (HFLC) diet that helps people lose weight and improve health (1).

The keto WOE is so much more than just a weightless plan. There are studies that have proven it to combat diabetes, cancer, seizure disorders, and even Alzheimer's Disease (2, 3, 4, 5).

Moving on…

So, what happens when you drastically reduce your carbohydrate intake and increase the amount of healthy fats that you eat? Your body goes into a metabolic state called ketosis. Ketosis involves the body producing ketones and using them for energy instead of sugar (carbs).

Ketosis is something that you want to have happen. Depending on your body, it can take anywhere from a few hours to a few days to reach a state of ketosis. Once you jumped over into ketosis territory, your body will begin the process of learning how to burn fat for energy once all the ketones have been used up. In addition, the fat in your liver will turn into ketones and these ketones can supply energy for your brain. Say goodbye to brain fog, people (6, 7)!

Many people who struggle with blood sugar problems such as diabetes and insulin resistance have noticed an extreme decrease in blood glucose levels. There are many benefits to having your blood sugar balanced (8).

Summary

The ketogenic diet is a healthy high fat, moderate protein, very low-carbohydrate WOE that balances blood sugars and naturally shifts the body's metabolism away from carbohydrates and plunges it into the land of ketones and fat.

Exploring the different Types of Ketogenic WOE's

You probably didn't know this but there are a few different ways to approach the ketogenic diet. Let's take a look at them:

- Standard Keto diet (SKD) – This is the type of keto WOE that most people start with as it is cut and dry and easy to follow and maintain. It is very high healthy fat, moderate in protein, and very low-carb. Normally, the diet follows a 75% fat, 20% protein, and 5% carbs ratio.
- Cyclical ketogenic diet (CKD): This WOE allows you to have times of higher carb eating. For example, you may have 5 very strict SKD days followed by 2 high-carbohydrate days. Some folks refer to this as "refeeding".
- Targeted ketogenic diet (TKD) – If you are an athlete or body builder, TKD may be the type of keto WOE that works best for you as it allows you to add carbs centered around your workouts.
- High-protein ketogenic diet – This type of keto WOE is pretty similar to a SKD, but it allows for more protein consumption. The ratio looks something like 60% fat, 35% protein, and 5% carbs.

Keep in mind, when choosing a ketogenic WOE, only the SKD and high-protein methods have been researched and studied extensively. The other keto diets mentioned are a bit more advanced and widely used in the athlete/body builder communities.

Overall, the SKD is the most researched and most recommended of the four.

At the end of the day, only you know the right ketogenic diet style to engage in. Perhaps, talking over the different styles with your doctor will be helpful, too. More than likely, unless you're an extreme athlete, the SKD will be your go-to.

CHAPTER 2
Let's Chat About Ketosis

Why is Being in Ketosis Important?

So, we touched briefly on ketosis in chapter 1 and now we will explore it a bit further. It's important that you have a good understanding of what ketosis is, how it works, and why you need your body to be in it while eating a ketogenic diet.

What is Ketosis?

As previously stated, ketosis is a metabolic state in which carbs no longer work as the main source of energy for the body. Instead, your body uses ketones and then fat for fuel.

When you stop feeding your body carbs (sugar) it has limited access to glucose, which it uses for fuel. You see, when there is glucose in your body you will always burn it first because when glucose levels become to high, it can be deadly. Your body is smart and knows just what to do to keep you alive. There are malfunctions in this process when someone is a diabetic.

Here's a fun fact. Babies are born in a state of ketosis. One might argue that being in ketosis is more natural than using carbs for fuel. I'd say that they are right since we come into the world this way (9). Ketosis also happens during pregnancy and when you are fasting.

In order to get yourself into a state of ketosis, you need to restrict your carbohydrate intake rather extremely. This means you should eat no more than 50 grams of carbs per day. Some folks need to keep their intake to around 20 grams of carbs while they ate first starting the keto diet.

You'll have to remove certain foods from your diet in order to make this happen. Toss out the candy, grains, sugar-laden soda pop, starchy vegetables, and fruit, to name a few.

As you decrease your carbohydrate intake, your insulin levels also decrease and fatty acids are released from your body fat reserves in quite hefty amounts.

Another interesting concept is that ketones can cross the blood-brain barrier and fatty acids cannot. Ketones give your brain a mega-boost of energy when glucose is not present. This is a very good thing.

Benefits of Being in Ketosis

Being in ketosis comes with many benefits and most of them are health and weight loss related. If you are dealing with certain health issues such as high blood pressure, diabetes, and fatty liver disease, being in ketosis can actually help reverse these ailments.

In addition to helping you combat serious health problems, being in ketosis can help you lose weight and maintain the loss. I don't know about you, but this aspect is one of my favorites parts of being in ketosis. Following a ketogenic diet can help you toss out those fat pants, forever.

Health

Diabetes – So, it is no wonder that following a ketogenic diet and being in a state of ketosis can help diabetics. The diet is all about restricting carbs (sugar) and nourishing the body with healthy fats. Since most diabetics practice carb restriction, anyway, the keto way of eating shouldn't be to hard for them. When these folks start adding healthy fats into the mix is when the magic happens.

Researchers conducted a 24-week study, in 2008, to understand and determine the effects of a low-carb diet on folks with type-2 diabetes (10). These people were also dealing with obesity. As the study concluded, subjects who followed the keto WOE saw marked improvements in their blood sugar levels and were even able to reduce their diabetes medication. The other test groups, who followed a low-glycemic diet, didn't have as good of results. Another study, performed in 2017, determined the ketogenic diet outshined a standard, low-fat diabetes diet over the course of 32 weeks in correlation to weight loss and A1c levels (11). Additionally, a 2013 review reports that the keto WOE can lead to impressive improvements in balancing blood glucose, lowering and stabilizing A1c levels, weight loss, and even help people get off their diabetes management medications more than any other diet (12).

Metabolic Syndrome – A very tough illness to beat, the signs of this syndrome include having a large midsection, high blood pressure, high triglyceride levels, low HDL levels, and high glucose levels. Unfortunately, this syndrome is linked with type 2 diabetes and cardiovascular disease.

Researchers at Bethel University of Minnesota conducted a study of three groups composed of adults with metabolic syndrome. One group followed the keto diet without exercise, the second ate a Standard American Diet (SAD) without exercise, and the third group followed a SAD diet with 30 minutes od exercise most days of the week.

The study concluded that the folks following the ketogenic diet with exercise had much more success than the other 2 groups did in terms of achieving weight loss and more effective against a large range of health disorders (13).

Brain issues – A common myth is that the brain needs 130 grams of carbohydrates to function. A report by the US Institute of Medicine's Food and Nutrition Board clearly debunks this myth and states that the brain can actually function on zero carbs (14).

Eating a ketogenic diet supply's energy for the brain by way of ketogenesis and gluconeogenesis (15).

One major issue of the brain is epilepsy and keto has shown to be a key component in easing the symptoms of this debilitating disorder. In fact, in 1924, the Classic Ketogenic Diet was created by doctors to help children suffering from epileptic seizures (16). This WOE is still used today to treat seizure disorders.

Cancer – Eating a ketogenic diet is known to weaken cancer cells. Studies have shown that sugar feeds cancer and creates an acidic environment within the body. When you consume a high-fat/low-carb diet you are essentially not giving cancer cells what they need to thrive. What happens? They die (17)!

Reduces inflammation – When your body is inflamed you can experience all sorts of things such as arthritic pain and autoimmune issues. Eating excess sugar produces high amounts of insulin within your body which raises inflammatory markers and triggers chronic disease, Nixing the sugar and following a keto WOE can reverse these problems and help you to feel better ([18](18)).

Cholesterol – So, you've probably been taught that fat makes you fat and causes heart disease and high cholesterol, right? Well, research has proven this to be a myth. In fact, research has shown that sugar(carbs) make you fat and cause health issues like high triglyceride levels. Now, if you combine both carbs and fat together in your diet then yes, you are creating a recipe for disaster. Removing the carbs and enjoying healthy fats by themselves will do the opposite ([19](19)).

Blood Pressure – A study was conducted involving a few test groups who all had high blood pressure and were put on various diets like The Zone, Ornish, and Atkins. It was concluded that the Atkins group saw the highest decrease in both systolic and diastolic blood pressure ([20](20)). Granted, this study didn't include the keto diet, but it did prove that a low-carb diet is successful in lowering blood pressure.

Fatty Liver Disease – There are a number of factors that play into fatty liver disease. If you struggle from nonalcoholic fatty liver disease your lifestyle is the biggest culprit to why you have the disease in the first place. Eating much and exercising too little are key players in the game of fatty liver disease. Turning to a low-fat diet to correct fatty liver disease has been shown to be counterproductive and ineffective. However, keto has displayed some promising results ([21](21)).

Lifestyle

How will the ketogenic diet affect your life? Well, we've already established that if you are dealing with certain health ailments eating a ketogenic diet can help bring you relief. You'll also notice other areas of your life improving such as less fatigue, clearer thinking, more energy, and stabilized moods.

Sounds good to me!

Weight-loss – The ketogenic diet has been proven time and time again to help people lose weight. Removing carbs from the diet and being in a state of ketosis encourages your body to burn fat for fuel. When you use your fat stores for fuel you are losing fat on your body. This will cause the much-coveted weight-loss effect leaving you with a trimmer body and smaller clothes.

Hunger management/appetite control – When you begin increasing healthy fats into your diet you'll find yourself becoming satiated quicker and for longer periods of time. Fat tastes good and is very satisfying. Sugar (carbs) on the other hand, gives you a burst of energy and satisfies your hunger pains for a brief time but shortly, you'll notice you are craving sugar again and begin to feel sluggish. This is called a "sugar crash". It is important to understand that fat nourishes and satisfies your body while sugar inflames and increases your cravings.

Energy – As aforementioned, carbohydrates give you a temporary burst of fuel but that energy is quickly followed by a crash. When you are in ketosis and are being fueled by healthy fat, you'll experience sustained energy throughout your day.

Mental clarity – When your body starts using ketones for fuel and then fat, you'll notice that your brain fog will lift. You'll experience clearer thinking, better decision making, and an overall crisper thought process ([22](22)).

You'll burn fat for fuel – As we've been discussing this entire book so far, the keto WOE allows your body to burn fat for fuel and when you tell glucose to take a hike, well, all sorts of great things happen. You'll find yourself feeling better across the entire board.

Mood stabilization – When we aren't eating a healthy diet and consuming high amounts of sugar, we can become aggravated, moody, and overly emotional. Have you ever heard the term "hangry"? It means you are angry because you are hungry. Being "hangry" is due to your body craving carbohydrates. When on a ketogenic diet you won't be craving sugar and you'll feel more satiated which will ultimately lead to having better moods. The inflammation in your body will also improve which again, leads to the stabilization of your emotions.

Is the Ketogenic Diet for You?

Honestly, that is a question you need to ask yourself. Taking in all of the information that I've supplied you thus far, does it seem that keto would be a good fit for you? Do you have any health issues that might make keto difficult or unsafe?

I highly recommend that you speak with your family doctor before beginning the ketogenic WOE. In most cases, a doctor is going to give you his or her blessing to go forward with a low-carb diet. Why? Because most health care professionals aren't in the business of pushing high-sugar diets on their patients.

Please, understand, that I am not your doctor and the information in this book is not meant to treat or diagnose your health problems.

Whatever issues you may have going on with your health, please, talk them over with your doctor and tell him or her why you think a keto WOE is good for you. Glean your doctor's input.

Keto may not be appropriate for the following people who have the following health issues:

- Diabetes
- Kidney disease
- Liver or pancreatic disease
- Pregnant or nursing mothers
- People who actively have or are recovering from an eating disorder
- People recovering from surgery
- People who are underweight
- Children under the age of 18

If anything on the list above applies to you, please, understand that this doesn't mean you are automatically exempt from following a keto WOE. It just means you really need to talk your condition and keto over with your doctor before you begin. I highly recommend you follow the advice of your health care provider.

Ketoacidosis

You may have heard some hype between the ketogenic diet and ketoacidosis. I am here to explain the difference between the two because they are nothing alike, at all (23).

We've already been talking about what ketosis is so let's recap. Ketosis is the presence of ketones in the body and it is not harmful. You get into a state of ketosis by restricting carbohydrate intake.

Ketoacidosis (DKA) is an extremely serious condition that affects people who suffer from type 1 diabetes mellitus. It is a life-threatening condition and requires immediate medical help due to the presence of dangerously high amounts of ketones and blood sugar levels. When this happens, your blood becomes too acidic, which changes the way your bodily organs work.

There are a few things that can lead a person who suffers from type 1 diabetes mellitus into a state of ketoacidosis and they include illness, not eating properly, or not getting enough insulin. Very rarely is ketoacidosis brought on by eating a low-carb diet, especially in a person who is not diabetic.

Ketoacidosis can also develop in folks who suffer from type 2 diabetes who have very little to no insulin production.

Ketosis = Safe

Ketoacidosis = Very Dangerous

Again, I cannot stress this enough, if you suffer from underlying health problems, especially any form of diabetes, please talk over the ketogenic diet with your doctor before starting.

Ketoacidosis is very rare, even in people who are diabetic, and it is pretty much non-existent in a person who does not have diabetes.

Keto Flu

You may or may not have heard of the keto flu. There is a good possibility that you are reading this right now and thinking, "The flu?? Why on earth would I do a diet plan that gives me the flu?"

Woah, hold your horses, pardner! The keto flu is not the "flu" at all. There are no viruses or bacteria involved whatsoever. You don't need medication or a trip to the doctor. Actually, a few swigs of pickle juice will probably due the trick.

I'm sure I've just confused you even more. Pickle juice?

Okay, here's the 411 on the keto flu. When you restrict carbohydrates your body sort of goes into a panic. For years, you've lovingly fed your bed sugar and your body got used to that relationship. All of a sudden, you stop with the cookies, cakes, and breads and your body doesn't quite know how to handle the breakup.

This is when, a new follower of keto, you begin to feel a little bit terrible. However, don't worry, these flu-like symptoms are temporary and will subside once your body adjusts to eating a low-carb diet.

Symptoms of the Keto Flue include:

- Craving sugar
- Feeling dizzy
- Not being able to think clearly

- Grouchiness
- Lack of concentration/focus
- Upset stomach

- Feeling nauseous
- Muscle cramps
- Feeling confused
- Not being able to sleep

Now, you may or may not experience these symptoms. Some folks only experience a few while others experience them all. Keto flu truly depends on the individual and their personal metabolic flexibility. Metabolic flexibility is simply how well you can adapt to using a different energy source such as carbs, or fats. Your genetics and lifestyle deeply impact your metabolic flexibility.

As you restrict carbohydrates, water and sodium are flushed out of the body which can leave you a bit parched. Dehydration can make you feel those dreaded flu-like symptoms. A great rule of thumb is to always drink plenty of water while begging the ketogenic diet (you always should, anyway). What about that pickle juice? Pickle juice contains a ton of sodium which helps replenish those electrolytes. Taking a few sips can help you feel better.

Tips for remedying symptoms of the keto flu:

- Drinking water with a pinch of unrefined salt
- Supplement your diet with sodium, magnesium, and potassium
- Eat more fat
- Exercise – low-intensity
- Meditate
- Get adequate sleep

Things you should not do:

- High-intensity workouts
- Consume high amounts of protein
- Stress over uncontrollable things
- Eat carbs/sugar

So, remember, the keto flu is not dangerous, and it will most likely happen to you as you begin to cut carbs from your plate. Keep in mind that this is a transition that your body is going through and it to shall pass. Use the tips above to remedy your symptoms and keep on ketoing.

CHAPTER 3
So....What Should We Do Next?

Welcome to chapter 3! If you are still with me then it is clear you are serious about your keto journey. I'm proud of you.

So, we've learned a lot about the keto WOE up to this point and now it is time to jump into the fat of the diet (no pun intended). In this chapter you will learn how to get started in the ketogenic lifestyle. We'll cover all the basics that you need to know in order to be successful.

You might be feeling a little overwhelmed with all the information and new terms you are learning but don't worry. By the time you finish this chapter you are going to be ready to start keto like a champ.

Let's go!

KETO IN A NUTSHELL

Let's refresh a bit and go over the basic tenants of keto, shall we?

We know that the ketogenic diet is high in healthy fats, moderate in protein, and very low in carbohydrates.

We know that once you begin the ketogenic diet and restricting your carbs your body will fall into ketosis.

We know that ketosis is safe and not at all what ketoacidosis is. Ketosis means there are ketones in your blood and you are now burning them for fuel instead of glucose.

We know that you may or may not feel symptoms of the "keto flu" when you are still starting out.

We know not to worry about the keto flu because we understand how to combat it.

We know that the ketogenic WOE leads to sustainable weight-loss, better health, and more energy.

What else do we know?

Keto is amazing ☺

KNOW YOUR BODY

The very first stepping stone to starting a ketogenic diet is knowing your body. You need to know where you're at in terms of health, weight, and measurements. The best way to do this is to schedule a full-body exam with your doctor.

You'll want to go over any pre-existing health issues with your doctor and discuss how starting keto will impact them. If you learn you have other health problems, discuss those, too.

Ask your doctor to perform blood work on you. You'll want a full lipid panel profile at this starting point. It's great to know your numbers and then have them rechecked in 6 months or so and compare your progress.

You'll want to calculate your Body Mass Index (BMI). You can do this by dividing your weight in pounds by your height in inches. Then, divide your answer by your height again to get your individual BMI. You can also follow this same formula in kilograms and meters. To make things even easier, you can find a BMI calculator on-line and simply input your stats and let the robots do the figuring for you.

Make sure to weight yourself and record your answer so you can keep track of your progress.

You'll want to get measurements of your body. This is very important for those times when you don't see the scale moving as much as you'd like it to be. Many times, folks will see massive differences in inch-loss versus scale lose.

Measure your hips, calf, thigh, wrist, and forearm. You can do this by using a seamstress tape measure. Or, if you know of a local gym, perhaps a trainer there can do it for you. Make sure to record your findings so you can compare progress at a later time.

If you are on a budget and the thought of going to the doctor's office makes you cringe due to high medical costs, I've got some solutions for you.

Does your employer offer medical insurance or a health incentive plan? If you don't have access to health insurance, make sure to ask your doctor's finance department if they offer a discount for cash-paying patients. Most of the time, you'll be given as much as a 60% discount.

There are also programs you can sign up for that offer cost-sharing. This means that you pay a monthly fee of x amount of dollars as do other people from around the country. When you go to the doctor's office you submit your bills to the program and your fees are paid for.

If all else fails, you can easily weigh and measure yourself at home. You won't be able to perform a full-body exam or give yourself bloodwork but at least you'll know some starting point numbers.

I do recommend that you try your best to get in to see your health care professional at some point, though. You want to be sure all your parts are functioning properly, especially when starting a new diet plan.

WHAT IS YOUR "WHY"

This next section is very important, and it is something I really want you to think about. What is your "why'? Why are you deciding to start the keto WOE? What has motivated you to kick bad eating habits and get healthier?

Perhaps, you have health conditions that you want to improve, or you aren't at a weight that is acceptable to you. Maybe, you want to get healthier, so you can play with your children/grandchildren with ease and not always be sore and tired.

Whatever your "why" is, I want you to write it down and keep it some place handy so whenever you feel like giving up you can return to your "why" and remember what this is all for. When I started keto, I kept my "why" posted on the refrigerator so that I could see it every day. I've even heard of people keeping a sticky note on their bathroom mirror.

Another good thing you can do is journaling. Write out your thoughts as to why you are changing your lifestyle. Once you establish your "why" you can then start to list out some goals. Make sure your goals are realistic and attainable. You and I both know that making a goal to lose 50 pounds (unless you are morbidly obese) in a month is not realistic. However, 10 is.

I really want you to wrap your head around your "why" and give it some good thought. Your "why" will be your motivating factor to keep ketoing on.

If you aren't into writing things down, that's okay! As long as you can remember why you are doing this and it helps keep you disciplined, you're good. Maybe you can tattoo your "why' on your body? Just kidding ☺

KETONE MONITORING SUPPLIES: WHICH DO YOU USE?

Believe it or not, there are ways to know the level of ketones swirling around in your body. So folks in the ketogenic community are die-hard users of these devices while some think they are unnecessary. I fall somewhere in between. I feel that if you have these monitors, great, if you don't, also great.

Now, I will say, knowing that you are in ketosis when you first start the ketogenic diet is a plus. It is motivating and gives you the comfort that this keto thing is really working.

There are <u>three types of monitors</u> in which you can test yourself for the presence of ketones:

- Blood
- Breath
- Urine

Blood monitors are highly accurate but they are expensive. Plus, you must poke yourself in order to use them. Most folks don't relish the idea of playing in their own blood. Many people in the diabetic community opt for blood monitors because it gives them a concise estimate of their blood glucose and ketone levels. It also helps them keep an eye out for ketoacidosis.

Pros – Most accurate ketone testing method

Cons – Expensive and not very pleasant to use

Breath ketone monitors measure the amount of acetone in the breath. Yes, acetone as in the main ingredient in nail polish remover. Your breath may smell of this for a period of time as your body adjusts to the low-carb lifestyle. Measuring breath acetone can tell you whether you are in mild ketosis or not. This device is useful for people trying to establish a baseline of ketosis without needing to know how deeply they're into it.

Pro- - Easy to use and affordable

Cons – Isn't as in-depth as a blood monitor

Measuring ketones in your urine is extremely affordable an easy. You simply urinate into a cup and hold the dipstick in the urine for a few seconds. The more purple the color is the higher the concentration of ketones are in your body. Urine sticks, just like breath monitors, can determine whether you are in ketosis or not, but they cannot determine how deeply like blood monitoring can.

Pros – Easy to use and cheap

Cons – You need to collect urine. Not as effective as blood monitoring

So, in the end, unless you are a diabetic, I wouldn't spend the money on a blood monitoring system. If anything, the breath or urine ways of monitoring will work just fine. Many people, myself included, prefer breath monitoring because it is less messy than urine testing.

Please, remember, that if you can't afford these ketone testing supplies or you simply don't want them that that is perfectly fine. You really don't need them in order to be successful on the ketogenic diet as there are clear signs and symptoms of being ketosis as we discussed in chapter 2.

MACROS

You may or may not have heard of "macros" before which is short for macronutrients. Macronutrients are the energy-giving properties of the foods that we eat and they fuel our bodies. Macros consist of fat, protein, and carbohydrates. When embarking on a keto diet journey, knowing your personal macros is important because you need to have the right balance of fats, proteins, and carbs in order to get into ketosis and to stay there. You want your body to be a fat-burning powerhouse.

Let me further break macros down for you.

Carbohydrates are the only macronutrient that you do not need for survival. Fats and proteins are considered to be essential for survival, but carbs are not. For someone who is just getting started on the keto WOE you should aim for no more than 20 grams of carbohydrates per day.

Keep in mind, that carbs aren't just sugary cakes, cookies, and candy. Carbs are in vegetables, fruit, wheat, and bread. You must keep an eye on your intake of all carbs in all foods.

When you look at a food label you re going to see carbohydrates listed. You will also see fiber listed. What you want to do is find the NET CARB count. To do this, subtract the carbs from the fiber and that is the number you use. Fiber that occurs naturally in a food does not impact your glycemic index, so it basically cancels out some of the total carb count.

Protein is important in a ketogenic diet as it helps you preserve your lean body mass. The amount of protein you need will depend on the amount of lean body mass you already have. Check out these general guidelines for protein intake per the Ketogasm website (24):

- 0.7 to 0.8 grams of dietary protein per pound of muscle to preserve muscle mass
- 0.8 to 1.2 grams of dietary protein per pound of muscle to gain muscle mass

Keep in mind, you DO NOT want to lose muscle mass. You want to lose fat. I know many of you are just looking to lose weight no matter how it happens but losing muscle mass is not the way.

Getting adequate protein is important in the ketogenic diet, however, you don't want to go overboard with it as to much protein can be stressful to the kidneys.

Find your daily protein percentage by multiplying your body weight by your body fat percentage. Then subtract your body fat weight from your total weight and that will give you your lean body mass. Next, take your lean body mass amount and multiply it by your protein requirement ratio and you'll find the grams of protein you need on a daily basis to maintain your muscle mass.

Fat is an essential component to the ketogenic lifestyle. It is the macronutrient that satisfies your hunger pangs due to be so satiating. When wanting to maintain your weight you need to eat enough fat to support your total daily fuel expenditure. To lose weight, you'll need to eat a fat deficit.

Putting it All Together

So, the best way to find your personal macros is by using a macronutrient calculator. You can find one at the Ketogains website. These calculators make it super simple to find your individual macros. All you have to do is put your weight and body fat percentage in and the calculator will do the rest.

Your MACROS Will Change

As you begin to lose weight you will need to adjust your macros. I, personally, would make these adjustments every two weeks. It is so important to keep track of your weight, so you know how to figure your macronutrients. As your size begins to shrink so will your macros.

FOODS YOU SHOULD MAKE FRIENDS WITH

When it comes to keto, there are a few staple foods that you really should keep on hand just help yourself stay satiated and to encourage ketosis. The following list isn't a must-have, but it does help. I like to think of these foods as "keto staples".

- Coconut oil – This oil is super nourishing for the body. It is purely fat and great for helping you to get into ketosis. You also may want to consider using MCT (medium chain triglycerides) oil which is a concentrated form of coconut oil that is high in Caproic, caprylic, capric, and lauric acids. These acids quickly turn into energy and metabolized in the body.
- Extra-virgin olive oil – Another oil that is high in healthy fat and great for using in homemade salad dressings and marinades. You don't want to use olive oil in high heat settings so save it for your favorite cold-recipes.
- Cheese – Cheese is probably one of my favorite keto-friendly foods. It's high in healthy fats, tastes wonderful, and very filling. You can use cheese in a variety of recipes. Feel free to consume any type of cheese you want including cream cheese. Keep in mind that processed cheese, like Velveeta, are not part of the keto equation as they contain sugar.
- Tree nut butter – Tree nut butters are an amazing source for both fat and protein. They taste great and are wonderful by the spoonful or in keto desserts. You can use peanut butter, but it needs to be

a natural peanut butter without added sugar. When using any nut butters make sure to keep an eye on the ingredients and net carb count.

- Cauliflower – When it comes to keto veggies, cauliflower is the real deal. This powerhouse veggie is very low in carbs and can be used to create all sorts of substitutes like rice, noodles, and even pizza crust! There are tons of recipes that show you how to do this. You can even make faux mashed potatoes with cauliflower.

- Cod liver oil – Cod liver oil is chock full of omega 3's and is great for keeping your heart healthy. I wouldn't use this oil in recipes or for straight up eating as it tastes extremely fishy. However, finding yourself a good cod liver oil supplement is a wise move to make for the added cardiovascular benefits.

- Kelp – The best and easiest way to incorporate kelp into your diet is when it is in a powdered form. You may think it is super fishy tasting, but it really isn't! It's great for sprinkling on salads and even into keto-approved smoothies. I like to add kelp to tomato soup. Sea kelp is a natural source of vitamins A, B1, B2, C, D, and E and includes minerals zinc, iodine, magnesium, potassium, copper, and calcium.

- Avocado – If you choose to be on a ketogenic diet then you pretty much have to like avocados. Kidding! However, avocados are an excellent source of fat and they are quite versatile. If you find yourself lacking in your fat macros just add an avocado to your plate and you'll be good.

- Mushrooms – Depending on the type of mushrooms you are consuming you can get a healthy dose of vitamin C out of the deal. Sautee mushrooms with garlic and onion in grass-fed butter for a amazing keto-friendly snack. Watch the amount of garlic and onions you use as these veggies are higher in carbs.

- Eggs – As any fellow follower of keto knows, eggs are a staple low-carb food. The contain the perfect balance of protein and fat. You can eat eggs every day while on the keto diet. Feel free to be liberal in the amount you consume.

- Dark chocolate – Yes! You can have chocolate on the keto diet! You should stick to a 90 to 99% cocoa ratio. This form of chocolate is actually very good for you. Now, it is going to be quite bitter but you can consume chocolate that is sweetened by stevia and you'll feel as if you are eating a "regular" candy bar.

- Bone Broth – Bone broth is ultra-nourishing for the body. You can purchase it at the grocery store or easily make your own. When you start feeling symptoms of the keto flu, warm yourself up a mug of bone broth and sip your symptoms away. Make sure to add pink Himalayan salt to the mix.

- Pork belly – Pork belly is fatty, delicious, and is what bacon is all about. Eat it with your eggs in the morning or make yourself a batch to snack on throughout the day. It is highly satiating.

- Berries – Although fruit is not ideal for a ketogenic diet, berries are. I don't want you to go overboard on them, but a handful of strawberries, blueberries, or blackberries here and there will do you no harm. They have a very low impact on the glycemic index. Plus, if you are feeling a craving for something sweet, berries can help satisfy the urge to reach for a donut.

- Grass-fed butter – You certainly may use corn-fed butter but grass-fed is the best. It tastes better and metabolizes differently within your body. Kerry Gold is an excellent brand to use. Yes, you can eat butter and lose weight. Imagine that!

When purchasing any foods, even the foods on the above list, it is very important to read labels. There are always going to be hidden carbs/sugars in certain foods that you never knew were there. For example, you purchase a bag of frozen strawberries and think you've got a glorious serving of nature's candy in your hand. You turn the bag over and see that the manufacturer added sugar to the berries to further sweeten them. Had you not checked you would have consumed added sugar and potentially kicked yourself out of ketosis.

Remember, you want to subtract the total carbs from the fiber content to know the net carbs that are in a food. Your goal is to keep it at 20 grams or less per day.

GETTING YOUR PANTRY PREPPED

You first need to determine whether you are a single or a family. This shouldn't be hard to determine, haha! If you are prepping for yourself, getting your pantry keto-ready is a bit simpler. However, if you are part of a family unit you need to either see if your family is able/wants to do keto with you or section off an area for your food.

When you have other people living with you and they aren't interested in keto you can't go tossing out all the carb-laden food. If you do that you're going to create a warzone within your home.

Prepping with a family will require more discipline on your part because you are going to have to live with non-keto foods in your home, however, I've done this myself and was successful. You can and will be successful, too!

So, as a family-prepper, if there are any carb-laden foods that are just yours, give them away. The same thing goes if you are single-prepper. If the food isn't half-eaten or spoiled, considering giving them to a family in need or donating to your local food pantry. There is no reason to throw away food that can help feed hungry bellies, no matter how carby it may be.

Once your pantry is cleared of non-keto foods, it is time to head to the grocery store. You can begin with the staple foods listed above or make your own low-carb list to work from. I like to sit down and look up keto recipes from some of my favorite keto websites. I'll then make a shopping list and meal plan for the week. Works like a charm! It always helps to have a list when going to the grocery store. You tell yourself that you are ONLY buying items from the list and you will not make any exceptions. This helps you to stay on task with keto-friendly foods. It also helps you stick to a budget.

TAKE A WALK AND GET A FEEL FOR WHICH RESTAURANT HAVE KETO OPTIONS

Or, you can drive, whichever tickles your fancy. I would opt for walking if possible because it is a way to get in some exercise.

Anyway...

You want to have a good idea of which eateries and cafes in your neighborhood are "safe zones" to eat at. Visit different establishments and ask them if you can have a menu. Scout the menu for keto-friendly options.

Honestly, I have found that every restaurant is going to have keto-options because you can MAKE them keto.

Let's say there is a small eatery that your family wants to go to and it sells primarily deep fried/battered food. Look for a chicken option. When you get your chicken you can simply peel away the breading and enjoy. Most places always have a side salad, too.

Did you know that fast food restaurants like McDonalds and Burger King allow you to order burgers without the bun? They'll typically warp your meat and toppings in a leaf of lettuce and give you a fork.

Now, don't get me wrong, you should not be eating like this all the time because these types of foods are not the healthiest but they will do when you're hungry and in a pinch.

4-WEEK BREAKDOWN OF BEGINNING YOUR KETO JOURNEY

WEEK 1

This is the starting point for your new keto journey. Congratulations! So, this week should feel pretty exciting for you. You'll undoubtedly be full of enthusiasm and drive. Perhaps, you may even experience a small twinge of fear because you've never done a low-carb diet before that requires you to eat lots of fat. That's okay and normal. I've experienced a bit of apprehension when I first started keto, myself.

As you begin to restrict carbohydrates you are most likely going to feel a lot of hunger pangs. In fact, you are going to crave carbs like crazy. This is normal. You see, most people are addicted to sugar. Yes, I said "addicted". So, like any addiction, there are going to be symptoms of withdrawal and cravings are one of them.

Tips to handle feelings of carb withdrawal and hunger:

- Add salt to your food as it replaces lost electrolytes and helps with dehydration. When you are thirsty you tend to have false food cravings. Make sure the salt is either sea or pink Himalayan. Mineral salt works well, too.
- Consume a tablespoon of coconut oil or MCT oil upon getting out of bed. This is pure, healthy fat that not only satiates your cravings but gives you an enormous burst of sustainable energy.
- Eat more butter! Butter is satiating and very nourishing for the body. Make sure you are consuming grass-fed if at all possible.
- Drink Bullet Proof Coffee (BPC) when hunger pangs strike. BPC is coffee made with MCT oil and butter. You place the hot coffee and oils in a blender and whip it into a frothy fat-filled drink that tastes absolutely lovely.
- When cravings strike, pop a few nuts in your mouth as they are known to help with hunger.
- Cheese is another great food to snack on when trying to beat the hunger beast.

Remember, keep cutting out the carbs and adding in good fats to your diet. Do not give in to your sugar cravings. All that will do is prolong your suffering and keep you stuck at square one.

WEEK 2

This is the week where you are going to probably see some results on the scale. Yay! Keep in mind that what you are seeing is not yet fat loss but water weight. When you restrict carbohydrates the stored glycogen in your fat cells is the first thing to leave your body. It comes out by way of water weight. You may even notice that you are urinating more during this week.

Now, if you aren't seeing any weight loss yet, that is also normal. Don't get upset or give up because your "whoosh" of water weight will surely come. Be patient and trust the process.

You may find yourself becoming familiar with the keto flu during week 2. Here are some tips to combating this pesky, but temporary, symptom:

- Make sure you are drinking an adequate amount of water and then drink some more.
- If you notice the keto flu is really being persistent, don't freak out. It just means your body is struggling to adapt to restricting carbs. This is normal, and many people experience a rough keto flu phase. It too shall pass.
- Make sure you are keeping your carbs at around 20 grams or less per day and following your fat macros. These things will help alleviate the keto flu.
- Make sure to follow all of your macros to avoid slipping into gluconeogenesis which will surely derail the fat burning train within your body.

Other physical symptoms that you may notice during week 2 are bad breath, cramps, fatigue, and waking up in the middle of the night to urinate. Here are some tips to help you deal with these symptoms:

- If you find that your breath isn't smelling all that fresh try chewing on mint leaves, taking a chlorophyll supplement, and regularly brushing your teeth and using a mouth rinse.
- Again, keep up with the salt intake so your electrolytes stay balanced. This will help with any cramps you are feeling. You may want to consider taking a magnesium/potassium supplement.
- If you are having trouble sleeping due to weird dreams, insomnia, and frequent urination, don't get upset. There are many people who deal with this when they start a low-carb diet. Sugar is seriously a beast to detox from and it does funny things to your body in the process. Try to not drink anything an hour before bed. Relax in a hot shower and turn off all screens and distraction before going to sleep for the night.
- Some folks complain of a "keto rash" especially in fat folds, groin area, and under the breasts. This is due to increased excretion of acetone and can be quite irritating. Use a powder or cornstarch on the areas until the rash clears up.

Remember, these symptoms are all temporary and will lessen and eventually disappear as you get deeper into your keto lifestyle.

WEEK 3

By now, you should be fairly acquainted with the daily needs of the keto diet. You'll find yourself having a good grasp on your macronutrient needs. In fact, you may feel as somewhat of a macro guru as you will begin to easily know the approximate amount of carbs, fats, and proteins in a meal. Look at you go!

Another great thing that comes with week 3 is your knowledge of knowing how to boost your fat intake whenever you feel that the day is passing and you are not getting your allotment. There is nothing wrong with adding a spoonful of butter or coconut oil to your food to increase your fat intake. At this point, you should have a "quick fat food" list in a handy place so you can easily utilize it.

WEEK 4

Hooray! You've soldiered on and reached week 4. Almost one month into your new keto WOE. That's awesome! At this point, for most people, the symptoms of the keto flu should be about gone. In fact, you are probably starting to feel pretty fine and dandy. I'm willing to bet the farm you are feeling more energized. Hiking up that steep hill has got nothing on you! Your focus is most likely better and you're reaping the benefits of mental clarity.

If you are not great around the kitchen, meaning, if you don't like to cook, your keto meals might be getting a bit repetitive at this point. Consider learning some new meals and being prepared with a stocked pantry of the items you need to make them. Weekly meal planning is quite helpful.

Lucky for you non-cook folks, this book is chock full of keto recipes and you are almost to that point. You'll find a meals for folks who are on-the-go and meals that take a more traditional cooking approach.

TROUBLESHOOTING COMMON ISSUES OF THE KETO DIET

So, you're not getting into ketosis. What are you doing wrong?

First of all, don't beat yourself up. You aren't "everyone". You are you. Some folks have a bit more of a struggle getting into ketosis than others and that's just life. However, there are a few questions to ask yourself:

"Am I watching my macros"?

"Am I watching for gluconeogenesis"?

"Am I watching for hidden carbs/sugars in my food?"

Please know that most people get into ketosis pretty quickly after 24 to 72 hours of carb restriction. You will most likely fall into this category.

What are net carbs and total carbs and which do you follow?

So, net carbs are carbs that are subtracted from the amount of natural fiber in a food. Many people use a net carb calculation because fiber is scientifically not a carbohydrate (25).

Total carbs is the number of carbs in a food that has not been subtracted by fiber or sugar alcohols. If you find yourself having trouble getting into ketosis, you can calculate your carb intake using the total number and then slowly switch back to the net carb method once you've been in ketosis for a while.

Is fat really good for you?

Yes. For years, we have been taught that fat makes you fat and saturated fat is basically the devil. This couldn't be further from the truth. Recent scientific studies have shown that fat is nourishing to the body and does not make you "fat". In fact, more research has shown that sugar makes you fat. When you combine fat and carbs together, this also makes you fat. Thus, that is why we've landed on the ketogenic diet.

If you are still concerned about saturated fats you can switch to eating only monounsaturated fats but let me warn you, this will significantly restrict the delicious foods you will be eating. Saturated fat is yummy and satiating.

Remember, keto is a high-fat diet and in order for it to work properly you need to consume your daily intake of fat.

Can you eat as much as you want?

Technically, yes. Keto is not a calorie counting type of diet. However, is also not a free-for-all, either. In the beginning, you may find yourself snacking on keto-approved foods all the time. This is normal. However, as you progress, you'll find you aren't as hungry as you were when eating a carb-heavy diet. In fact, most folks only eat 2 meals a day!

Try to stay within your macros and you'll be fine.

Why can't you eat 50 grams of carbs a day like Bob and still remain in ketosis?

Simply put, you aren't Bob. Everyone is different and has their own carb intake needs. You may only be able to tolerate 20 grams and Bob can tolerate 50 grams of carbs because of the state of metabolic damage that you are in.

There is a light at the end of the tunnel, though. The longer you remain in ketosis and eventually become fat adapted, you will be able to consume more carbs without being kicked out of ketosis.

Why haven't you lost weight yet?

If you haven't lost any weight, please don't stress about it. I'm willing to bet you have lost inches and your clothes fit better. Your body, at this point in time, may even be perfectly balanced and doesn't want to lose any weight.

Consider the health benefits you are seeing. Keto isn't all about weight loss, it's about getting your body out of a state of sugar addiction and becoming healthier over the long run.

Now, if it is obvious that you need to lose weight and you haven't done so yet, you may not fully be in ketosis, especially if your lack of weight loss is accompanied by constant keto flu symptoms.

Why is your cholesterol out of whack?

Many folks will see a significant increase in their cholesterol numbers when they first start keto. Both the HDL (good) and LDL (bad) tend to rise. I know this may worry you but it will even out and improve the longer you ar eon a ketogenic diet. When you see your cholesterol, especially the LDL, going up this signifies that your body is healing. Keep in mind that sugar is very inflammatory, and cholesterol is what tries to control the inflammation. Decreasing carbs is a shock to the system, initially, so the inflammation rises a bit. Depending on how bad your metabolic damage is, you may see a rise in cholesterol for a few months before it levels out.

YOU MADE IT! 1 MONTH IN TO KETO!

Congratulations! You have cleared your first month of keto. You craved carbs, combated the keto flu, and even saw weeks where the scale refused to move yet you kept ketoing on. Great for you!

You are now well prepped for the keto lifestyle and armed with a wealth of information.

This is the time where you need recipes to keep you going and not becoming bored with the basic keto foods you've been eating over the past 30 days. The recipes in the next chapter will help you to sustain your newfound ketogenic lifestyle.

Remember, if you have one of those days and eat a donut, dust yourself off, and realize it isn't the end of the world. You may fall out of ketosis for a short period of time but you can and will readapt quickly.

You've got this.

CHAPTER 4
All Planned Out And Ready!

28 Day Meal Plan for Ketosis

The ketogenic diet is an increasingly popular diet. So many people around the world have found success in weight loss through the keto lifestyle, and now you can too! The key to making this diet work is to monitor your macros carefully- the keto lifestyle consists of a diet that is high in fat, moderate in protein, and low in carbs. Because carbs are limited, it's also very important to keep your diet as nutritionally diverse as possible- this will ensure you're getting a balance of nutrients, in order to stay healthy and stick to this plan long term.

This meal plan will help you as you begin your journey into the keto lifestyle! For the next four weeks, you'll have your meals and snacks carefully planned out in order to provide you with a healthy, nutritionally diverse diet that adheres to the strict rules of the keto diet.

If you take a quick look at the meal plan, you'll see that every day includes three meals plus one snack, dessert, or drink to enjoy at your discretion. You'll also find that each recipe lists the calories and macros and that each day has a total. Remember, the meal plan is based on a daily intake of 1500 to 2,000 calories (give or take 100 calories) and an approximate macronutrient ratio of 70% to 80% fat, about 10% to 20% protein, and 5% to 10% carbohydrates.

In order to achieve ketosis, it's important to monitor carb intake carefully. Try to stay within 30 grams of net carbs a day (give or take a gram or two). Curious about the difference between gross carb count and net carb count? In order to easily calculate the net carbs in a recipe, subtract the insoluble fiber from the total carbohydrate and total fiber counts. Next, take a look at the sugar alcohol content- if the total count of sugar alcohols exceed 5 g, subtract half of that number from the total carb count to yield net carbs.

Protein intake is also quite important, and should be measured carefully. While some meal plans stress low protein intake, it's best to introduce yourself slowly to the keto lifestyle by keeping your protein in balance- you can still achieve ketosis with higher protein levels at first, and your body will naturally adjust to a point where it doesn't need or crave as much protein. You'll also find that your appetite will reduce the longer your body is in ketosis- this is a great sign! Listen to your body, and only eat as much as your body needs.

Intermittent fasting is a great way to jolt your body into ketosis, and one of the cornerstones of the keto lifestyle. While this meal plan provides you with food options daily, feel free to fast one day a week if you're able to, or skip a meal here and there in order to introduce yourself to the concept. While fasting, remember to consume plenty of water, and help yourself to a cup of bone broth if you're feeling hungry.

Pay close attention to the shopping list- as you may have noticed, we've given you a few substitution options. While the majority of these items can all be found in grocery and health food stores, we wanted to ensure that you had viable alternative options in the event you can't find something. Each of the substitution options listed can be used in the exact same quantity and application as the original ingredient item.

To save you time and money, some of the protein and produce items are can also be carried over into the following week- for example, if you only need 4 oz of chicken in one week, but 8 oz the week after, it makes sense to purchase it all in one shot. Remember with meat especially, it's usually less expensive to purchase in bulk and portion and freeze it to be used over a longer period of time.

Without further ado, here are EIGHT 7-day meal plans to get you started!

TRADITIONAL MEAL PLAN

This meal plan is for folks who have time to cook and like to be in the kitchen. Of course, it is for everyone else, too. You'll find the recipes to be concise and easy to make. Plus, these meals are totally delicious if I do say so myself!

Save time and money on your keto diet by doing the following:

- Intermittent fasting- If you're not hungry, don't eat! While this may seem like a simple enough premise, it is something to keep in mind as intermittent fasting aids in raising your ketone levels. The recipes and meal recommendations in this guide are here to give you options as you begin your keto journey, but don't feel obligated to eat just because the plan is telling you to do so (LISTEN to your body!)

- Meal prep- Look over your meal plan every week, as well as your shopping list, and figure out what you can prep ahead of time to save yourself time during the week. Many of these recipes can be prepped ahead of time and kept on hand to enjoy at your convenience. Dinner leftovers make fast, easy lunches, and breakfast can be a repeat of your favourite recipe (if you love keto lattes in the morning, stick with that!)

- The recipes in this plan are made to empower you to make your own food choices! Particularly in the dinner section (because, let's face it- dinner is usually the one meal we all struggle with!), you will find an assortment of side dish recipes that are meant to be eaten in conjunction with a protein, and usually one or two other sides as well. The meal plan is a guideline, but as you become more comfortable with it, feel free to make small swaps here and there as you see fit (just make sure to track the macros!)

- Many of these recipes come with add-on options (such as added sour cream in the quesadillas recipe), with individual macros listed below the overall nutritional info. If you choose to use the add-on items, make sure to adjust the macros as needed.

Week 1 Traditonal Meal Plan

Day	Breakfast	Lunch	Dinner	Snack/Dessert	Calories/Macros
1	Cheesy Scrambled Eggs 424 cal 39.8 fat 15.3 protein 1.9 carbs	Salmon, spinach and goat cheese Salad 311 cal 17.5 g fat 24 g protein 11 g carbs	4 oz Baked Salmon with warm mushrooms and brown butter 650 cal 54 g fat 40 g protein 6 g carbs	2 oz macadamia nuts 241 cal 25,4 g fat 2.7 g protein 1 g carbs	Calories: 1626 Fat: 136.7 g Protein: 82 g Net Carbs: 19.9 g
2	Dairy Free Keto Pumpkin Spice Latte 190 cal 18 g fat 6 g protein 0.9 g carbs	Green Goddess Avo Salad 905 cal 75.5 g fat 32 g protein 10 g carbs	Eggplant Parmesan 385 cal 28.1 g fat 22.5 g protein 12.3 g carbs	FASTING PERIOD Intermittent fasting is a cornerstone of the keto diet, and helps your body achieve ketosis (water allowed)	Calories: 1480 Fat: 121.6 g Protein: 60.5 g Net Carbs: 23.2 g
3	Greek Style Scrambled Eggs 404 cal 37.8 g fat 15.3 g protein 1.9 g carbs	Eggplant Parmesan (leftover) 385 cal 28.1 g fat 22.5 g protein 12.3 g carbs	4 oz Steak (cooked to your liking) with Cauliflower Goat Cheese Mash 785 cal 60.1 g fat 56 g protein 4.6 g carbs	FASTING PERIOD Intermittent fasting is a cornerstone of the keto diet, and helps your body achieve ketosis (water allowed)	Calories: 1574 Fat:126 g Protein: 93.8 g Net Carbs: 18.8 g

4	Western Scrambled Eggs 498 cal 43.8g fat 23.4g protein 2,9 g carbs	Beef and Avocado Lettuce Wraps 454 cal 37 fat 21 protein 6 carbs	1 serving lemon and thyme chicken legs with 1 serving Bacon Parmesan Asparagus 639 cal 61.8 g fat 65.6 protein 6.6 g carbs	4 stalks celery, ¼ bell pepper and 1 serving Tahini 89 cal 8 g fat 2.6 g protein 1 g carb	Calories: 1680 Fat: 150.6 g Protein: 112.6 g Net Carbs: 16.5 g
5	Bacon Egg and Avo Sandwich 899 cal 83.9 g fat 24.2 g protein 4.1 g carbs	1 serving lemon and thyme chicken legs with 1 cup greens, ½ oz pecans, and 1 serving Strawberry Balsamic Dressing 599 cal 53 g fat 30,5 g protein 0.9 g carbs	Bacon Wrapped Cod 323 cal 27.6 fat 17.5 protein 0.7 carbs	**FASTING PERIOD** Intermittent fasting is a cornerstone of the keto diet, and helps your body achieve ketosis (water allowed)	Calories: 1821 Fat: 164.5 g Protein: 72.2 g Net Carbs: 18.8 g
6	Coconut Chia Pudding 451 cal 42 g fat 6.6 g protein 8 g carbs	Leftover Bacon Wrapped Cod with 1 serving Bacon Parmesan Asparagus 583 cal 54.4 fat 52.6 protein 6.7 carbs	Pesto Chicken Casserole 501 cal 37.6 g fat 38 g protein 4.6 g carbs	1 oz pecans 197 cal 23.3 g fat 3 g protein 1.1 g carbs	Calories: 1732 Fat 157.3 g Protein: 100.2 g Net Carbs: 20.4 g

| 7 | Dairy Free Mocha Latte

190 cal

18 g fat

6 g protein

0.9 g carbs | Eggplant Parmesan

(leftover)

385 cal

28.1 g fat

22.5 g protein

12.3 g carbs | 4 oz Steak (cooked to your liking) with Cauliflower Goat Cheese Mash and Bacon Parmesan Asparagus

1045 cal

86.9 g fat

91.1 g protein

10.6 g carbs | FASTING PERIOD

Intermittent fasting is a cornerstone of the keto diet, and helps your body achieve ketosis

(water allowed) | Calories: 1620

Fat 133 g

Protein:119.6 g

Net Carbs: 23.8 g |

Week 2 Traditional Meal Plan

Day	Breakfast	Lunch	Dinner	Snack/Dessert	Calories/Macros
8	Double Egg Breakfast Sandwich

607 cal

53 fat

30,2 protein

2.4 carbs | Keto Quesadillas

330 cal

21.5 fat

29.7 protein

4.1 carbs | Southwest Chicken Chili

410 cal

23.1 fat

28.9 protein

7 carbs | Coconut Chia Pudding

451 cal

42 g fat

6.6 g protein

8 g carbs | Calories: 1798

Fat: 139.6 g

Protein: 95.4 g

Net Carbs: 22.5 g |

9	Strawberry Smoothie with 1 Breakfast Roll and 1 tbsp almond butter 737 cal 53 fat 33.5 g protein 8.3 g net carbs	Southwest Chicken Chili (leftover) 410 cal 23.1 fat 28.9 protein 7 carbs	Asian Style Beef Salad 603 cal 22 g fat 85.2 g protein 5 g carbs	FASTING PERIOD Intermittent fasting is a cornerstone of the keto diet, and helps your body achieve ketosis (water allowed)	Calories: 1750 Fat: 98.1 g Protein: 147.6 g Net Carbs: 20.3 g
10	1 serving Cinnamon Roll Donuts 160 cal 11.8 g fat 3.2 g protein 1.2 g carbs	Asian Style Beef Salad (leftover) 603 cal 22 g fat 85.2 g protein 5 g carbs	Middle Eastern Halloumi 700 cal 53.2 g fat 33.7 g protein 15 g carbs	Coconut Matcha Latte 255 cal 28.8 g fat 3.4 g protein 3 g carbs	Calories: 1718 Fat: 115.8 g Protein: 125.3 g Net Carbs: 24.2 g
11	Dairy Free Keto Latte 190 cal 18 fat 6 g protein 0.9 g carbs	Italian Chopped Salad 790 cal 66 g fat 47 protein 5.9 carbs	Coconut Curry Shiratake Noodles 557 cal 41.7 g fat 33.7 g protein 13 g carbs	1 serving Cinnamon Roll Donuts 160 cal 11.8 g fat 3.2 g protein 1.2 g carbs	Calories: 1697 Fat: 137.5 g Protein: 89.9 g Net Carbs: 21 g

12	Goat Cheese Pancakes 425 cal 39 fat 14 protein 5 carbs	Coconut Curry Shiratake Noodles (leftover) 557 cal 41.7 g fat 33.7 g protein 13 g carbs	Lemon and Thyme Chicken Leg with Mushrooms and Brown Butter (plus optional side of greens) 879 cal 74.8 g fat 48.5 g protein 6 g carbs	FASTING PERIOD Intermittent fasting is a cornerstone of the keto diet, and helps your body achieve ketosis (water allowed)	Calories: 1861 Fat: 155.5 g Protein: 96.2 g Net Carbs: 24 g
13	Keto Dairy Free Vanilla Latte 190 cal 18 g fat 6 g protein 0.9 g carbs	Lemon and Thyme Chicken Leg with Mushrooms and Brown Butter (Left over) With ½ cup greens 879 cal 74.8 g fat 48.5 g protein 6 g carbs	Creamy Bacon and Spinach Zucchini Noodles 770 cal 65 fat 37.6 protein 12 g carbs	FASTING PERIOD Intermittent fasting is a cornerstone of the keto diet, and helps your body achieve ketosis (water allowed)	Calories: 1839 Fat: 157.8 g Protein: 92.1 g Net Carbs:18.9 g
14	Keto Dairy Free Pumpkin Spice Latte plus 1 egg cooked to your liking 235 cal 23 g fat 11.5 g protein 0.9 g carbs	Creamy Bacon and Spinach Zucchini Noodles 770 cal 65 fat 37.6 protein 12 g carbs	Taco Night 860 cal 77.6 fat 54.5 protein 3.9 carbs	FASTING PERIOD Intermittent fasting is a cornerstone of the keto diet, and helps your body achieve ketosis (water allowed)	Calories: 1865 Fat: 165.6 g Protein: 103.6 g Net Carbs: 16.8 g

					Week 3 Traditional Meal Plan

Week 3 Traditional Meal Plan

Day	Breakfast	Lunch	Dinner	Snack/Dessert	Calories/Macros
15	Western Scrambled Eggs 498 cal 43.8 g fat 23.4 g protein 2.9 g carbs	Burrito Bowl (using leftover taco meat) 545 calories 32 g fat 48.6 g protein 11 g carbs	Keto Cabbage Rolls 405 cal 16.4 g fat 53.6 g protein 7 g carbs	2 oz Almonds 328 cal 28.4 g fat 12 g protein 4 g carb	Calories: 1776 Fat: 120.6 g Protein: 137.6 g Net Carbs: 24.9 g
16	Halloumi Shakshouka with Keto Dairy Free Vanilla Latte 350 cal 29.8 g fat 9.2 g protein 2.1 g carbs	Keto Cabbage Rolls (left over) 405 cal 16.4 g fat 53.6 g protein 7 g carbs	Asian Style Beef Salad 603 cal 22 g fat 85.2 g protein 5 g carbs	3 oz prosciutto with 2 oz mozzarella 283 cal 14.8 g fat 33.6 g protein 3 g carb	Calories: 1641 Fat: 83 g Protein: 181.6 g Net Carbs: 18.1 g
17	Dairy Free Mocha Latte 190 cal 18 g fat 6 g protein 0.9 g carbs	Asian Style Beef Salad (leftover) 603 cal 22 g fat 85.2 g protein 5 g carbs	Bacon Wrapped Cod with Mushrooms and Brown Butter, and Bacon Parmesan Asparagus 1083 cal 101.4 g fat 70.6 g protein 12.7 carbs	FASTING PERIOD Intermittent fasting is a cornerstone of the keto diet, and helps your body achieve ketosis (water allowed)	Calories: 1876 Fat: 141.4 g Protein: 161.8 g Net Carbs: 18.5 g

18	Strawberry Smoothie 150 cal 14 fat 0.1 g protein 1.4 g net carbs	Bacon wrapped cod with ½ cup greens and bacon parmesan asparagus 626 cal 54.4 g fat 52.6 g protein 6.7 g carbs	Shiratake Carbonara 720 cal 67 g fat 33.9 g protein 4.7 g carb	Coconut Matcha Latte 255 cal 28.8 g fat 3.4 g protein 3 g carbs	Calories: 1751 Fat:164.2 g Protein: 89.1 g Net Carbs: 15.8 g
19	Greek Style Scrambled Eggs 404 cal 37.8 fat 15.3 protein 1.9 carbs	Keto Cabbage Rolls (leftover) 405 cal 16.4 g fat 53.6 g protein 7 g carbs	Roulade of Chicken 700 cal 63.8 g fat 72.9 g protein 3.6 g carbs	FASTING PERIOD Intermittent fasting is a cornerstone of the keto diet, and helps your body achieve ketosis (water allowed)	Calories: 1509 Fat: 112.8 g Protein: 90.5 g Net Carbs: 21.3 g
20	Dairy Free Keto Pumpkin Spice Latte 190 cal 18 g fat 6 g protein 0.9 g carbs	1 serving Chicken Roulade (leftovers) with ½ cup spinach and 1 serving Creamy Poppy seed dressing 937 cal 90.6 fat 73.9 protein 4.6 g carbs	Keto Pizza 761 cal 52 g fat 70 g protein 7 carbs	FASTING PERIOD Intermittent fasting is a cornerstone of the keto diet, and helps your body achieve ketosis (water allowed)	Calories: 1888 Fat: 160.6 g Protein: 149.9 g Net Carbs: 12.5 g
21	Smoked salmon, cream cheese and greens breakfast sandwich 539 cal 53 g fat 35.6 g protein 5.7 g carbs	Keto Cabbage Rolls (leftover) 405 cal 16.4 g fat 53.6 g protein 7 g carbs	4 oz steak with Cauliflower Goat Cheese Mash 785 cal 59.8 g fat 56 g protein 4.6 g net carb	FASTING PERIOD Intermittent fasting is a cornerstone of the keto diet, and helps your body achieve ketosis (water allowed)	Calories: 1729 Fat: 129.2 g Protein:145.2 g Net Carbs: 17.3 g

Week 4 Traditional Meal Plan

Day	Breakfast	Lunch	Dinner	Snack/Dessert	Calories/Macros
22	Double Egg Sandwich 607 cal 53 g fat 30.2 g protein 2.4 g carbs	Keto Quesadillas with 3 tbsp sour cream 407 cal 29.1 g fat 30.8 g protein 5.6 g carbs	Shiratake Carbonara (leftover) 720 cal 67 g fat 33.9 g protein 4.7 g carb	4 stalks celery, ¼ bell pepper and 1 serving Tahini 89 cal 8 g fat 2.6 g protein 1 g carb	Calories: 1823 Fat: 157.1 g Protein: 97.5 g Net Carbs:13.7 g
23	Swiss Omelette 425 cal 39 g fat 14 g protein 5 g carbs	Keto Pizza (leftover) 761 cal 52 g fat 70 g protein 7 carbs	1 serving lemon and thyme chicken legs with 1 serving Bacon Parmesan Asparagus 639 cal 61.8 g fat 65.6 protein 6.6 g carbs	FASTING PERIOD Intermittent fasting is a cornerstone of the keto diet, and helps your body achieve ketosis (water allowed)	Calories: 1825 Fat: 152.8 g Protein: 149.6 g Net Carbs: 18.6 g
24	Cheesy Chicken Breakfast Burrito 830 cal 75.2 g fat 50.3 g protein 3.5 g carbs	½ cup greens with 2 strips bacon and 1 serving Creamy Onion Poppyseed dressing 446 cal 42.7 g fat 15.5 g protein 1.7 g carbs	Pesto Chicken Casserole 501 cal 37.6 g fat 38 g protein 4.6 g carbs	FASTING PERIOD Intermittent fasting is a cornerstone of the keto diet, and helps your body achieve ketosis (water allowed)	Calories: 1777 Fat: 155.5 g Protein: 103.8 g Net Carbs: 9.8 g

25	Mushroom, Spinach and Goat Cheese Frittata 316 cal 27 fat 16.4 protein 2.4 carbs	Italian Chopped Salad 790 cal 66 g fat 47 g protein 5.9 g carbs	Oysters Rockefeller with optional side of greens 700 cal 55.6g fat 60.9 g protein 13 g carbs	FASTING PERIOD Intermittent fasting is a cornerstone of the keto diet, and helps your body achieve ketosis (water allowed)	Calories: 1806 Fat: 148.6 g Protein: 119 g Net Carbs: 21.3 g
26	Dairy Free Keto Mocha Latte 190 calories 18 g fat 6g protein 0.9 g carbs	Leftover Mushroom, Spinach and Goat Cheese Frittata with ½ cup greens and 1 serving Strawberry Balsamic Dressing 536 cal 52 fat 16.4 protein 2.7 carbs	Coconut Curry Shiratake noodles with 1 serving Lemon and Thyme Chicken (leftover) 936 cal 69.5 g fat 64.2 g protein 13 g carbs	FASTING PERIOD Intermittent fasting is a cornerstone of the keto diet, and helps your body achieve ketosis (water allowed)	Calories: 1662 Fat: 139.5 g Protein: 86.6 g Net Carbs: 16.6 g
27	Cheesy Scrambled Eggs 424 cal 39.8g fat 15.3 g protein 1.9 g carbs	Pesto Chicken Casserole (leftover) 501 cal 37.6 g fat 38 g protein 4.6 g carbs	Pork Chops with Mushrooms 805 cal 73.4g fat 45.6 g protein 3.4 g carb	FASTING PERIOD Intermittent fasting is a cornerstone of the keto diet, and helps your body achieve ketosis (water allowed)	Calories: 1730 Fat: 150.8 g Protein: 98.9 g Net Carbs: 10.9 g

28	Double Egg Breakfast Sandwich 607 cal 53g fat 30.2 g protein 2.4 g carbs	Pork Chops with Mushrooms (leftover) 805 cal 73.4g fat 45.6 g protein 3.4 g carb	Eggplant Parmesan 385 cal 28.1 g fat 22.5 g protein 12.3 g carbs	FASTING PERIOD Intermittent fasting is a cornerstone of the keto diet, and helps your body achieve ketosis (water allowed)	Calories: 1797 Fat: 154.5 g Protein: 98.3g Net Carbs: 18.1 g

QUICK KETO MEAL PLAN

If you're a busy bee and don't have a lot of time to spend in the kitchen or on prep work, this quick keto meal plan will work wonders for you and your schedule. Get ready to be wowed with food, my friend.

Week 1 Quick Meal Plan					
Day	**Breakfast**	**Lunch**	**Dinner**	**Snack/Dessert**	**Calories/Macros**
1	Blue Smoothie 189 cal 16.6 fat 3.1 protein 1 carbs	Loaded Avocado Salad 430 cal 35.5 g fat 13.2 g protein 8 g carbs	3 oz Baked Salmon with leftover Loaded Avocado Salad 540 cal 41 g fat 29.7 g protein 8 g carbs	Caprese Rolls with Prosciutto 95 cal 4 g fat 12.5 g protein 1 g carbs	Calories: 1254 Fat: 149.9 g Protein: 58.5 g Net Carbs: 18 g
2	Coconut smoothie bowl 726 cal 69.4 g fat 11.4 g protein 6 g carbs	Keto Lunchables 590 cal 37.6 g fat 28.6 g protein 6 g carbs	Lettuce Wrapped Chicken Fajitas 320 cal 20 g fat 26.2 g protein 4 g carbs	FASTING PERIOD Intermittent fasting is a cornerstone of the keto diet, and helps your body achieve ketosis (water allowed)	Calories: 1636 Fat: 127 g Protein: 66.2 g Net Carbs: 16 g

3	Microwave Scrambled Eggs 394 cal 35.7 g fat 17.4 g protein 0.1 g carbs	Salmon and Avocado Nori Rolls 380 cal 29.6 g fat 20.6 g protein 3.5 g carbs	Coconut Lime Noodles and Tofu 303 cal 14.2 g fat 28.9 g protein 9.1 g carbs	2 oz pecans 390 calories 40 g fat 6 g protein 2 g carbs	Calories: 1467 Fat: 119.5 g Protein: 72.9 g Net Carbs: 14.7 g
4	Green Smoothie 350 cal 34g fat 4.1 g protein 1.5 g carbs	1 serving Cream of Broccoli Soup with easy green salad 478 cal 47 fat 3.3 protein 3.1 carbs	Cheesy Chicken Bake 488 cal 22.3 g fat 34 protein 9.3 g carbs	Beef Broth 273cal 28.6 g fat 4.9 g protein 0.9 g carbs	Calories: 1589 Fat: 131.9 g Protein: 46.3 g Net Carbs: 14.8 g
5	Microwave Scrambled Eggs with your choice of inclusions* 394 cal 35.7 g fat 17.4 g protein 0.1 g carbs *Macros will vary slightly dependent upon inclusions	Leftover Coconut Lime Noodles 303 cal 14.2 g fat 28.9 g protein 9.1 g carbs	1 serving Cream of Broccoli Soup With Easy Green Salad 478 cal 51.1 fat 3.3 protein 3.1 carbs	2 Servings Almond Coconut Fat Bomb 400 cal 40 g fat 6 g protein 4 g carbs	Calories: 1575 Fat: 141 g Protein: 55.6 g Net Carbs: 16.3 g

6	Nut Butter Smoothie Bowl 183 cal 13.3 fat 8.6 protein 0.1 carbs	Thai Chicken Salad 303 cal 14.2 fat 28.3 protein 9.1 carbs	Avocado BLT 540 cal 46.1 g fat 18.3 g protein 5.6 g carbs	Veggie Sticks and Tahini 89 cal 8 g fat 2.6 g protein 1 g carb	Calories: 1591 Fat 146.4 g Protein: 36.2 g Net Carbs: 10.8 g
7	Chicken Parm Fritatta 600 cal 31 g fat 45 g protein 9.3 g carbs	FASTING PERIOD Intermittent fasting (water allowed) *Note- if you don't think you can make it through the day without lunch, have your snack here and fast later	Salmon Putanesca 600 cal 30.3 g fat 72.4 g protein 8 g net carbs	2 servings Guacamole Deviled Eggs 390 cal 34 g fat 14 g protein 6 g carbs	Calories: 1590 Fat 95.3 g Protein:131.4 g Net Carbs: 23.3 g

Week 2 Quick Meal Plan

Day	Breakfast	Lunch	Dinner	Snack/Dessert	Calories/Macros
8	Blue Smoothie 189 cal 16.6 fat 3.1 protein 1 carbs	Salmon Putanesca with Easy Green Salad 846 cal 50.6 fat 72.8 protein 8.1 carbs	Ham and Swiss Cheese Crustless Quiche 566 cal 43.2 fat 36.3 protein 5.6 carbs	Coconut Matcha Fat Bomb 100 cal 11.5 g fat 0.2 g protein 2 g carbs	Calories: 1701 Fat: 121.9 g Protein: 112.4 g Net Carbs: 16.7 g

9	Leftover Ham and Swiss Crustless Quiche 566 cal 43.2 fat 36.3 protein 5.6 carbs	Tuna Salad Lettuce Wraps 466 cal 24.2 g fat 48.1 g protein 7.1 g net carbs	Chicken a la king 494 cal 36.9 g fat 29.1 g protein 4.3 g carbs	Beef Broth 273cal 28.6 g fat 4.9 g protein 0.9 g carbs	Calories: 1799 Fat:132.9 g Protein: 118.4 g Net Carbs: 17.9 g
10	Matcha Smoothie Bowl 691 cal 67.9 g fat 12.9 g protein 8 g carbs	Cream of Broccoli Soup 232 cal 22.8 fat 2.9 protein 3 carbs	Portobello Burger 485 cal 30 fat 48.6 protein 2 carbs	Caprese Rolls with Prosciutto 95 cal 4 g fat 12.5 g protein 1 g carbs	Calories: 1503 Fat: 124.7 g Protein: 76.9 g Net Carbs: 14 g
11	Green Smoothie 350 cal 34 fat 4.1 g protein 1.5 g carbs	Caprese Salad 534 cal 52.2fat 16.6 protein 3 carbs	Thai Chicken Salad 303 cal 14.2 g fat 28.9 g protein 9.1 g carbs	2 Servings Almond Coconut Fat Bomb 400 cal 40 g fat 6 g protein 4 g carbs	Calories: 1587 Fat: 140.4 g Protein: 55.6 g Net Carbs: 17.6 g
12	Easy Eggs Benedict 366 cal 32.8 fat 11.5 protein 5 carbs	Keto Lunchables with your choice of inclusions 590 cal 37.6 g fat 28.6 g protein 6 g carbs	Shrimp Stir Fry 600 cal 56g fat 30.6 g protein 7 g carbs	FASTING PERIOD Intermittent fasting is a cornerstone of the keto diet, and helps your body achieve ketosis (water allowed)	Calories: 1556 Fat: 126.4 g Protein: 70.7 g Net Carbs:18 g

13	Microwave Scrambled Eggs with your choice of inclusions 394 cal 35.7 g fat 17.4 g protein 0.1 g carbs	Leftover Shrimp Stir Fry 600 cal 56g fat 30.6 g protein 7 g carbs	Middle Eastern Style Stuffed Tomatoes 400 cal 33 fat 22.9 protein 5 g carbs	2 servings Coconut Matcha Fat Bombs 200 cal 23 g fat 0.4 g protein 4 g carbs	Calories: 1594 Fat: 147.7 g Protein: 71.3 g Net Carbs: 16.1 g
14	Nutty Coffee Plus 3 Pieces Bacon 476 calories 39.6 g fat 26.6 g protein 2.1 carbs	Leftover Middle Eastern Stuffed Tomatoes 400 cal 33 fat 22.9 protein 5 g carbs	Ma Po Tofu 449 cal 30.1 fat 35.1 protein 6 carbs	Caprese Rolls with Prosciutto 95 cal 4 g fat 12.5 g protein 1 g carbs	Calories: 1420 Fat: 106.7 g Protein: 97.1 g Net Carbs: 14.1 g

Week 3 Quick Meal Plan

Day	Breakfast	Lunch	Dinner	Snack/Dessert	Calories/Macros
15	Scotch Eggs 442 cal 46 g fat 25 g protein 0 g carbs	Easy green salad with 4 oz baked salmon 396 calories 35.3 g fat 22.4 g protein 0.1 g carbs	Bacon-butter cod with parmesan crusted cauliflower 273 cal 20 g fat 23 g protein 2 g carbs	2 oz Almonds 328 cal 28.4 g fat 12 protein 4 g carb	Calories: 1439 Fat:129.7 g Protein: 82.4 g Net Carbs: 6.1 g

16	Keto Lemon Tea Plus 1 egg any way and 3 pieces bacon 622 cal 55.6 g fat 27.3 g protein 4.2 g carbs	Leftover Butter-Bacon Cod with parmesan crusted cauliflower 273 cal 20 g fat 23 g protein 2 g carbs	Cheesy Mushrooms with easy green salad 370 cal 43.8 g fat 1.9 g protein 0.3 g carbs	Beef Broth 273cal 28.6 g fat 4.9 g protein 0.9 g carbs	Calories: 1538 Fat: 141 g Protein: 57.1 g Net Carbs: 7.4 g
17	Coconut Smoothie 638 cal 57.4 g fat 7.2 g protein 9 g carbs	Leftover Cheesy Mushroom with Easy green salad 370 cal 43.8 fat 1.9 g protein 0.3 carbs	Cream of Broccoli Soup 232 cal 22.8 fat 2.9 protein 3 carbs	Veggie Sticks and Guacamole 294 cal 30 g fat 12 g protein 4.2 g carbs	Calories: 1534 Fat: 154 g Protein: 24 g Net Carbs: 26.4 g
18	Easy Eggs Benedict 366 cal 32.8 fat 11.5 protein 5 carbs	Chicken BLT Salad 734 cal 52.5 g fat 45.1 g protein 9 g carbs	Bacon-Tomato-Cheddar Soup 270 cal 21.9 g fat 12.2 g protein 1 g carb	2 servings Prosciutto Mozzarella and Basil rolls 190 calories 8 g fat 25 g protein 2 g carbs	Calories: 1560 Fat: 115.2 g Protein: 93.8 g Net Carbs: 17 g
19	Blue Smoothie plus 1 egg and 3 slices bacon 560 cal 44.8 fat 29.8 protein 2.2 carbs	Thai Chicken Salad 303 cal 14.2 fat 28.3 protein 9.1 carbs	Pesto Pasta 646 cal 53.8 g fat 32.4 g protein 10 g carbs	FASTING PERIOD Intermittent fasting is a cornerstone of the keto diet, and helps your body achieve ketosis (water allowed)	Calories: 1509 Fat: 112.8 g Protein: 90.5 g Net Carbs: 21.3 g

20	Keto Lemon Tea 251 cal 27.4 g fat 0.6 g protein 3 g carbs	Leftover pesto pasta 646 cal 53.8 g fat 32.4 g protein 10 g carbs	Cheesy Meatballs 331 cal 20.6 g fat 40.1 g protein 10 carbs	2 oz pecans 390 calories 40 g fat 6 g protein 2 g carbs	Calories: 1618 Fat: 141.8 g Protein: 79.4 g Net Carbs: 25 g
21	Microwave Scrambled Eggs with choice of inclusions 394 cal 35.7 g fat 17.4 g protein 0.1 g carbs	Leftover Cheesy Meatballs 331 cal 20.6 g fat 40.1 g protein 10 carbs	Chicken, spinach and goat cheese salad 700 cal 51.8 g fat 45.3 g protein 3 g net carb	Beef Broth 273cal 28.6 g fat 4.9 g protein 0.9 g carbs	Calories: 1698 Fat: 136.7 g Protein: 107.7 g Net Carbs: 14 g

Week 4 Quick Meal Plan

Day	Breakfast	Lunch	Dinner	Snack/Dessert	Calories/Macros
22	Green Smoothie 350 cal 34g fat 4.1 g protein 1.5 g carbs	Southwest Chicken Avocado Salad 800 cal 53.1 g fat 41.9 g protein 5 g carbs	Bacon-Tomato-Cheddar Soup 270 cal 21.9 g fat 12.2 g protein 1 g carb	Caprese Rolls with Prosciutto 95 cal 4 g fat 12.5 g protein 1 g carbs	Calories: 1515 Fat: 113 g Protein: 70.7 g Net Carbs: 8.5 g
23	Keto Lemon Tea 251 cal 27.4 g fat 0.6 g protein 3 g carbs	Easy green salad with 4 oz baked salmon 396 calories 35.3 g fat 22.4 g protein 0.1 g carbs	Baked Cod with lemony asparagus 554 cal 26 g fat 81 g protein 1.3 g carbs	2 servings Coconut Matcha Fat Bombs 200 cal 23 g fat 0.4 g protein 4 g carbs	Calories: 1401 Fat: 111.7 g Protein: 111.4 g Net Carbs: 8.4 g
24	Asparagus and Goat Cheese Omelette 694 cal 59.7 g fat 35 g protein 4.5 g carbs	Leftover Baked Cod with lemony asparagus 554 cal 26 g fat 81 g protein 1.3 g carbs	Bacon-Tomato-Cheddar Soup 270 cal 21.9 g fat 12.2 g protein 1 g carb	Veggie Sticks and Tahini 89 cal 8 g fat 2.6 g protein 1 g carb	Calories: 1607 Fat: 115.6 g Protein: 130.8 g Net Carbs: 7.8 g

25	Easy Eggs Benedict 366 cal 32.8 fat 11.5 protein 5 carbs	Keto Lunchables with your choice of inclusions 590 cal 37.6 g fat 28.6 g protein 6 g carbs	Shrimp Stir Fry 600 cal 56g fat 30.6 g protein 7 g carbs	FASTING PERIOD Intermittent fasting is a cornerstone of the keto diet, and helps your body achieve ketosis (water allowed)	Calories: 1556 Fat:76.4 g Protein: 70.7 g Net Carbs: 18 g
26	Nutty Coffee 168 calories 15.8 g fat 5.5g protein 2.1 carbs	Leftover Shrimp Stir Fry 600 cal 56g fat 30.6 g protein 7 g carbs	Asparagus, goat cheese and smoked salmon salad 466 cal 31.6 g fat 41.9 g protein 2.3 g carbs	2 servings Guacamole Deviled Eggs 390 cal 34 g fat 14 g protein 6 g carbs	Calories: 1624 Fat: 117.4 g Protein: 92 g Net Carbs: 17.4 g
27	Matcha Smoothie Bowl 691 cal 67.9 g fat 12.9 g protein 8 g carbs	Easy green salad with 4 oz baked salmon 396 calories 35.3 g fat 22.4 g protein 0.1 g carbs	Bacon-Tomato-Cheddar Soup 270 cal 21.9 g fat 12.2 g protein 1 g carb	1 serving coconut matcha fat bombs 100 cal 10.3 g fat 0.2 g protein 2 g net carbs	Calories: 1457 Fat: 135.4 g Protein: 47.7 g Net Carbs: 11.1 g
28	Southwest style eggs 546 cal 35 g fat 26 g protein 12 g carbs	Chicken and Avocado Nori Wraps 657 cal 50.5 g fat 33 g protein 9 g carbs	Baked Cod with lemony asparagus 554 cal 26 g fat 81 g protein 1.3 g carbs	Veggie Sticks and Tahini 89 cal 8 g fat 2.6 g protein 1 g carb	Calories: 1846 Fat: 119.5 g Protein: 142.6 g Net Carbs: 23.3 g

CHAPTER 5
Oh Something's Cookin

Traditional Meal Plan Recipes

Breakfast

Cheesy Scrambled Eggs

Scrambled eggs and cheese are the ultimate comfort food.

Serving: 1

Serving Size: whole recipe

Prep Time: 5 minutes

Cook Time: >5 minutes

Ingredients

2 eggs, beaten

1 oz butter

1 oz shredded cheddar cheese

Instructions

Beat the eggs with a pinch of salt and pepper.

Preheat a small pan over medium heat, and melt in the butter

Pour in the eggs, and stir constantly for 3 minutes, until cooked through

Add in the cheese, and stir for another minute.

Nutrition: 424 calories, 39.8 g fat, 15.3 g protein, 1.9 g net carbs

Strawberry Smoothie

This smoothie is so easy to make, and a low calorie way to start your morning. Enjoy on its own, or as a beverage with your favourite breakfast food. It also makes a great snack any time of the day!

Serving: 1

Serving Size: whole recipe

Prep Time: 5 minutes

Cook Time: 0 minutes

Ingredients

2 frozen strawberries, thawed slightly

¾ almond milk

¼ tsp erythritol (optional)

1 tbsp coconut oil

Instructions

Blend together all ingredients until smooth. Serve immediately.

Nutrition: 150 calories, 14 g fat, 0.1 g protein, 1.4 g net carbs

Greek Style Scrambled Eggs

These eggs are creamy, delicious, and have a yummy mediterranean twist!

Serving: 1

Serving Size: whole recipe

Prep Time: 5 minutes

Cook Time: >5 minutes

Ingredients

2 eggs, beaten

1 tsp dried oregano

1 oz butter

1 oz feta

Instructions

Beat the eggs with a pinch of salt and pepper, and the oregano.

Preheat a small pan over medium heat, and melt in the butter

Pour in the eggs, and stir constantly for 3 minutes, until cooked through

Add in the feta, and stir for another minute.

Nutrition: 404 calories, 37.8 g fat, 15.3 g protein, 1.9 g net carbs

Smoked Salmon and Goat Cheese Eggs

This is an elegant, low car, high flavour breakfast! Enjoy with a few slices of cucumber or your favourite low carb bread!

Serving: 1

Serving Size: whole recipe

Prep Time: 5 minutes

Cook Time: >5 minutes

Ingredients

2 eggs, beaten

1 oz butter

1 oz goat cheese

2 oz smoked salmon

Instructions

Beat the eggs with a pinch of salt and pepper

Preheat a small pan over medium heat, and melt in the butter

Pour in the eggs, and stir constantly for 3 minutes, until cooked through

Add in the goat cheese, and stir for another minute.

Slice the salmon into thin strips, and toss with the eggs at the last minute. Serve immediately

Nutrition: 524 calories, 44.3 g fat, 30.3 g protein, 1.2 g net carbs

Dairy Free Keto Pumpkin Spice Latte

Is there anything more satisfying than a PSL? Only the satisfaction of knowing this one is ketogenic!

Serving: 1

Serving Size: whole recipe

Prep Time: >5 minutes

Cook Time: 0 minutes

Ingredients

2 eggs

1 tbsp coconut oil

1 cup hot coffee or boiling water

1 tsp pumpkin pie spice

1 tsp stevia or erythritol (optional)

Instructions

Blend the eggs, coconut oil and pumpkin spice (and sweetener, if using) in a blender for 20 seconds, to mix

Add the coffee, and blend for another minute or so

Serve immediately

Nutrition: 190 calories, 18 g fat, 6 g protein, 0.9 g net carbs

Dairy Free Keto Vanilla Latte

This vanilla latte is so easy to make, and the perfect start to your morning!

Serving: 1

Serving Size: whole recipe

Prep Time: >5 minutes

Cook Time: 0 minutes

Ingredients

2 eggs

1 tbsp coconut oil

1 cup hot coffee or boiling water

1 tsp vanilla extract

1 tsp stevia or erythritol (optional)

Instructions

Blend the eggs, coconut oil and vanilla (and sweetener, if using) in a blender for 20 seconds, to mix

Add the coffee, and blend for another minute or so

Serve immediately

Nutrition: 190 calories, 18 g fat, 6 g protein, 0.9 g net carbs

Dairy Free Keto Mocha Latte

If you're not a fan of coffee with your hot chocolate, use boiling water instead. Add a bit of cream for extra richness, if you like.

Serving: 1

Serving Size: whole recipe

Prep Time: >5 minutes

Cook Time: 0 minutes

Ingredients

2 eggs

1 tbsp coconut oil

1 cup hot coffee or boiling water

¼ tsp vanilla extract

1 tbsp cocoa powder

1 tsp stevia or erythritol (optional)

Instructions

Blend the eggs, coconut oil, vanilla, and cocoa (and sweetener, if using) in a blender for 20 seconds, to mix

Add the coffee, and blend for another minute or so

Serve immediately

Nutrition: 190 calories, 18 g fat, 6 g protein, 0.9 g net carbs

Chocolate Almond Smoothie

This caffeine free drink is full of great fat, and makes a great breakfast or snack!

Serving: 1

Serving Size: whole recipe

Prep Time: >5 minutes

Cook Time: 0 minutes

Ingredients

½ cup almond milk

1 tbsp coconut oil

2 tbsp almond butter

2 tbsp cocoa powder

1 tsp stevia or erythritol (optional)

Instructions

Blend all ingredients until smooth. Serve immediately

Nutrition: 370 calories, 33 g fat, 8 g protein, 5 g net carbs

Coconut Raspberry Smoothie

This caffeine free drink is full of great fat, and makes a great breakfast or snack!

Serving: 1

Serving Size: whole recipe

Prep Time: >5 minutes

Cook Time: 0 minutes

Ingredients

½ cup coconut milk

1 tbsp coconut oil

¼ cup frozen raspberries

1 tsp stevia or erythritol (optional)

Instructions

Blend all ingredients until smooth. Serve immediately

Nutrition: 408 calories, 42.3 g fat, 3 g protein, 6 g net carbs

Coconut Smoothie

This caffeine free drink is full of great fat, and makes a great breakfast or snack!

Serving: 1

Serving Size: whole recipe

Prep Time: >5 minutes

Cook Time: 0 minutes

Ingredients

½ cup coconut milk

1 tbsp coconut oil

½ cup ice

¼ tsp vanilla extract

1 tsp stevia or erythritol (optional)

Instructions

Blend all ingredients until smooth. Serve immediately

Nutrition: 408 calories, 42.9 g fat, 5 g protein, 3.7 g net carbs

Western Scrambled Eggs

Ham, cheese and tomato with eggs- the perfect start to your day!

Serving: 1

Serving Size: whole recipe

Prep Time: 5 minutes

Cook Time: >5 minutes

Ingredients

2 eggs, beaten

1 tsp dried thyme

1 oz butter

1 oz shredded cheddar cheese

1 oz ham, cubed

½ tomato, diced

1 tbsp red onion, diced (optional)

Instructions

Beat the eggs with a pinch of salt and pepper, and the thyme.

Preheat a small pan over medium heat, and melt in the butter

Add in the ham and tomato (and onion, if using), sauteing for 1 minute or so

Pour in the eggs, and stir constantly for 3 minutes, until cooked through

Add in the cheese, and stir for another minute.

Nutrition: 498 calories, 43.8 g fat, 23.4 g protein, 2.9 g net carbs

Mushroom, spinach and goat cheese frittata

This frittata is loaded with greens and good fat! This recipe serves two; enjoy this frittata for lunch the next day if you like- it's great hot or cold!

Serving: 2

Serving Size: Half recipe

Prep Time: 5 minutes

Cook Time: 15 minutes

Ingredients

4 eggs, beaten

¼ cup cream

1 tsp dried thyme

1 oz butter

1 oz goat cheese

1 handful spinach

½ cup sliced mushrooms

Instructions

Preheat oven to 350F

Beat the eggs and cream with a pinch of salt and pepper, and the thyme.

Preheat a small pan over medium heat, and melt in the butter

Add in the spinach and mushrooms with a pinch of salt, sauteing for 1 minute or so. Remove pan from heat.

Pour in the eggs, and top with the cheese. Transfer the pan to the oven, and bake 10-12 minutes. Store Leftovers in the fridge for up to 4 days.

Nutrition: 316 calories, 27 g fat, 16.4 g protein, 2.4 g net carbs

Bacon, Egg and Avo Breakfast Sandwich

This sandwich uses two halves of an avocado for the bun- adding a ton of great fat! This is a high calorie meal, so intermittent fasting will be important later in the day.

Serving: 1

Serving Size: whole recipe

Prep Time: 5 minutes

Cook Time: 15 minutes

Ingredients

1 egg

1 oz butter

1 avocado, sliced in half

1 tsp sesame seeds (for garnish)

2 slices bacon, cooked

1 slice tomato (optional, but delicious)

1 small handful arugula or 1 leaf of romaine

Instructions

Preheat a small pan over medium heat.

Melt in the butter, and crack in the egg. Cook to desired doneness.

Lay the lettuce, tomato (if using), and bacon onto one half of the avocado. Top with the egg, and close the sandwich. Sprinkle the top half of avocado with the sesame seeds, and enjoy immediately.

Nutrition: 899 calories, 83.9 g fat, 24.2 g protein, 4.1 g net carbs

Double Egg Breakfast Sandwich

This sandwich uses two fried eggs instead of bread- giving you ALL of the good stuff, NONE of the carbs!

Serving: 1

Serving Size: whole recipe

Prep Time: 5 minutes

Cook Time: >10 minutes

Ingredients

2 eggs

1 oz butter, room temperature

1 oz ham or 2 slices bacon, cooked

2 oz shredded cheddar cheese

1 slice tomato

Instructions

Preheat oven to 350F

Grease a 2 sections of a cupcake tin with the butter, and crack an egg into each one (Prep tip- if you want to make this sandwich all week, or want eggs available pre-cooked for the week, fill all 12 slots! Cooked eggs will last for a week in the fridge!)

Bake for 5-7 minutes, until the eggs are firm. Carefully pop the eggs out of the moulds, and lay them onto a plate.

Lay the cheese on top of the first egg, then top with the ham and tomato. Close with the second egg. Serve immediately.

Nutrition: 607 calories, 53 g fat, 30.2 g protein, 2.4 g net carbs

Coconut Chia Pudding

This creamy chia pudding is so easy to prep, and really delicious!

Serving: 2

Serving Size: Half recipe

Prep Time: 5 minutes

Cook Time: >5 minutes

Ingredients

1 oz chia seeds

1 cup coconut milk

3 tbsp unsweetened coconut flakes

¼ tsp cinnamon

Instructions

Mix all ingredients together and pour into two small mason jars or sealed containers

Allow to sit in the fridge overnight

Will keep in the fridge for up to 1 week

Nutrition: 451 calories, 42 g fat, 6.6 g protein, 8 g net carbs

Ricotta Cheese Pancakes

These pancakes are the best way to start a day! Add blueberries, strawberries, or coconut for a fun twist! These pancakes can also be made with cottage cheese, goat cheese or cream cheese, if you prefer to switch it up!

Serving: 1

Serving Size: 2-3 pancakes

Prep Time: 5 minutes

Cook Time: >10 minutes

Ingredients

1 egg

2 oz Ricotta

¼ tbsp psyllium husk flour

½ oz coconut oil

1 tbsp erythritol, optional

Instructions

Beat together all ingredients, and allow to sit for a minute to thicken

Preheat a small pan over medium high heat, and melt in the coconut oil

Spoon in a dollop of pancake batter, and cook 1-2 minutes per side.

Continue until all the batter has been used up. Serve warm

Nutrition: 425 calories, 39 g fat, 14 g protein, 5 g net carbs

Swiss Omelette

Gooey cheese and ham make this omelette a delicious way to start any day!

Serving: 1

Serving Size: whole recipe

Prep Time: 5 minutes

Cook Time: 5 minutes

Ingredients

2 eggs

3 tbsp heavy cream

2 tbsp butter

1 oz ham, cubed or cut into ribbons

2 oz swiss cheese

Instructions

Beat together the eggs and cream with salt and pepper

Preheat a pan over medium heat and melt in the butter

Add in the egg mixture, and allow to cook for 3 minutes.

Flip, and cook for another minute. Lay the cheese and ham onto the top of the omelette, and carefully fold it over so that the good stuff is tucked inside. Cover the pan, and cook for 1 more minute

Nutrition: 425 calories, 39 g fat, 14 g protein, 5 g net carbs

Cheesy Chicken Breakfast Burrito

This recipe uses leftover Lemon and Thyme Chicken Legs with cheese, Low Carb Tortillas, salsa and eggs! What a great way to start a morning!

Serving: 1

Serving Size: whole recipe

Prep Time: 10 minutes

Cook Time: 5 minutes

Ingredients

1 egg, beaten

 2 tbsp salsa

1 oz butter

1 oz shredded cheddar cheese

 1 serving Keto Tortilla

1 Serving Lemon and Thyme Chicken, shredded

Instructions

Beat the eggs and salsa together with a pinch of salt and pepper.

Preheat a small pan over medium heat, and melt in the butter

Pour in the eggs, and stir constantly for 3 minutes, until cooked through

Lay the chicken onto the tortilla, and spoon the eggs over top.

Top with the cheese, and fold the burrito. Serve immediately.

Nutrition: 830 calories, 75.2 g fat, 50.3 g protein, 3.5 g net carbs

Keto Breakfast Rolls

Sometimes, you just want a soft piece of bread to start your day off right. These rolls are beautifully fluffy, and low carb! Toast them and spread some butter or nut butter for a convenient breakfast on the go, or fill them with your favourite breakfast foods to make a delicious sandwich! These can also be formed into bagels if you like.

Serving: 4

Serving Size: 1 bun

Prep Time: 15 minutes

Cook Time: 16 minutes

Ingredients

½ cup almond flour

½ cup psyllium husk fiber

1 ½ tsp xantham gum

1 egg, beaten

3 tbsp cream cheese

1 ½ cups mozzarella, shredded

1 oz butter, melted

Instructions

Preheat oven to 375F

Melt together the cream cheese and mozzarella in the microwave for 1 minute.

Meanwhile mix together the almond flour, psyllium husk and xantham gum, and beat in the egg.

Mix in the melted cheeses, stirring well until a dough has formed.

Form the dough into 4 balls, and lay onto a baking sheet lined with parchment

Brush the dough balls with the melted butter, and bake in the oven for 15 minutes.

Store leftover buns in an airtight container in the fridge for up to a week, and reheat in a 350F oven for 2-3 minutes.

Nutrition: 489 calories, 50 g fat, 30 g protein, 5.5 g net carbs

With 1 tbsp almond butter: 98 calories, 9 g fat, 3.4 g protein, 1.4 g net carbs

With 1 egg (cooked how you like): 63 calories, 4.4 g fat, 5.5 g protein, 0.3 g net carbs

Smoked salmon, cream cheese and greens breakfast sandwiches

These breakfast sandwiches are a great way to start the day! Use whatever greens you have on hand or like best- kale, romaine, spinach or arugula are all great options. Feel free to add a slice of tomato for a little added nutritional value.

Serving: 1

Serving Size: whole recipe

Prep Time: 10 minutes

Cook Time: 2 minutes

Ingredients

1 serving Breakfast Rolls

1/2 tbsp cream cheese

1 oz smoked salmon

Small handful greens

Instructions

Slice the breakfast roll in half, and toast for 2 minutes or so

Spread the cream cheese over the breakfast roll, and layer on the greens and salmon. Close the sandwich, and serve immediately.

Nutrition: 539 calories, 53 g fat, 35.6 g protein, 5.7 g net carbs

Coconut Matcha Latte

This latte is easy to prepare, and so so yummy! For an iced latte, just blend with ice! Because of the low caffeine content, this is a great option for the late afternoon or evening as a snack, if you're trying to watch your caffeine intake!

Serving: 1

Serving Size: whole recipe

Prep Time: 10 minutes

Cook Time: 0 minutes

Ingredients

½ tbsp erythritol

1 tbsp matcha powder

4 oz coconut milk

½ cup boiling water

Instructions

Mix all ingredients together until smooth. Serve hot, or chill for an iced latte.

Nutrition: 255 calories, 28.8 g fat, 3.4 g protein, 3 g net carbs

Halloumi Shakshouka

Shakshouka is a middle eastern dish consisting of eggs, herbs and a richly flavoured tomato sauce. We've added halloumi for an added hit of flavour and good fat.

Serving: 1

Serving Size: whole recipe

Prep Time: 5 minutes

Cook Time: >10 minutes

Ingredients

1 egg

1 tbsp tomato paste

1 tsp dried oregano

3 tbsp beef or chicken broth

1 tbsp butter

1 oz halloumi, cubed

1 tbsp fresh parsley

Instructions

Preheat oven to 350F

Grease a small ramekin (small enough to comfortably hold the egg) with the butter

Mix together the broth, tomato paste and oregano. Spoon half the mixture into the ramekin, and then crack in the egg. Top with the remaining tomato mixture

Layer the halloumi cubes gently around the egg, making sure not to crack the yolk

Bake for 5-10 minutes, until the egg white is set and the yolk is still runny. Top with parsley and serve warm.

Nutrition: 160 calories, 11.8 g fat, 3.2 g protein,1.2 g net carbs

Cinnamon Roll Donuts

You can have donuts on the keto diet! Try these beautiful pastries with a coffee, or with a keto latte!

Serving: 6

Serving Size: 1 donut

Prep Time: 10 minutes

Cook Time: 15 minutes

Ingredients

½ cup erythritol

2 eggs

½ cup almond milk

¾ cup almond flour

½ cup psyllium husk fiber

1 tbsp cinnamon

1 tbsp baking powder

2 tbsp butter, melted

Instructions

Preheat oven to 350F

Mix together the eggs, almond milk, cinnamon, baking powder, erythritol, almond flour and psyllium husk.

Stir in the melted butter.

Grease a donut pan with a bit of butter or cooking spray, and pour the batter into the pan.

Bake for 18-20 minutes, until the donuts are set in the center. Allow to cool for 5-10 minutes, then turn out of the pan. Store leftovers in an airtight container in the fridge for up to 5 days, or freeze for up to 3 months. Reheat in the microwave for 1-2 minutes.

Nutrition: 160 calories, 11.8 g fat, 3.2 g protein,1.2 g net carbs

Lunch

Green Goddess Avo Salad

This salad is so fast and easy! The avocado dressing is only good for a day, so just make what you need at the time! This is a high calorie meal! Make sure that you fast at some point today!

Serving: 1

Serving Size: whole recipe

Prep Time: 10 minutes

Cook Time: 0 Minutes

Ingredients

2 strips bacon, cooked and chopped into bits

2 cherry tomatoes, halved

½ cup romaine, chopped

1 egg, hardboiled

1 tbsp pumpkin seeds

For the dressing:

2 tbsp olive oil

½ avocado, mashed

1 tbsp white wine vinegar

1 tsp onion powder

Instructions

Make the dressing- In a blender, puree all ingredients until smooth. Adjust the consistency with a bit more oil if needed, and season with salt and pepper

Toss the dressing with the rest of the ingredients. Serve immediately, or keep in the fridge for up to 24 hours.

Nutrition: 905 calories, 75.5 g fat, 32 g protein, 10 g net carbs

Salmon, spinach and goat cheese Salad

This salad is a deliciously simple way to get a ton of nutrients and vital fats during a busy weekday

Serving: 1

Serving Size: whole recipe

Prep Time: 10 minutes

Cook Time: 0 Minutes

Ingredients

2 oz smoked salmon

½ cup spinach

1 oz goat cheese

3 cherry tomatoes, halved

1 tbsp pumpkin seeds

Instructions

Toss all ingredients together. If you wish, drizzle with a bit of avocado oil and a pinch of salt and pepper. Serve immediately.

Nutrition: 311 calories, 17.5 g fat, 24 g protein, 11 g net carbs

Beef and avocado lettuce wraps

These lettuce wraps are absolutely delicious, and so easy to make! To save time, prep your beef up to 3 days in advance!

Serving: 1

Serving Size: 4 bundles

Prep Time: 10 minutes

Cook Time: 10 Minutes

Ingredients

2 oz beef, sliced thinly

1 tbsp soy sauce (gluten free)

¼ tsp ginger

1 red chili, chopped finely

1 tbsp avocado oil

For the wraps:

4 romaine leaves

½ avocado, diced

¼ red onion, sliced

Instructions

Marinate the beef in the soy sauce, ginger, and chilis for at least 5 minutes.

Preheat a pan over medium high heat. Drizzle in the oil, and add the beef and marinade. Toss constantly for 5-10 minutes, until the beef has cooked through. Allow to cool. Store cooked beef in the fridge for up to 3 days.

Make the wraps- Lay the lettuce leaves out, and spoon in the beef, avocado and red onion. Roll up, and enjoy immediately.

Nutrition: 454 calories, 37 g fat, 21 g protein, 6 g net carbs

Keto Quesadillas

These quesadillas use Keto Tortillas for a quick, satisfying keto-friendly lunch. This is a basic quesadilla recipe (tortilla and cheese), although you can certainly make it your own by adding any of your favourite ingredients (taco meat, chicken, bacon, jalapenos, smoked salmon and cream cheese- the possibilities are endless!)

Serving: 1

Serving Size: whole recipe

Prep Time: 10 minutes

Cook Time: 6 Minutes

Ingredients

2 servings Keto Quesadillas (found in dinner recipes)

3 oz cheddar cheese

For serving:

Sour cream

Salsa

Instructions

Preheat oven to 375F

Lay one tortilla onto a baking sheet lined with parchment. Cover with cheese (and any other fillings you like), and top with the second tortilla. Bake in the oven for 6 minutes, until the cheese melts and the tortillas are golden. Slice into 4 equal pieces, and serve immediately.

Nutrition: 330 calories, 21.5 g fat, 29.7 g protein, 4.1 g net carbs

With 3 tbsp sour cream: 77 calories, 7.6 g fat, 1.1 g protein, 1.5 g carbs

Italian Chopped Salad

This salad is so big and full of all sorts of great ingredients! You'll want to eat it everyday!

Serving: 1

Serving Size: whole recipe

Prep Time: 10 minutes

Cook Time: 0 Minutes

Ingredients

3 oz mozzarella cheese, shaved or cut into chunks

3 oz proscuitto

1 egg, hardboiled

1 tomato, cut into wedges

1 cup arugula (or any other green)

6 olives

2 tbsp olive oil

1 tbsp balsamic vinegar

Handful basil

Instructions

Toss all ingredients together. Serve immediately.

Nutrition: 790 calories, 66 g fat, 47 g protein, 5.9 g net carbs

Keto Creamy Onion Poppyseed Dressing

The problem with store bought salad dressings is that they're often loaded with sugar and other preservatives. Making your own ensures that you can control exactly what's going into it. Make a batch and keep it in the fridge for whenever you need a delicious dressing or dip

Serving: 8

Serving Size: 2-3 tbsp

Prep Time: 10 minutes

Cook Time: 0 Minutes

Ingredients

¼ onion, diced

1 tsp garlic powder

1 tbsp dijon mustard

1 cup olive oil

3 tbsp poppy seeds

Instructions

In a blender, or using an immersion blender, puree together all ingredients except the poppy seeds. Mix in the seeds, and season with salt and pepper. Store in an airtight container in the fridge for up to 2 weeks.

Nutrition: 237 calories, 26.8 g fat, 1 g protein, 1 g net carbs

With ½ cup greens (spinach, arugula, or romaine) and 2 strips bacon, crumbled: 209 calories, 15.9 g fat, 14.5 g protein, 0.7 g net carbs

Keto Strawberry Balsamic Dressing

The problem with store bought salad dressings is that they're often loaded with sugar and other preservatives. This dressing is slightly sweet, slightly tangy, and goes really well with spinach and goat cheese.

Serving: 8

Serving Size: 2-3 tbsp

Prep Time: 10 minutes

Cook Time: 0 Minutes

Ingredients

2 large strawberries (frozen is fine)

2 tbsp balsamic vinegar

1 tsp dried basil

½ tbsp dijon

1 cup olive oil

Instructions

Blend together all ingredients until smooth and creamy. Season with salt and pepper.

Nutrition: 220 calories, 25.2 g fat, 0 g protein, 0.3 g net carbs

Dinner

Warm mushrooms and brown butter

Serve this mushroom side with your favourite protein (it goes amazingly well with red meat, but is also delicious with fish or chicken!). Any leftovers are delicious on top of spinach for a healthy salad the next day

Serving: 2

Serving Size: Half recipe

Prep Time: 5 minutes

Cook Time: >10 Minutes

Ingredients

3 cups mushrooms, sliced

3 oz butter

2 tbsp dried thyme

3 tsp garlic powder

1 tsp onion powder

3 tbsp heavy cream

Instructions

Preheat a medium pan over medium high heat.

Melt in the butter, and add in the thyme, garlic, and onion powder. Reduce the heat to medium low, and cook the butter until it foams and begins to darken in colour, about 3 minutes.

Add the mushrooms with a pinch of salt, and saute well for 5 minutes until they have begun to cook down.

Serve over your favourite protein. Refrigerate any leftovers in an airtight container for up to 4 days- this is delicious hot or cold!

Nutrition: 500 calories, 47 g fat, 18 g protein, 6 g net carbs

Plus 4 oz steak: 226 cal, 5.7 g fat, 41 g protein, 0 g carbs

Plus salmon: 150 cal, 7 g fat, 22 g protein, 0 g carbs

Asian Style Beef Salad

This salad is packed with flavour and really delicious! It makes an awesome dinner, and an even better lunch the next day!

Serving: 2

Serving Size: Half recipe

Prep Time: 15 minutes

Cook Time: 10 Minutes

Ingredients

For the Beef:

1 tbsp sesame oil

1 tbsp fish sauce

1 tbsp ginger

2 tsp chili flakes (or as much or as little as you like)

1 tsp tamari

1 lb steak (such as flank steak or rib eye), thinly sliced

For the sesame aioli:

1 tbsp mayo

1 tsp sesame oil

1 tsp avocado oil

½ lime, juice and zest

For the salad:

3 cherry tomatoes, halved

½ cucumber, spiralized or cut into thin strips

1 carrot, spiralized or cut into thin strips

1 cup iceberg lettuce, finely chopped

3 green onions, sliced

Handful fresh cilantro

Instructions

Cook the beef- Toss the beef with the rest of the ingredients, and allow to marinate for 5-10 minutes

Preheat a medium pan over medium high heat.

Add the beef with the marinade, and toss well for 10 minutes, until fully cooked.

Make the aioli- Mix all ingredients together until smooth.

Make the salad- Toss together all ingredients. Toss in the warm beef. Drizzle with the aioli, and toss once more to combine.

Nutrition: 603 calories, 22 g fat, 85.2 g protein, 5 g net carbs

This pureed cauliflower is the perfect substitute for mashed potatoes! In this recipe, the cauliflower is enhanced with creamy goat cheese and roasted garlic, but you can easily keep this simple with just cream and butter, or mix in some bacon and cheddar cheese for a delicious comfort food experience. Serve this decadent side with a piece of protein (steak, chicken or fish all work great with this) and a serving of greens for a complete meal that will please everyone!

Serving: 4

Serving Size: Half recipe

Prep Time: 5 minutes

Cook Time: 40 Minutes

Ingredients

1 head cauliflower, chopped

1 cup heavy cream

6 oz goat cheese

4 oz butter

1 head garlic

¼ cup olive oil

Instructions

Preheat oven to 400F. Lay the head of garlic in a small, oven safe container.

Slice the top off the head of garlic (leaving the cloves intact), and pour the oil all over it. Sprinkle with a pinch of salt. Roast 15 minutes, until fragrant and soft, then allow to cool while you move on to the next step.

In a large pot, bring 4 cups of water to a boil. Boil the cauliflower for 5 minutes, until soft. Drain, and set aside.

Preheat a large sized sauce pan over medium heat. Pop the roasted garlic cloves out of their skin, and add it to the pan with the butter. Stir constantly until the butter has melted completely, then add in the cream and the cauliflower, continuing to stir for 5 minutes.

Using an immersion blender or food processor, puree the cauliflower until completely smooth.

Continue to cook over medium heat for another 10 minutes, until the mixture has thickened. Stir in the goat cheese, and season with salt and pepper. Keep leftovers in an airtight container in the fridge for up to 7 days.

Nutrition: 559 calories, 54.1 g fat, 15 g protein, 4.6 g net carbs

Plus 4 oz steak: 226 cal, 5.7 g fat, 41 g protein, 0 g carbs

Plus 4 oz salmon: 150 cal, 7 g fat, 22 g protein, 0 g carbs

Plus 1 roasted chicken leg, skin on: 553 cal, 15.7 g fat, 30.5 g protein, 0 carbs

Plus 1 chicken breast, skin on: 193 cal, 7.6 g fat, 29.2 g protein, 0 carbs

Lemon and Thyme Roasted Chicken Legs

This chicken dish so easy to make, but impressive enough to serve to guests! The juicy, high fat dark meat is perfect for the ketogenic diet, so enjoy these as often as you like! If you're a fan of breasts, this method will work great for that too! Chicken legs are considered the thigh and drum attached.

Serving: 4

Serving Size: 1 leg

Prep Time: 5 minutes

Cook Time: 45 Minutes

Ingredients

4 large chicken legs, bone in skin on

1 bunch fresh thyme, chopped

2 cloves garlic, minced

¼ cup butter, softened

1 lemon, zested and cut into wheels

Instructions

Preheat oven to 350F. Prepare a roasting pan by laying down the lemon wheels, then placing the chicken thighs over top.

Mix together the thyme, garlic, lemon zest and butter.

Lift the skin slightly from the meat of the chicken, and stuff the butter mixture under the skin. Continue until all 4 chicken thighs are done

Season the top of the skin with salt and pepper, then bake the chicken for 35-40 minutes, until completely cooked through. Serve with your favourite sides. Leftovers will keep in the fridge for up to 4 days.

Nutrition: 379 calories, 27.8 g fat, 30.5 g protein, 0.6 g net carbs

Bacon Wrapped Cod

This recipe is really easy and delicious! Serve with your favourite sides for a complete, beautiful meal.

Serving: 2

Serving Size: 1 fillet

Prep Time: 5 minutes

Cook Time: 20 Minutes

Ingredients

2 4 oz fillets cod

4 strips bacon

Instructions

Preheat oven to 350F

Pat the cod dry, and season with salt and pepper. Wrap two slices of bacon around each fillet, and lay them onto a baking sheet lined with parchment.

Bake 20 minutes. Serve with your favourite sides. Leftovers will keep in the fridge for up to two days.

Nutrition: 323 calories, 27.6 g fat, 17.5 g protein, 0.7 g net carbs

Bacon-Parmesan Roasted Asparagus

This yummy side dish is the perfect addition to any meal, but also makes a great lunch or snack on its own. Asparagus gives you the greens you need, without a lot of extra carbs.

Serving: 4

Serving Size: 3 spears

Prep Time: 5 minutes

Cook Time: 22 Minutes

Ingredients

12 asparagus spears, trimmed

4 slices bacon

¼ cup olive oil

1 tsp garlic powder

½ cup parmesan, grated

Instructions

Preheat oven to 400F

Bring a large pot of salted water to a boil, and blanch the asparagus for 1 minute. Transfer to an ice bath.

Lay the asparagus out onto a baking sheet lined with parchment, and drizzle with oil. Toss together the garlic and parmesan, and sprinkle over the asparagus evenly.

Divide the stalks into bundles of 3, and wrap each bundle with a strip of bacon. Bake for 20 minutes.

Nutrition: 260 calories, 26.8 g fat, 35.1 g protein, 6 g net carbs

This recipe is fast, easy, and delicious! It can be eaten on its own, but also makes a great side! Serve with your favourite protein for a complete meal. This is a high calorie item, so make sure you incorporate intermittent fasting in your day as well!

Serving: 2

Serving Size: Half of recipe

Prep Time: 15 minutes

Cook Time: 25 Minutes

Ingredients

4 strips bacon, diced

½ cup heavy cream

2 cloves garlic, minced

½ cup parmesan, grated

¼ cup olive oil

4 zucchinis, spiralized

Instructions

Preheat a large pan over medium heat. Add in the olive oil and bacon, and cook until bacon is cooked through, about 2 minutes. Add in the garlic, and saute for another minute.

Pour in the cream, and reduce heat to low. Allow to simmer for 10 minutes.

Add in the zucchini noodles, and toss well to combine. Cook for about 10 minutes until cooked through. Serve immediately or keep leftovers in a container in the fridge for up to 3 days.

Nutrition: 770 calories, 65 g fat, 37.6 g protein, 12 g net carbs

This is such a comforting meal! If you want to switch it up, swap out chicken for sausage, pork, or anything else. If you have previously cooked chicken from another recipe, save yourself time by using that instead of raw chicken thighs!

Serving: 4

Serving Size: about 1 cup

Prep Time: 15 minutes

Cook Time: 45 Minutes

Ingredients

12 oz chicken thighs, bones removed and diced into small pieces

½ onion, diced

1 tsp dried thyme

1 tsp dried basil

1 oz butter

3 oz pesto (jarred is fine- just read the ingredients to make sure there are no added sugars!)

1 cup heavy cream

½ red pepper, diced

2 oz parmesan cheese

2 oz mozzarella cheese

Instructions

Preheat oven to 400F

Preheat a dutch oven or ovensafe pan over medium high heat, and melt in the butter. Add in the chicken with a pinch of salt and pepper, and the basil and thyme. Cook for 5-10 minutes, until all sides are browned

Mix together the pesto, cream, and diced red bell pepper

Pour the mixture in with the chicken, and top with the cheeses

Bake covered for 35-40 minutes. Serve warm with a side of greens. Leftovers will last in the fridge for up to a week.

Nutrition: 501 calories, 37.6 g fat, 38 g protein, 4.6 g net carbs

Southwest Chicken Chili with Avocado Cream

This white chili leaves out the legumes and focuses on meat and flavour! If you have leftover cooked chicken from a previous recipe, save yourself time by using it in the recipe instead of uncooked thighs. You can swap out chicken for beef or pork if you like. The avocado cream is delicious on top of this recipe, but also makes a great topper for salads, or an alternative to mayo!

Serving: 4

Serving Size: about 1 cup

Prep Time: 5 minutes

Cook Time: 40 Minutes

Ingredients

½ lb chicken thighs, skinless, boneless and diced

½ lb chicken breasts, skinless, boneless and diced

2 tbsp olive or avocado oil

1 onion, diced

3 cloves garlic, minced

1 tbsp cumin

2 tbsp chili powder

1 tsp cinnamon

½ tbsp dried oregano

2 jalapenos, diced (optional)

1 bell pepper, diced

1 8 oz can diced tomatoes

1 cup chicken stock

Handful cilantro, for garnish

For the avocado cream:

1 avocado, mashed

¼ cup heavy cream

Instructions

Preheat a large pot over medium high heat.

Drizzle in the oil, and add in the chicken, spices, salt and pepper. Brown the chicken on all sides (about 10 minutes), then remove from the pan.

Add in another drizzle of oil, and toss in the peppers, onion and garlic. Stir well for 3-5 minutes. Add the chicken back in, along with the diced tomatoes and stock. Bring to a boil, then reduce heat to low. Let simmer for 20-25 minutes, stirring occasionally.

Make the avocado cream- mash the avocado well, and combine with the cream in a small bowl. Beat with a whisk until smooth. Taste, and season with salt and pepper.

To serve, pour the chili into a bowl and top with a bit of cilantro (optional) and a big scoop of avocado cream. Serve immediately. Leftover chili will keep in the fridge for up to a week, avocado cream will keep in the fridge for 1 day.

Nutrition: 410 calories 23.1 g fat, 28.9 g protein, 7 g net carbs

Roulade of chicken with ricotta, spinach and lemon cream

This might sound fancy, but it's super easy to put together! Impress your guests, or just enjoy this all by yourself on a weeknight! Serve with a side of asparagus, or a green salad. You can also swap out the ricotta for goat cheese or cream cheese, if you prefer. This is a high calorie meal, so make sure you incorporate fasting in your day.

Serving: 2

Serving Size: 1 breast

Prep Time: 10 minutes

Cook Time: 30 Minutes

Ingredients

2 6 oz boneless skinless chicken breasts

1 cup spinach

1 oz ricotta cheese

1 tbsp butter, softened

1 tbsp olive oil

1 tbsp thyme

For the cream:

½ cup heavy cream

1 oz parmesan

1 lemon, zest only

Instructions

Preheat oven to 350F

Cut an incision through the center of the breast (making sure not to go all the way through!), and then run your knife under each side so that the breast opens like a book

In a small bowl, mix together the butter, ricotta, and spinach, and season with a pinch of salt and pepper

Spoon the filling into the center of each chicken breast, and fold the sides back up to close

Brush the chicken with the olive oil, and sprinkle on the thyme, as well as some salt and pepper. Bake for 30 minutes

While the chicken is baking, add the cream and lemon zest to a small saucepan and warm it over medium heat, stirring constantly for 3-5 minutes.

Reduce the heat to low, and cook for another 15 minutes, stirring occasionally. Stir in the cheese and keep warm until ready to serve.

To serve, slice the chicken breasts into 3 or 4 equal sized medallions. Spoon the sauce over top. Serve warm or cold. Leftovers will keep in the fridge for up to a week

Nutrition: 700 calories 63.8 g fat, 72.9 g protein, 3.6 g net carbs

Keto Pizza

Pizza nights can still happen on the keto diet! This crust is made with cheese instead of flour, making it deliciously decadent and keto friendly! This is a basic recipe for pepperoni pizza, but you can also add whichever toppings you like- as long as they're keto friendly, and you make sure to take the extra macros into consideration.

Serving: 2

Serving Size: Half Pizza

Prep Time: 10 minutes

Cook Time: 30 Minutes

Ingredients

For the crust:

4 oz mozzarella

4 oz parmesan

6 eggs

For the topping:

4 oz mozzarella, shredded

¼ cup Low carb tomato sauce (check the label, make sure it's sugar free)

1 oz Pepperoni

Instructions

Preheat oven to 425F

Make the crust- In a bowl, mix together the parm, mozzarella, and eggs. Lay the mixture out onto a baking sheet or pizza stone lined with parchment, flattening it into a large circle- for personal size pizzas, just make two equal sized circles

Bake for 10 minutes, until the cheese has melted and it resembles a crust. Carefully remove the crust from the oven, making sure not to disturb it. Let it cool for at least 5-10 minutes

Spread the sauce and toppings on top of the crust, and return to the oven for another 10 minutes. Allow to cool for 5 minutes before slicing. Leftovers will last in the fridge for up to a week.

Nutrition: 761 calories 52 g fat, 70 g protein, 7 g net carbs

Burrito Bowl

Everybody knows the best part of a burrito bowl is the meat and cheese anyway, so leave those beans and rice out and replace them with MORE of the good stuff! If you really need rice, cauliflower rice is a great addition to this meal. If you have leftover beef from Taco night, feel free to use it in this recipe!

Serving: 2

Serving Size: Half recipe

Prep Time: 10 minutes

Cook Time: 30 Minutes

Ingredients

1/2 lb ground beef

1 tbsp onion powder

1 tbsp garlic powder

1 tsp cayenne (or as much as you like)

½ tbsp cumin

½ tbsp oregano

3 oz shredded cheddar cheese

6 green onions, sliced

Handful cilantro, chopped

½ bell pepper, diced

½ avocado, sliced

Instructions

Preheat a pan over medium high heat

Add in the beef and spices with some salt, and cook until the beef has cooked through- about 10 minutes

Add in the bell pepper, and toss well.

Spoon the mixture into two bowls, and top with the cheese, green onions, cilantro and avocado. Serve with your favourite salsa if you like.

Nutrition: 545 calories 32 g fat, 48.6 g protein, 11 g net carbs

Keto Cabbage Rolls

This Eastern European classic dinner is a surefire hit! Cabbage, loaded with ground beef and pork, and topped with a rich beefy tomato sauce, this recipe is low cal and high flavour!

Serving: 4

Serving Size: 3 rolls

Prep Time: 10 minutes

Cook Time: 1 hour 30 Minutes

Ingredients

1 lb ground beef

½ lb ground pork

1 tbsp onion powder

1 tbsp garlic powder

1 tsp cayenne (or as much as you like)

12 large cabbage leaves

1 egg

For the sauce:

1 can diced tomatoes

1 cup beef stock

½ tbsp onion powder

1 tsp worchestershire sauce

1 tsp oregano

2 tbsp butter

Instructions

Preheat oven to 350F

Make the sauce- In a large saucepan, combine all ingredients and bring to a boil. Reduce heat to low, and simmer for 15 minutes. Puree with an immersion blender, or transfer to a blender or food processor until smooth.

Bring a large pot of water to a boil

Boil the cabbage leaves for 3 minutes, until tender, then drain.

Combine the beef, pork, seasonings, and egg in a bowl. Season with salt and pepper.

Lay the cabbage leaves out evenly into a roasting pan.

Spoon the meat mixture into the center of each leaf, and roll it up.

Cover the rolls with the sauce, and cover the roasting pan. Bake for 75 minutes.

Nutrition: 405 calories, 16.4 g fat, 53.6 g protein, 7 g net carbs

Pork Chops with Mushrooms

These easy pork chops are delicious, and go great with asparagus, cauliflower puree, or a simple salad. This is a high calorie meal! Make sure you fast at some point during the day!

Serving: 2

Serving Size: 1 pork chop

Prep Time: 10 minutes

Cook Time: 45 Minutes

Ingredients

2 6 oz pork chops

1 cup mushrooms, chopped

6 stems fresh thyme, leaves removed and chopped

3 tbsp butter

3/4 cup heavy cream

1 clove garlic, minced

1 oz parmesan

Handful fresh parsley, chopped

Instructions

Preheat oven to 350F

Make the sauce- Preheat a large pan over medium heat. Melt in the butter, and add the mushrooms, garlic and thyme. Saute for 2 minutes or so, until the mushrooms begin to cook down- be careful not to burn the butter!

Add in the cream, and stir for 5 minutes. Reduce heat to low, and simmer for 20 minutes. Stir in the parmesan during the last minute of cooking.

Meanwhile, roast the pork- Pat the pork chops dry, and lay them on a baking sheet lined with parchment. Season both sides with salt and pepper, and bake for 30 minutes.

Spoon the sauce over the pork chops. Garnish with chopped parsley. Leftovers will keep in the fridge for up to a week.

Nutrition: 805 calories, 73.4 g fat, 45.6 g protein, 3.4 g net carbs

Low Carb Tortillas

These tortillas are perfect for tacos and wraps, and are keto friendly! Make a big batch and freeze them individually, so that you can have a low carb mexican meal any time you like!

Serving: 6

Serving Size: 1 tortilla

Prep Time: 10 minutes

Cook Time: 5 Minutes

Ingredients

3 egg whites

1 whole egg

4 oz cream cheese

1 tbsp psyllium husk fiber

1 tbsp coconut flour

Instructions

Preheat oven to 400F

Whip the egg whites until fluffy.

Beat together the cream cheese and the whole egg. Add in the flours, continuing to beat well. Fold in the egg whites.

Divide the mixture into 6 equal sized balls. Lay the balls out onto a baking sheet lined with parchment, and press them down to flatten them.

Bake for 5 minutes, until the tortilla has started to brown. Allow to cool fully before handling. Leftovers will keep in the fridge for up to two weeks, or in the freezer for 5 months.

Nutrition: 95 calories, 7.6 g fat, 4.5 g protein, 1.3 g net carbs

Keto Taco Night

These tortillas are perfect for tacos and wraps, and are keto friendly! Make a big batch and freeze them individually, so that you can have a low carb mexican meal any time you like!

Serving: 2

Serving Size: 2 tacos

Prep Time: 10 minutes

Cook Time: 45 Minutes

Ingredients

3/4 lb ground beef

2 tbsp olive or avocado oil

½ onion, diced

1 tsp garlic powder

2 tsp cumin

2 tsp chili powder

2 tsp oregano

½ tsp cinnamon

Toppings:

½ cup iceberg lettuce, shredded

½ cup cheddar cheese, shredded

Salsa

½ avocado, diced

Handful cilantro, chopped

4 servings Keto Tortillas

Instructions

Preheat a pan over medium high heat

Drizzle in the oil, and add in the onion, seasonings, and a pinch of salt. Saute until the onions become fragrant, about 5 minutes

Add in the beef. Stir well to combine, and cook completely- about 10 minutes.

To serve, spoon the filling out into the center of each taco. Top as desired, and eat immediately

Nutrition: 860 calories, 77.6 g fat, 54.5 g protein, 3.9 g net carbs

Oysters Rockefeller

This New Orleans classic has made a big comeback lately- mainly because it is ABSOLUTELY delicious! Oysters are baked with cream, butter, cheese, bacon and spinach for a high fat, high flavour seafood option.

Serving: 2

Serving Size: 6 oysters

Prep Time: 10 minutes

Cook Time: 25 Minutes

Ingredients

4 strips bacon, diced

1 tbsp butter

½ cup heavy cream

½ cup spinach

1 jalapeno, diced

1 clove garlic, minced

1 tsp thyme

12 oysters, shucked

2 oz parmesan, shredded

2 oz mozzarella, shredded

Instructions

Preheat broiler to 550F

Preheat a pan over medium heat. Melt in the butter, and cook the bacon until just cooked, about 2 minutes. Add in the thyme, garlic, and cook for another 2 minutes or so.

Add the cream and the jalapeno, and stir well for 3 minutes. Add in the spinach, tossing well to combine. Cook on medium until the spinach has cooked down and the liquid has reduced down a bit, about 6 minutes

Spoon the mixture into the oysters, and top with the cheese. Broil for 10 minutes, until the cheese is bubbling. Serve immediately.

Nutrition: 700 calories, 55.6 g fat, 60.9 g protein, 13 g net carbs

Shiratake Carbonara

Shiratake noodles are a miraculously delicious low carb noodle! This creamy carbonara recipe is easy to make, and delicious

Serving: 2

Serving Size: Half recipe

Prep Time: 10 minutes

Cook Time: 15 Minutes

Ingredients

12 strips bacon, diced

2 tbsp butter

1 tsp thyme

1 tbsp diced onion

¼ onion, diced

1 egg yolk

1 cup heavy cream

2 oz parmesan cheese

1 8 oz package shiratake noodles

Instructions

Preheat a pan over medium heat. Melt in the butter, and cook the bacon until just cooked, about 2 minutes. Add in the thyme, onion and garlic, and cook for another 2 minutes or so.

Add the cream and stir well for 1 minute. Whisk in the egg yolks one at a time, mixing well between each addition.

Add in the noodles, and toss well to combine. Allow to cook for 3-5 minutes, until the noodles have absorbed the sauce. Toss in the cheese, and season with salt and pepper. Leftovers will keep in the fridge for up to a week.

Nutrition: 720 calories, 67 g fat, 33.9 g protein, 4.7 g net carbs

Coconut Curry Shiratake Noodles

These noodles are creamy, spicy and really yummy!

Serving: 2

Serving Size: Half recipe

Prep Time: 10 minutes

Cook Time: 15 Minutes

Ingredients

1 tbsp avocado oil

6 oz chicken thighs, boneless, skinless, diced

1 8 oz can coconut milk

1 tbsp curry powder

2 red chilies (or as many as you like)

1 tsp ginger

1 clove garlic, minced

1 8 oz package bean sprouts

Handful cilantro

1 lime, juice and zest

½ bell pepper, sliced thinly

6 green onions, sliced thinly

1 8 oz package shiratake noodles

Instructions

Preheat a large pan over medium heat. Drizzle in the oil, and add the chicken with a pinch of salt. Cook until brown on all sides, about 5 minutes.

Add in the garlic, ginger, chilies, and curry powder, and stir well. Add in the coconut milk, and bring to a boil, then reduce heat to low and simmer for 10 minutes until the mixture has thickened

Add in the shiratake noodles, tossing well to combine. Add in the bell pepper and bean sprouts. Toss well. Squeeze in the lime juice, and toss in the cilantro and green onions. Serve warm. Leftovers will keep in the fridge for up to a week.

Nutrition: 557 calories, 41.7 g fat, 33.7 g protein, 13 g net carbs

Middle Eastern Style Halloumi

Halloumi is a middle eastern cheese that is slightly salty and perfectly melty. Crispy cucumbers, red onion and tomatoes make this a perfectly rounded dinner.

Serving: 1

Serving Size: whole recipe

Prep Time: 10 minutes

Cook Time: 5 Minutes

Ingredients

For the halloumi:

4 oz wedge of halloumi

½ tsp cumin

¼ tsp sumac

¼ tsp coriander

¼ tsp cinnamon

¼ tsp turmeric

For the salad:

2 tbsp red onion, diced

½ cucumber, diced

1 roma tomato, diced

Handful parsley, chopped finely

1 serving Tahini

Instructions

Preheat broiler to 500F

Mix the spices together and rub them into both sides of the cheese

Lay the halloumi out onto a baking sheet lined with parchment, and broil for 3-4 minutes, until golden and soft.

Toss together the red onion, cucumber, tomato and parsley. Spoon the tahini over top. Lay the halloumi on top, and serve immediately

Nutrition: 700 calories, 53.2 g fat, 33.7 g protein, 15 g net carbs

Tahini

Tahini is a creamy, flavourful sauce that can be used on salads, sandwiches, or as a dip!

Serving: 4

Serving Size: 2-3 tbsp

Prep Time: 10 minutes

Cook Time: 0 Minutes

Ingredients

Handful parsley, roughly chopped

1 clove garlic

1 lemon, juice and zest

¼ cup tahini paste

¼ cup water

Instructions

Puree all ingredients until smooth. Season with salt.

Keep in an airtight container in the fridge for up to a week.

Nutrition: 89 calories, 8.1 g fat, 2.5 g protein, 1.3 g net carbs

Eggplant Parmesan

This delicious vegetarian keto recipe is super rich and delicious! Use the same method to make chicken parmesan too!

Serving: 4

Serving Size: 1-2 pieces eggplant

Prep Time: 10 minutes

Cook Time: 45 Minutes

Ingredients

1 large eggplant, sliced into medallions

3 tbsp olive oil

4 oz shredded mozzarella

5 oz parmesan

1 cup marinara sauce (make sure it's low carb!)

1 tbsp garlic powder

1 tbsp onion powder

1 tbsp dried thyme

1 tbsp dried oregano

Fresh parsley, chopped

Instructions

Preheat oven to 450F

Brush the eggplant medallions with oil, and season with salt, pepper and the seasonings. Lay the medallions into a roasting pan.

Top the medallions evenly with half of the parmesan, and bake for 5 minutes

Remove from the oven, and reduce the oven temp to 375

Pour the marinara sauce over the eggplant. Top with the rest of the cheese, and cover with tinfoil. Bake for 40 minutes. Finish with parsley.

Nutrition: 385 calories, 28.1 g fat, 22.5 g protein, 12.3 g net carbs

Weekly Shopping List

*Note- It can be more economical to purchase meat items in bulk. Portioning out your meat items and freezing them will save time and money later.

Pantry Staples For the Month:

Almond Milk- 6 L

Curry Powder- 1 package, about 300g

Cumin- 1 package, about 300g

Ground Ginger- 1 package, about 300g OR 1 root

Onion Powder 1 package, about 300g

Garlic Powder 1 package, about 300g

Cinnamon 1 package, about 300g

Pumpkin Pie Spice- 1 pack, about 300g

Dried Italian herbs 1 package, about 300g

Turmeric-   1 package, about 300g

Sumac-   1 package, about 300g

Coriander-   1 package, about 300g

Poppyseeds- 1 package, about 300g

Baking powder

Tahini- 1 jar

Sugar Free Sriracha Sauce- 1 bottle

Gluten Free Tamari or soy sauce - 1 bottle

Vanilla extract

Pesto- 2 jars

Salsa- 1 jar

Olives- 2 jars

Tomato Paste- 2 jars

Marinara sauce (sugar free)- 2 jars

Balsamic vinegar- 1 bottle

Fish sauce- 1 bottle

Coconut oil

Sesame oil- 1 bottle

Coffee- 1 lb

Avocado Oil

Olive Oil

Salt

Pepper

Beef Stock- either 3L prepared, or bouillon cubes

Chicken Stock- either 3L prepared, or bouillon cubes

Pecans 6 oz

Almonds 6 oz

macadamia nuts 6 oz

Chia Seeds 16 oz

Coconut flour- 8 oz

Matcha powder- 4 oz

Unsweetened coconut flakes- 1 package

Cocoa powder- 1 can

Psyllium Husk Fiber- 8 oz

Erythritol- 8 oz

Frozen strawberries- 1 bag

Week 1 Shopping List

Seafood, Meat and Eggs:

Eggs- 2 dozen

Salmon- 4 oz

Smoked Salmon- 1 lb

Bacon- 1 lb

Steak- 12 oz

Chicken Legs- 1 package (about 1 lb)

Ham- 1 package (about 6 oz)

Cod- 2x 4 oz fillets

Dairy Products:

Feta Cheese- 8 oz

Goat Cheese- 8 oz

Cheddar cheese- 1 lb

Butter- 1 lb

Heavy Cream- 1 L

Mozzarella- 6 oz

Parmesan Cheese- 12 oz

Produce:

Spinach- 1 lb

Mushrooms- 1 lb

Avocados- 4

1 eggplant

Asparagus- 1 bunch

Cauliflower- 1 head

3 lemons

1 head romaine

1 bell pepper

1 head garlic

1 package red chilies

2 roma tomatoes

1 lb carrots

1 red onion

Yellow onions- 1 lb

Celery- 1 head

Week 2 Shopping List

Meat and Eggs:

Chicken thighs- 1 lb

Chicken Legs- 1 lb

Ground beef- 1 lb

Prosciutto- 8 oz

Bacon- 1 lb

Eggs- 1 dozen

Dairy Products:

Halloumi- 1 lb

Ricotta Cheese- 8 oz

Produce:

2 roma tomatoes

1 Pint Cherry Tomatoes

3 lemons

2 Avocados

2 jalapenos

1 bell pepper

1 bunch cilantro

1 lime

1 red onion

1 bunch parsley

Kalamata olives- 1 lb

1 bunch arugula

1 bunch fresh thyme

4 zucchinis

1 head garlic

Week 3 Shopping List

Meat and Eggs:

Ground beef- 1 lb

Ham- 4 oz

Bacon- 2 lbs

Eggs- 2 dozen

Prosciutto- 8 oz

Pepperoni- 1 lb

Steak- 12 oz

Cod- 2 4 oz fillets

Chicken Breasts- 1 package (2 lbs)

Smoked salmon- 1 lb

Dairy Products:

Feta Cheese- 1 lb

goat cheese - 8 oz

Halloumi- 1 lb

Cheddar Cheese- 1 lb

Cream cheese- 16 oz

Mozzarella- 1 lb

Cream- 1 L

Sour cream- 8 oz

Butter- 1 lb

Swiss cheese- 8 oz

Produce:

Cabbage- 1 head

1 Package Fresh Basil

2 roma tomatoes

Asparagus 1 bunch

1 package cherry tomatoes

1 Lime

1 red onion

1 Bunch Cilantro

1 head romaine lettuce

2 lemons

½ lb Spinach

2 jalapenos

Mushrooms- 1 lb

1 bunch green onions

Cauliflower-1 Head

Mixed greens

Week 4 Shopping List

Meat and Eggs:

Chicken Breast-1 lb

Eggs- 1 dozen

Chicken thighs- 1 pack, about 2 lbs

Chicken thighs- 1 lb

Bacon 1 lb

Oysters- 12 individual (purchase on or before the day you plan on using them)

Prosciutto- 8 oz

Cod- 6 oz

Ham- 8 oz

Pork chops- 8 oz

Dairy Products:

Goat Cheese- 8 oz

Heavy Cream- 8 oz

Butter 1 lb

Mozzarella- 1 lb

Produce:

1 bunch Asparagus

3 Avocados

1 package spinach

1 Package Fresh Basil

1 Head Cauliflower

1 eggplant

3 zucchini

Mushrooms- 1 lb

3 Bell Peppers

1 Cucumber

1 Tomato

1 pint cherry tomatoes

4 Onions

2 lemons

1 lime

1 bunch green onions

BREAKFAST

Coconut Smoothie Bowl

Mix in your favorite nuts and seeds to add valuable fat, texture and flavor! Be mindful of how many berries you add, so that you don't consume too many carbs

Serving: 1

Serving Size: whole recipe

Prep Time: 5 minutes

Cook Time: 0 minutes

Ingredients

1 can coconut cream

1 lime, juice and zest

¼ cup fresh raspberries

¼ cup chopped almonds

2 tbsp chia seeds

1 tbsp stevia or erythritol, optional

Instructions

Mix together the coconut, lime, and stevia (if using).

Top with the almonds, raspberries and chia seeds. Serve immediately, or store in an airtight container in the fridge for up to 12 hours.

Nutrition: 726 calories, 69.4 g fat, 11.4 g protein, 6 g net carbs

Microwave Scrambled Eggs

Using the microwave, you can have delicious scrambled eggs in less than 5 minutes! Greasing your ramekin or bowl before cracking in the eggs adds a nice bit of fat and keeps the eggs from sticking. Add in your favourite ingredients, including sliced mushrooms, chopped pepper or tomato, spinach, cheese or bacon, and enjoy!

Serving: 1

Serving Size: whole recipe

Prep Time: 5 minutes

Cook Time: 3-5 minutes, depending on add-ins

Ingredients

1 tbsp butter or olive oil

3 eggs, beaten

2 tbsp heavy cream

Salt and pepper, to taste

Instructions

Grease a microwave safe bowl well with the butter or oil

Beat together the eggs, cream and seasonings. If you're adding in any extra ingredients, do so now.

Cover the bowl with a plate or a lid (make sure it's microwave safe!), and pop into the microwave.

Cook on high for 2 minutes. Give it a quick stir, and cook at 1 minute intervals until cooked through.

Nutrition: 394 calories, 35.7 g fat, 17.4 g protein, 0.1 g net carbs

Green Smoothie

Getting your greens has never been more delicious! If you have a hard time with green smoothies, try freezing the avocado and adding some crushed ice, to make a smoothie bowl instead! Top with a few berries and nuts for a touch of sweetness and texture if you desire.

Serving: 1

Serving Size: whole recipe

Prep Time: 5 minutes

Cook Time: 0 minutes

Ingredients

1 Cup of Spinach

1/2 Avocado

¼ Cup Coconut Milk

1 Tablespoon Chia Seeds

Instructions

Pour the coconut milk into a high speed blender or food processor

Add in the rest of the ingredients, and puree until smooth. Drink immediately.

Nutrition: 350 calories, 34 fat, 4.1 g protein, 1.5 g net carbs

Chicken Parm Frittata

Use leftover Cheesy Chicken Bake to make this quick, easy frittata in a flash!

Serving: 2

Serving Size: Half of recipe

Prep Time: 1 minute

Cook Time: 12 minutes

Ingredients

1 serving Cheesy Chicken Bake (found in dinner recipes)

2 eggs, beaten

Instructions

Preheat oven to 400F

Mix together the eggs and chicken mixture in an oven safe dish or ramekin large enough to fit everything comfortably.

Bake for 12 minutes, until cooked through. Serve immediately, and store any leftovers in an airtight container for up to 7 days.

Nutrition: 600 calories, 31 g fat, 45 g protein, 9.3 g net carbs

Nut Butter Smoothie Bowl

This nutty smoothie bowl is decadently delicious and full of good fat to fuel your morning!

Serving: 1

Serving Size: about 1 cup

Prep Time: 5 minutes

Cook Time: 0 minutes

Ingredients

2 tbsp Almond butter

1 Cup Almond milk

¼ cup ice

1 Tbsp Hemp Seeds

1 tbsp chia seeds

1 tbsp walnuts

Instructions

In a blender, puree together the ice, almond butter and almond milk until smooth.

Spoon the mixture into a bowl, and top with the hemp, walnuts and chia seeds. Serve immediately.

Nutrition: 183 calories, 13.3g fat, 8.6 g protein, 0.1 g net carbs

Blue Smoothie

This vibrant blue smoothie is just the thing to get you going in the morning! Spirulina powder is a great way to supplement your diet with a bit more green power, and also contains fiber, making it a welcome addition to this breakfast treat!

Serving: 1

Serving Size: about 1 cup

Prep Time: 5 minutes

Cook Time: 0 minutes

Ingredients

½ cup frozen blueberries

1 cup almond milk

1 tbsp coconut oil

1 tbsp spirulina

1 tsp stevia or erythritol, optional

Instructions

In a blender, puree everything together until smooth. Serve immediately.

Nutrition: 189 calories, 16.6 g fat, 3.1 g protein, 1 g net carbs

Easy Eggs Benedict

These eggs bennys are the easiest thing you've ever made, and oh-so-delicious! Serve them on top of a slice of ham, or your favourite keto-friendly bread for a delectable treat that's ready in minutes!

Serving: 1

Serving Size: whole recipe

Prep Time: 5 minutes

Cook Time: 7 minutes

Ingredients

2 eggs

2 tbsp mayo

1 tbsp olive oil

1 tbsp lemon juice

¼ tsp cayenne

Instructions

Preheat broiler to 500F

To poach the eggs, fill a regular coffee mug with ¼ cup water. Crack in one egg, and cover the cup with a plate or lid. Microwave on high for 50 seconds. Scoop out your perfectly poached egg, and set it aside. Repeat with the second egg.

Meanwhile, whisk together the mayo, olive oil, lemon and cayenne. Place the poached eggs on top of keto-friendly toast, ham, or avocado. Drizzle the hollandaise over the the eggs, and broil for 3-5 minutes. Serve immediately.

Nutrition: 366 calories, 32.8g fat, 11.5g protein, 5 g net carbs

Matcha Smoothie Bowl

This smoothie bowl is exotic and delicious! If you wish, add a bit of spirulina to really amp up the colour and add an extra dose of green power!

Serving: 1

Serving Size: whole recipe

Prep Time: 5 minutes

Cook Time: 0 minutes

Ingredients

2 tsp matcha powder

1 cup coconut milk

1 tbsp chia seeds

1 tbsp coconut flakes

2 tbsp almond slivers

2 tsp spirulina (optional)

Instructions

Mix the coconut milk and matcha together in a bowl. Stir in the spirulina, if using.

Top with the chia seeds, coconut flakes and almonds. Serve immediately or refrigerate overnight.

Nutrition: 691 calories, 67.9 g fat, 12.9 g protein, 8 g net carbs

Nutty Coffee

A spin on Bulletproof coffee, this flavourful coffee is the perfect thing if you're craving something a bit different

Serving: 1

Serving Size: about 1 ½ cups

Prep Time: 5 minutes

Cook Time: 0 minutes

Ingredients

1 tbsp almond butter

1 tsp cinnamon

1 tsp butter, melted

1 cup freshly brewed coffee

¼ cup almond milk

Instructions

Blend together all ingredients until smooth.

Nutrition: 168 calories, 15.8 g fat, 5.5 g protein, 2.1 g net carbs

Scotch Eggs

Scotch eggs are traditionally soft-boiled eggs that have been coated in sausage and breading, and deep fried! The perfect Scotch egg is gooey in the center, and crispy on the outside with a thick coating of perfectly seasoned sausage all around.

Serving: 4

Serving Size: 1 egg

Prep Time: 5 minutes

Cook Time: 10 minutes

Ingredients

½ lb ground pork

2 tsp nutmeg

1 tsp dried thyme

Salt and pepper, to taste

4 eggs

1 cup ground pork rinds

6 cups oil, for frying

Instructions

Soft boil the eggs- In a medium sized saucepan with 1 cup of water in the bottom, boil the eggs for 4 minutes. Transfer to an ice bath, and allow to cool. Peel carefully, making sure not to break the eggs.

Mix together the pork, nutmeg, thyme, salt and pepper. Carefully mould the pork mixture around the soft boiled eggs, and roll the mixture in the ground pork rinds.

Pour the oil into a large pot and bring to a temperature of 350f on the stove, using a candy thermometer. Roll the sausage-coated eggs in the pork rinds, and fry for 2-4 minutes, until the eggs begin to float. Remove from heat, drain on a paper towel, and serve immediately.

Nutrition: 442 calories, 46g fat, 25g protein, 0g net carbs

Coconut Smoothie

Coconut and citrus zest come together in this simple smoothie

Serving: 1

Serving Size: Whole Recipe

Prep Time: 5 minutes

Cook Time: 0 minutes

Ingredients

1 cup coconut cream

½ cup crushed ice

1 orange, juice and zest

1 lime, juice and zest

Instructions

In a blender, combine all ingredients until smooth. Serve immediately

Nutrition: 638 calories, 57.4 g fat, 7.2 g protein, 9 g net carbs

Keto Lemon Tea

Classic warm lemon tea is amped up with the addition of coconut oil for a keto morning beverage

Serving: 1

Serving Size: Whole Recipe

Prep Time: 5 minutes

Cook Time: 0 minutes

Ingredients

2 tbsp coconut oil

1 cup boiling water

1 lemon, juice and zest

Instructions

Combine all ingredients, and let sit for 5 minutes. Drink warm.

Nutrition: 251 calories, 27.4 g fat,0.6 g protein, 3 g net carbs

Asparagus Goat Cheese Omelette

This elegant omelette comes together super fast!

Serving: 1

Serving Size: Whole Recipe

Prep Time: 5 minutes

Cook Time: 8 minutes

Ingredients

2 tbsp butter

3 eggs, beaten

¼ cup cream

2 oz goat cheese

2 stalks asparagus, sliced

Instructions

Preheat a pan over medium heat

Beat the eggs and cream with a pinch of salt and pepper

Melt the butter into the pan, then add the asparagus. Pour in the egg mixture

Reduce heat to low, and cook until almost completely cooked through, about 5 minutes.

Flip, and cook the other side for 3 minutes. Top with goat cheese. Serve immediately.

Nutrition: 694 calories, 59.7 g fat, 35 g protein, 4.5 g net carbs

Southwest style eggs

This fun egg recipe combines southwest flavours for a zesty kick to your morning!

Serving: 1

Serving Size: Whole Recipe

Prep Time: 5 minutes

Cook Time: 5 minutes

Ingredients

2 eggs, beaten

¼ cup cream

1 tbsp butter

6 cherry tomatoes, halved

1 tsp cumin

½ tsp chili powder

½ tsp oregano

4 green onions, sliced

¼ cup cheddar cheese, grated

Instructions

Beat the eggs and cream with the seasoning.

Preheat a pan over medium heat, and melt in the butter. Pour in the egg mixture, and cook 2-3 minutes, stirring to scramble. Add in the tomatoes, green onion and cheese, and continue to mix for another 2 minutes.

Serve immediately

Nutrition: 546 calories,35 g fat, 26 g protein, 12 g net carbs

LUNCH

Loaded Avocado Salad

Creamy, salty, and oh-so-satisfying! This avo salad is the perfect midday meal for a busy day!

Serving: 2

Serving Size: 1/2 recipe

Prep Time: 10 minutes

Cook Time: 0 Minutes

Ingredients

2 strips bacon, cooked and chopped into bits

½ avocado, chopped

1 jalapeno, diced (optional)

6 cherry tomatoes, halved

½ cup romaine, chopped

¼ cup blue cheese, crumbled

2 tbsp olive oil

1 tbsp pumpkin seeds

Instructions

Drizzle the oil over the romaine. Toss with the rest of the ingredients. Season with salt and pepper.

Nutrition: 430 calories, 35.5 g fat, 13.2 g protein, 8 g net carb

Keto Lunchables

Just like those compartmentalized lunches you had as a kid, this easy lunch is perfectly portable, easy to put together, and full of all your favourite things! Mix up the contents, but keep the proportions the same in order to maintain your macros.

Serving: 1

Serving Size: Whole recipe

Prep Time: 10 minutes

Cook Time: 0 Minutes

Ingredients

2 oz (about ½ a small breast) cooked chicken breast, sliced

1 hard boiled egg, sliced in half

1 pickle, sliced

4 broccoli florets

4 cauliflower florets

6 grape tomatoes

3 tbsp ranch dressing

*Suggested alternatives- ¼ red pepper, sliced, 4 baby carrots, guacamole, nuts, 2 oz cheese, cooked bacon or ham

Instructions

Place all the individual pieces into their own compartments or individual containers. Nibble and dip as you like.

Nutrition: 590 calories, 37.6 g fat, 28.6 g protein, 6 g net carbs

Salmon and Avocado Nori Rolls

Nori is a delicious, low cal option for wrapping all your favourite foods! Avocado adds a nice amount of good fat, although you can also use a bit of cream cheese for a different flavour profile! Serve alongside some tamari and wasabi for a delectable asian lunch!

Serving: 1

Serving Size: Whole recipe

Prep Time: 10 minutes

Cook Time: 0 Minutes

Ingredients

3 oz cooked salmon

½ avocado, mashed lightly

1 tbsp Sesame seeds

¼ cucumber, cut into sticks (about 4-6 pieces)

1 nori sheet

Instructions

Spread the avocado evenly over the nori sheet.

Flake the salmon over top, and top with the sesame seeds. Lay the cucumber sticks evenly down the side of the sheet. Gently roll the sheet, starting around the cucumber and working up to the other end, to create a maki roll.

Slice into 6 even pieces. Serve with a bit of tamari and wasabi.

Nutrition: 380 calories, 29.6 g fat, 20.6 g protein, 3.5 g net carbs

Smoked salmon Rolls

Smoked salmon and cream cheese are a match made in heaven! These little rolls make an excellent appetizer, but are also great on top of a light green salad for a delicious lunch or light dinner option

Serving: 1

Serving Size: Whole recipe

Prep Time: 10 minutes

Cook Time: 0 Minutes

Ingredients

5 oz smoked salmon

¼ cup cream cheese, softened

Instructions

Spread the cream cheese as evenly as you can over the smoked salmon strips. Roll into pinwheels. Serve immediately, or store in an airtight container in the fridge for up to 1 day.

Nutrition: 368 calories, 26.3g fat, 30 g protein, 1.5 g net carbs

Easy Green Salad

Because of the heart-healthy olive oil, this salad provides an extra boost of fat while also contributing to your daily intake of greens. Perfect for a quick snack, or to add on to any lunch or dinner!

Serving: 1

Serving Size: Whole recipe

Prep Time: 5 minutes

Cook Time: 0 Minutes

Ingredients

1 cup mixed greens (such as baby romaine, baby kale, spinach, or arugula)

Dressing:

2 tbsp olive oil

1 tsp dijon mustard

1 tsp balsamic vinegar

Instructions

Whisk together the oil, dijon and balsamic. Pour the dressing over the greens, and toss well. Season with salt and pepper. Serve immediately

Nutrition: 246 calories, 28.3g fat, 0.4 g protein, 0.1 g net carbs

Tuna Salad Lettuce Wraps

Fast, easy and so delicious! These lettuce wraps have it all!

Serving: 1

Serving Size: Whole recipe

Prep Time: 10 minutes

Cook Time: 0 Minutes

Ingredients

1 can tuna, drained

2 tbsp mayo

1 stalk celery, diced

¼ red pepper, diced

2 tbsp red onion, diced

Salt and pepper, to taste

4 large romaine leaves

Instructions

Mix together all ingredients, except the romaine leaves.

Spoon the mixture into the leaves, and roll into bundles.

Serve immediately, or store in an airtight container in the fridge for up to 1 day.

Nutrition: 466 calories, 24.2 g fat, 48.1 g protein, 7.1 g net carbs

Caprese Salad

This salad is light, quick, and delicious!

Serving: 1

Serving Size: Whole recipe

Prep Time: 3 minutes

Cook Time: 0 Minutes

Ingredients

1 tomato, sliced

2 oz mozzarella, sliced

Handful basil, chopped

3 tbsp olive oil

Handful arugula

1 tbsp balsamic vinegar

Instructions

Arrange the mozzarella, tomato, and basil onto a plate so that each ingredient overlaps each other.

Drizzle with the olive oil and balsamic. Top with the arugula. Serve immediately or keep in an airtight container in the fridge for a day.

Nutrition: 534 calories, 52.2 g fat, 16.6 g protein, 3 g net carbs

Chicken BLT Salad

A classic sandwich in salad form! Delicious!

Serving: 1

Serving Size: Whole recipe

Prep Time: 5 minutes

Cook Time: 0 Minutes

Ingredients

2 oz cooked chicken, sliced

2 strips bacon, cooked and diced

6 cherry tomatoes, cut in half

1 cup romaine lettuce

¼ cup cheddar cheese, grated

3 tbsp ranch dressing

Instructions

Toss together all ingredients. Serve immediately, or store in an airtight container in the fridge for up to 3 days

Nutrition: 734 calories, 52.5 g fat, 45.1 g protein, 9 g net carbs

Chicken and avocado nori wraps

Nori adds valuable greens and replaces grain-based wraps for this chicken sandwich

Serving: 1

Serving Size: Whole recipe

Prep Time: 5 minutes

Cook Time: 0 Minutes

Ingredients

2 oz cooked chicken, sliced

2 strips bacon, cooked and diced

¼ red pepper, sliced thinly

½ avocado, mashed

1 tbsp hot mustard

2 romaine leaves, chopped

Instructions

Spread the avocado onto the nori sheet. Add in the rest of the ingredients, and roll like a burrito. Serve immediately , or store in the fridge for up to a day.

Nutrition: 657 calories, 50.5 g fat, 33 g protein, 9 g net carbs

DINNER

Lettuce Wrapped Chicken Fajitas

Precooked chicken breasts make this a quick, easy dinner to throw together!

Serving: 1

Serving Size: Whole recipe

Prep Time: 5 minutes

Cook Time: 10 Minutes

Ingredients

4 oz cooked chicken breast

1 tbsp olive oil

¼ red pepper, sliced

¼ red onion, sliced

1 tsp garlic powder

1 tsp cumin

1 tsp chili powder

1 tsp oregano

1 tsp salt

3 large romaine leaves

1 serving Guacamole (*see snack recipes)

3 tbsp salsa

Cilantro, for garnish

Instructions

Preheat a medium pan over medium high heat.

Drizzle in the oil, and add in the peppers, onion, and seasonings. Saute for about 5 minutes.

Add in the chicken breast, and continue to saute for another 5 minutes.

To serve, scoop the chicken and veg into a lettuce leaf, and top with salsa and guac. Garnish with cilantro leaves

Nutrition: 320 calories, 20 g fat, 26.2 g protein, 4 g net carbs

Coconut Lime Noodles and Tofu

Shiritake noodles are low carb and absolutely delicious! Helloooo, keto friendly noodle dishes!

Serving: 2

Serving Size: Half recipe

Prep Time: 5 minutes

Cook Time: 10 Minutes

Ingredients

2 tbsp vegetable oil

1 tsp curry powder

1 tsp cayenne pepper

¼ tsp ground ginger

1 tsp garlic powder

1 lb tofu, diced

1 8oz package shiratake noodles

1/2 can coconut cream

1 tbsp sesame seeds

1 lime, juice and zest

2 tbsp tamari

1 jalapeno, sliced thinly

Handful cilantro, chopped

Instructions

Preheat a medium pan over medium high heat.

Drizzle in the oil, and add in the spices along with the tofu. Toss well for 2 minutes, making sure the tofu is evenly coated on all sides.

Add in the coconut cream and lime juice, and mix well. Add in the noodles straight away, tossing well to combine

Add in the jalapeno, cilantro, tamari, and sesame seeds. Continue to cook for another 5-7 minutes or so, until the sauce has thickened.

Nutrition: 370 calories, 31 g fat, 16 g protein, 4 g net carbs

Low Carb Marinara Sauce

Most store bought marinara sauces are loaded with sugar, making them a no-go for the ketogenic diet. Luckily, this tasty marinara sauce is easy to make, super flavourful, and low carb! Use it on veggie noodles, chicken parm, or on anything else you like!

Serving: 4

Serving Size: ¼ cup

Prep Time: 5 minutes

Cook Time: 0 Minutes

Ingredients

1 8oz can crushed tomatoes

2 tbsp dried oregano

1 tbsp dried basil

2 cloves garlic, chopped

½ onion, diced

Salt and pepper, to taste

Handful fresh basil and parsley, chopped

3 tbsp olive oil

Instructions

In a blender or food processor, puree everything together until smooth. Transfer to an airtight container, and store in the refrigerator for up to 5 days. When ready to use, pour desired amount into a saucepan and bring to a boil. Reduce heat to low, and simmer for 5 minutes.

Nutrition: 169 calories, 11.3 g fat, 3.8 g protein, 8 g net carbs

Cheesy Chicken Bake

Using precooked chicken makes this meal come together in a snap! Use homemade marinara sauce to avoid any sugars and additives.

Serving: 2

Serving Size: Half of recipe

Prep Time: 2 minutes

Cook Time: 10 Minutes

Ingredients

2 tbsp olive oil

1 8 oz chicken breast, cooked and sliced

1 tsp dried thyme

1 tsp dried basil

1 tsp dried oregano

1 tsp garlic powder

Salt and pepper, to taste

2 servings marinara sauce (about ½ cup)

¼ cup parmesan cheese

½ cup mozzarella cheese

Instructions

Preheat broiler to 550F.

Toss together the chicken, oil, and seasonings in an oven-proof container. Pour the marinara over top, and cover with cheese.

Broil for 10 minutes, until the cheese is bubbling. Serve warm.

Nutrition: 488 calories, 22.3 g fat, 34 g protein, 9.3 g net carbs

Cream of Broccoli Soup

This soup is a snap to make in a high powered blender! Make a big batch if you like- it'll keep for up to a week in the fridge, and up to 3 months in the freezer!

Serving: 6

Serving Size: 1 cup

Prep Time: 5 minutes

Cook Time: 10 Minutes

Ingredients

½ head broccoli, chopped

½ onion, diced

3 cloves garlic, chopped

½ tsp ground nutmeg

1 tsp dried thyme

3 cups heavy cream

2 cups chicken stock

¼ cup grated parmesan

Instructions

Puree all ingredients together in a high speed blender until smooth.

Transfer the portion you're using immediately to a saucepan big enough to hold it comfortably. Keep the rest in an airtight container in the fridge for up to 14 days, or freeze in individual portions for up to 3 months.

Cook over medium-high heat for 10 minutes, until heated through.

Nutrition: 232 calories, 22.8 g fat, 2.9 g protein, 3 g net carbs

Avocado BLT

Avo buns are all the rage, and this easy sandwich is satisfying and fun to eat!

Serving: 1

Serving Size: whole recipe

Prep Time: 5 minutes

Cook Time: 0 Minutes

Ingredients

1 avocado. Sliced in half

2 strips bacon, cooked

1 slice tomato

1 ring red onion

1 leaf romaine lettuce

½ tbsp mayo

½ tbsp dijon mustard

½ tsp sesame seeds

Instructions

Using the avocado as your "bun", spread on the mayo and mustard, and layer in the bacon, tomato, onion, and lettuce.

Close the sandwich, and sprinkle sesame seeds on top of the avocado bun for a fun look! Slice in half, and serve immediately.

Nutrition: 540 calories, 46.1 g fat, 18.3 g protein, 5.6 g net carbs

Salmon Putanesca

Who doesn't love flavourful tomatoes, olives and herbs over a good quality piece of fish? Purchase wild, sustainably caught salmon.

Serving: 2

Serving Size: 1 piece fish

Prep Time: 5 minutes

Cook Time: 15 Minutes

Ingredients

2 3 oz fillets salmon

8 cherry tomatoes, halved

2 oz anchovies, finely chopped

6 kalamata olives, pitted and chopped

1 tbsp olive oil

Handful fresh basil and parsley

Salt and pepper, to taste

Instructions

Preheat oven to 375F

Preheat a small pan over medium heat, Drizzle in the olive oil and add in the anchovies, tomatoes, olives, and herbs. Saute for about 3 minutes.

Lay the fish onto a baking sheet lined with parchment, and season with salt and pepper. Spoon the tomato mixture evenly over both pieces of fish, and bake for 10-12 minutes, until the fish is cooked through. Serve warm, and keep any leftovers in a tightly sealed container in the fridge for up to 2 days.

Nutrition: 600 calories, 30.3 g fat, 72.4 g protein, 8 g net carbs

Ham and Swiss Cheese Crustless Quiche

What's the difference between a frittata and a crustless quiche? Not much, actually! But you can definitely impress your friends and family with this fancy sounding name, and make an awesome one pan meal while you're at it!

Serving: 2

Serving Size: Half recipe

Prep Time: 5 minutes

Cook Time: 11 Minutes

Ingredients

1 tbsp butter

4 oz ham, cubed

4 oz swiss cheese, grated

4 eggs, beaten

1 tbsp mayo

¼ cup heavy cream

¼ cup spinach

Salt and pepper, to taste

Instructions

Preheat oven to 375F

Preheat a medium sized, oven safe pan over medium heat on the stovetop. Melt in the butter, and saute the spinach for 1 minute. Remove from heat.

Beat together the eggs, mayo, cream, salt and pepper. Pour the mixture over the spinach, and add in the rest of the ingredients.

Transfer the pan to the oven, and bake for 10-12 minutes until cooked through.

Nutrition: 566 calories, 43.2 g fat, 36.3g protein, 5.6 g net carbs

Chicken a la King

Have you ever had this vintage dish? It's creamy and comforting, and the perfect way to end your day! Cooked chicken breasts make this dish come together super fast! Eat on its own, or serve alongside a green salad if you like

Serving: 1

Serving Size: Whole recipe

Prep Time: 5 minutes

Cook Time: 15 Minutes

Ingredients

1 tbsp butter

4 oz cooked chicken breast, sliced

3 oz mushrooms, sliced

1 clove garlic, minced

¼ onion, diced

½ carrot, diced

½ cup heavy cream

¼ red pepper, diced

Instructions

Preheat a medium sized pan over medium high heat. Melt in the butter, and saute the mushrooms, carrot, garlic and onion with a pinch of pepper. Add in the cream, and stir well.

Add in the chicken and red pepper, stirring well for 3-5 minutes.

Reduce heat to medium low, and simmer another 10 minutes or so, until the sauce has thickened slightly and a stew-like consistency is achieved. Serve warm.

Nutrition: 494 calories, 36.9 g fat, 29.1 g protein, 4.3 g net carbs

Portobello Burger

This yummy burger uses two portobello mushrooms as the bun!

Serving: 1

Serving Size: Whole recipe

Prep Time: 5 minutes

Cook Time: 15 Minutes

Ingredients

¼ lb ground beef

1 egg

1 tsp garlic powder

Salt and pepper to taste

1 oz mozzarella cheese, grated

1 tomato slice

1 ring red onion

Handful arugula or 1 romaine leaf

2 portobello caps

1 tbsp oil

Instructions

Preheat oven to 375f

Brush the mushrooms with oil, and season with salt and pepper.

Mix together the beef, egg, garlic, salt and pepper. Form into a patty.

Lay the patty alongside the mushroom caps on a baking sheet lined with parchment. Bake 15 minutes.

Lay the cooked patty on top of one of the mushroom caps. Top with the cheese, tomato, onion and greens. Close the burger with the remaining cap. Serve warm.

Nutrition: 485 calories, 30 g fat, 48.6 g protein, 2 g net carbs

Shrimp Stir Fry

This stir fry uses guilt-free shiratake noodles, along with delicious shrimp and a variety of keto friendly veg for a really yummy dinner or lunch option!

Serving: 2

Serving Size: Half recipe

Prep Time: 5 minutes

Cook Time: 10 Minutes

Ingredients

2 tbsp sesame oil

1 orange, juice and zest

2 tbsp tamari

1 tbsp ginger

1 tbsp sesame seeds

2 cloves garlic, minced

3 red chilies, finely sliced

3 tbsp coconut oil

¼ onion, sliced finely

1 celery stalk, finely sliced

6 oz oyster mushrooms, torn

½ red pepper, sliced

12 jumbo shrimp, peeled and deveined

1 8oz package shiratake noodles

Instructions

Rinse the noodles well in a colander, and pat dry.

Preheat a wok or medium sized pan over medium high heat. Melt in the coconut oil, and add in the onion, celery, mushrooms and peppers. Saute for 2 minutes, until softened slightly. Add in the shrimp, and continue to saute for another 3 minutes.

Drizzle in the sesame oil, and add in the garlic, ginger, tamari and orange. Toss well for 2 minutes.

Add the shiratake noodles, and toss well. Continue cooking for another 5 minutes until the sauce has thickened slightly and coats the noodles. Serve warm, and store any leftovers in an airtight container for up to 3 days.

Nutrition: 600 calories, 56 g fat, 30.6 g protein, 7 g net carbs

Middle Eastern Style Stuffed Tomatoes

Ground beef, pine nuts, tomatoes and a drizzle of decadent tahini! What else could you want in a dinner?

Serving: 2

Serving Size: 1 tomato

Prep Time: 5 minutes

Cook Time: 15 Minutes

Ingredients

2 tbsp olive oil

¼ lb ground beef

¼ onion, diced

1 tsp garlic powder

1 tsp cumin

1 tsp coriander powder

1 tsp turmeric

1 tsp chili powder

2 tbsp pine nuts

Handful parsley, chopped

2 tomatoes, cut in half through the center (to make 4 shells)

¼ cup tahini (found in snack recipes)

Instructions

Preheat the oven to 450F.

Preheat a medium pan over medium high heat. Drizzle in the oil, and add the onion and seasonings. Saute for 1 minute, then add in the beef. Continue cooking for 5-7 minutes, until the beef is cooked through.

Lay the tomatoes onto a baking sheet, and spoon in the beef. Bake for 5 minutes.

To serve, drizzle with tahini and top with parsley.

Nutrition: 400 calories, 33 g fat, 22.9 g protein, 5 g net carbs

This spicy Szechuan dish incorporates bright flavours and tofu and ground beef. Eat on its own, or serve on top of a bed or shiratake noodles or cauliflower rice

Serving: 2

Serving Size: Half Recipe

Prep Time: 5 minutes

Cook Time: 15 Minutes

Ingredients

1 lb silken tofu

100 g ground beef

1 tbsp sesame oil

3 red chilies, finely chopped

2 tbsp tamari

1 cup beef stock

2 tbsp coconut oil

3 green onions, finely sliced

1 tsp ginger

2 cloves garlic, minced

¼ cup broccoli florets, steamed

Instructions

Mix together the beef and sesame oil with a pinch of salt, and set aside.

Dice the tofu into cubes, and submerge in boiling water with a pinch of salt. Set aside.

Preheat a wok over medium high heat. Melt in the coconut oil, then fry the beef for about 3 minutes. Spoon the beef onto a plate and set aside.

Drizzle in a bit more sesame oil, and add the green onion, ginger, garlic and chilies. Saute for 2 minutes until fragrant.

Add the beef stock and tofu, and bring to a boil. Add the beef back in, and cook for another 8 minutes, stirring well until the liquid has evaporated slightly. Add the tamari. Taste, and adjust seasoning as needed.

Serve with broccoli florets, and some cauliflower rice if you like.

Nutrition: 449 calories, 30.1 g fat, 35.1 g protein, 6 g net carbs

Bacon Butter Cod

This cod is deliciously decadent, and very easy to prepare! Serve with an easy green salad, or with a serving of parmesan crusted cauliflower for a complete meal.

Serving: 2

Serving Size: Half Recipe

Prep Time: >1 minute

Cook Time: 20 Minutes

Ingredients

2 4 oz fillets cod

4 strips bacon, diced

2 tbsp butter

1 tsp dried thyme

Salt and pepper to taste

Instructions

Preheat oven to 350F

Pat the cod dry, and season with salt and pepper. Bake for 15-20 minutes.

Meanwhile, preheat a small pan over medium heat. Cook the bacon and butter together, stirring constantly for about 3 minutes until the bacon is fully cooked. Add in the thyme, and continue to cook for another minute or so, being careful not to burn the bacon or the butter.

Once the fish has cooked, spoon the butter-bacon mixture over top. Serve immediately.

Nutrition: 323 calories, 27.6 g fat, 17.5 g protein, 0.7 g net carbs

Parmesan Roasted Cauliflower

This yummy side dish is the perfect addition to any meal, but also makes a great lunch or snack on its own. Swap out the cauliflower for broccoli if you're looking to incorporate a bit more green into your diet.

Serving: 2

Serving Size: Half Recipe

Prep Time: 5 minutes

Cook Time: 15 Minutes

Ingredients

½ head cauliflower, cut into florets

¼ cup olive oil

1 tsp salt

1 tsp garlic powder

½ cup parmesan, grated

Instructions

Preheat oven to 400F

Toss together all ingredients. Lay onto a baking sheet lined with parchment, and bake for 15 minutes. Serve warm, or keep in an airtight container in the fridge for up to a week.

Nutrition: 260 calories, 26.8 g fat, 35.1 g protein, 6 g net carbs

Cheesy Mushrooms

These mushrooms are easy, quick and delicious!

Serving: 2

Serving Size: Half Recipe

Prep Time: 5 minutes

Cook Time: 15 Minutes

Ingredients

2 portobello mushroom caps

¼ cup mozzarella cheese, shredded

1 tbsp olive oil

1 cup spinach

1 tbsp butter, room temp

Instructions

Preheat oven to 400F

Brush the mushrooms with the oil, and season with a bit of salt and pepper.

Mix together the butter and spinach, and press the mixture into the center of the mushroom caps.

Top with the cheese, and bake for 15 minutes. Serve warm.

Nutrition: 124 calories, 13.5 g fat, 1.5 g protein, 0.2 g net carbs

Bacon-tomato-cheddar soup

This soup is so rich and satisfying, you'll want to have it every night!

Serving: 4

Serving Size: 1 cup

Prep Time: 5 minutes

Cook Time: 15 Minutes

Ingredients

¼ onion, diced

1 can crushed tomatoes

1 tbsp dried thyme

1 cup chicken stock

1 cup cream

1 clove garlic

½ cup cheddar cheese, grated

2 tbsp butter

4 strips bacon, diced

Instructions

In a blender, puree together the tomato, garlic, chicken stock, onion and thyme.

In a large saucepan over medium heat, melt the butter and fry the bacon for 1 minute. Add the tomato mixture, and bring to a boil.

Reduce the heat to low, and simmer for 10 minutes. Add the cream, and simmer for another 2-3 minutes. Stir in the cheese. Serve immediately.

Nutrition: 270 calories, 21.9 g fat, 12.2 g protein, 1 g net carbs

Pesto Pasta

A super easy pesto on top of zucchini noodles is the perfect quick dinner for a busy weeknight!

Serving: 2

Serving Size: Half of recipe

Prep Time: 5 minutes

Cook Time: 10 Minutes

Ingredients

3 cups basil

2 cloves garlic

¼ cup pine nuts

½ cup parmesan, grated

¼ cup olive oil

4 zucchinis, spiralized

Instructions

In a blender, puree together the basil, garlic, pine nuts, parm and oil.

Preheat a large pan over medium heat. Add in the pesto and zucchini noodles, and toss well to combine. Cook for about 10 minutes until cooked through. Serve immediately or keep leftovers in a container in the fridge for up to 3 days.

Nutrition: 646 calories, 53.8 g fat, 32.4g protein, 10 g net carbs

Cheesy Meatballs

This dish is so fast to make, and really yummy! Serve it with Marinara for a quick, satisfying meal. Make a big batch in advance, and freeze them for a quick, satisfying meal any time!

Serving: 2

Serving Size: 4 meatballs

Prep Time: 5 minutes

Cook Time: 15 Minutes

Ingredients

¼ lb ground beef

¼ lb ground pork

1 tbsp garlic powder

1 tbsp dried oregano

1 tbsp dried thyme

1 egg, beaten

½ cup mozzarella, shredded

2 servings Low Carb Marinara Sauce

Instructions

Preheat oven to 375F

Mix together all ingredients except the marinara. Form into 8 balls, and lay on a baking sheet lined with parchment.

Bake for 10-12 minutes

Meanwhile, warm the sauce in a large pan over medium high heat

Once the meatballs have cooked, transfer to the pan with the sauce and cook together for 3-5 minutes

Nutrition: 331 calories, 20.6 g fat, 40.1 g protein, 10 g net carbs

Thai Chicken Salad

This salad comes together quickly, and can be made up to five days in advance!

Serving: 2

Serving Size: Half recipe

Prep Time: 10 minutes

Cook Time: 0 Minutes

Ingredients

6 oz cooked chicken, shredded

1 carrot, grated

½ cucumber, grated or spiralized

1 jalapeno, finely sliced

3 green onions, finely sliced

2 tbsp mayo

1 tbsp curry powder

2 tbsp coconut cream

1 tsp garlic powder

1 tsp ginger

½ cup bean sprouts

1 tsp sesame oil

Instructions

Whisk together the curry powder, garlic, ginger, mayo and coconut cream. Add in all the other ingredients, and toss well to combine. Store in an airtight container for up to 5 days.

Nutrition: 303 calories, 14.2 g fat, 28.9 g protein, 9.1 g net carbs

Southwest Chicken Avocado Salad

This fun salad is so yummy and healthy! You'll love it!

Serving: 1

Serving Size: whole recipe

Prep Time: 5 minutes

Cook Time: 0 Minutes

Ingredients

4 oz cooked chicken breast, sliced

¼ cup cheddar cheese, grated

1 avocado, diced

¼ red pepper, diced

6 cherry tomatoes, halved

1 jalapeno, diced

1 lime, juice and zest

1 tsp garlic powder

1 tsp cayenne

Instructions

Mix together all ingredients, tossing well to combine. Serve immediately, or keep in the fridge for up to 6 hours.

Nutrition: 800 calories 53.1 g fat, 41.9 g protein, 5 g net carbs

Baked Cod with Lemony Asparagus

A one pan meal that is easy, tasty and healthy!

Serving: 2

Serving Size:half recipe

Prep Time: >1 minutes

Cook Time: 20 Minutes

Ingredients

2 4 oz fillets cod

1 tsp thyme

8 stalks asparagus, trimmed

3 tbsp olive oil

Salt and pepper, to taste

1 lemon, juice and zest, PLUS

1 lemon, cut into wheels

Instructions

Preheat oven to 350F

Sprinkle the thyme and some salt and pepper over the fish

Lay the lemon wheels down on a baking sheet lined with parchment. Lay the fish on top of the lemon wheels.

Toss the asparagus in the oil, salt and pepper and lemon zest and juice. Lay it beside the fish on the baking sheet.

Bake 20 minutes. Serve immediately, and refrigerate any leftovers for 1 day.

Nutrition: 554 calories 26 g fat, 81 g protein, 1.3 g net carbs

Asparagus, smoked salmon and goat cheese salad

The perfect healthy salad to end your day

Serving: 1

Serving Size: whole recipe

Prep Time: 10 minutes

Cook Time: 0 Minutes

Ingredients

6 oz smoked salmon

1 oz goat cheese

6 stalks asparagus, sliced

Handful arugula

1 lemon, juice and zest

1 tbsp olive oil

Instructions

Mix the lemon juice, zest and olive oil together

Add in the arugula, and toss well to combine

Mix in the goat cheese, asparagus and salmon.

Serve immediately

Nutrition: 466 calories 31.6 g fat, 41.9 g protein, 2.3 g net carbs

SNACKS

Veggie Sticks and Guacamole

This creamy guac is loaded with fat and nutrients! Double up on the recipe and keep it in an airtight container in the fridge for up to 2 days, so that you can have it on-hand for whenever a craving strikes! Veggie sticks add a boost of nutrition, and are perfect for dipping.

Serving: 1

Serving Size: Whole Recipe

Prep Time: 10 minutes

Cook Time: 0 Minutes

Ingredients

½ avocado

1 lime, zest and juice

3 tbsp cilantro, chopped

½ jalapeno, diced

1 clove garlic, minced

Veggies:

¼ red pepper, cut into strips

1 stalk celery, cut into sticks

2 baby carrots, cut in half

Instructions

Preheat oven to 185C/375F. Wash and dry the kale fully, and chop it into large pieces. Toss it with the oil, and the rest of the ingredients.

Lay the dressed kale onto a baking sheet lined with parchment paper. Bake for 30 minutes, until crispy and fragrant.

Allow to cool fully. Portion the kale chips into two airtight containers, and store up to a week at room temperature.

Nutrition: 240 calories, 20.1 g fat, 4 g protein, 3.6 g net carbs

Almond Coconut Fat Bombs

Fat bombs are easy and fun to make! Although they do need time to set in the freezer, they take no time at all to whip up. These fat bombs contain coconut, almonds and chocolate.

Serving: 12

Serving Size: 1 fat bomb

Prep Time: >5 minutes

Cook Time: 1 Minute

Ingredients

¼ cup almond butter

¼ cup coconut oil

2 tbsp erythritol

¼ cup unsweetened coconut flakes

2 tbsp cocoa powder

Instructions

Mix together the coconut oil and almond butter in a microwave safe bowl, and microwave on high for 1 minute.

Stir in the rest of the ingredients.

Pour into 12 individual cupcake papers, and freeze for at least 10 minutes. Allow the fat bomb to come to room temperature before eating. Store fat bombs in a ziplock bag or airtight container in the freezer for up to 6 months.

Nutrition: 200 calories, 20 g fat, 3 g protein, 2 g net carbs

Tahini with veggie sticks

Tahini is a delicious middle eastern sauce made with sesame paste (also called tahini), garlic, lemon and herbs. Use it on top of anything that needs a boost of flavour and fat, or as a dip for veggies for a satisfying snack

Serving: 4

Serving Size: 3 tbsp

Prep Time: 10 minutes

Cook Time: 0 Minutes

Ingredients

3 tbsp tahini paste

1 lemon, juice and zest

1 clove garlic

Handful parsley, chopped

Salt, to taste

½ cup water

Veggies:

¼ red pepper, cut into strips

1 stalk celery, cut into sticks

2 baby carrots, cut in half

Instructions

In a blender or food processor, combine all ingredients until smooth.

Transfer to an airtight container and keep in the fridge for up to 7 days. Serve with your favourite veggies for a guilt free, full fat snack!

Nutrition: 89 calories, 8 g fat, 2.6 g protein, 1 g net carbs

Guacamole Deviled Eggs

Serving: 6

Serving Size: 2 Pieces

Prep Time: 10 minutes

Cook Time: 0 Minutes

Ingredients

6 Eggs, hardboiled

1 Avocado, mashed

1 Tbsp lime juice

1 jalapeno, diced

Salt and pepper to taste

Instructions

Peel the eggs, and slice in half. Remove the yolks, and transfer to a bowl with the rest of the ingredients. Set the whites aside for a moment.

Mash together the yolks, avocado, jalapeno and lime juice with the salt and pepper. If you like, add a pinch of cayenne.

Spoon the filling into the eggs. Eat immediately, or keep in an airtight container in the fridge for up to a week.

Nutrition: 195 calories, 17g fat, 7g protein, 3g net carbs

Caprese rolls with prosciutto

These simple rolls are the perfect snack to make on a busy evening! Because of the classic combination of salty, creamy and herby, they also make a great topping for a simple salad.

Serving: 1

Serving Size: 4 Pieces

Prep Time: 10 minutes

Cook Time: 0 Minutes

Ingredients

50 g sliced prosciutto

25 g mozzarella, sliced

4 large basil leaves

1 small tomato, sliced

1 tsp balsamic vinegar

Instructions

Lay the prosciutto out onto a plate or cutting board.

Layer the mozzarella over top, followed by the basil. Roll the prosciutto to form a wheel, so the cheese and basil are inside the meat.

Slice in half, and lay each piece on top of a slice of tomato.

Drizzle with balsamic. Serve immediately, or refrigerate up to 48 hours.

Nutrition: 95 calories, 4g fat, 12.5g protein, 1 g net carbs

Coconut Matcha Fat Bombs

Matcha powder is rich in antioxidants, and tastes fantastic! You'll love this asian inspired fat bomb!

Serving: 12

Serving Size: 1 fat bomb

Prep Time: 15 minutes

Cook Time: 0 minutes

Ingredients

½ cup coconut oil

½ cup coconut cream

1 tsp matcha powder

1 tbsp powdered stevia

¼ tsp salt

½ tsp vanilla extract

For the topping:

2 tbsp coconut flakes

1 tbsp matcha powder

Instructions

In a bowl, combine the coconut flakes and 1 teaspoon of matcha powder, and set aside.

In another bowl, beat together the rest of the ingredients using a hand mixer, or combine in a standing mixer using the whisk attachment until light and fluffy.

Spoon out 12 equal sized scoops onto a baking sheet lined with parchment. Roll each scoop into a ball, and drop into the coconut-matcha topping. Roll around until completely covered.

Freeze for at least 20 minutes, and keep in the freezer for up to 6 months.

Lt the fat bomb sit at room temperature for 15 minutes before eating.

Nutrition: 100 calories, 11.5 g fat, 0.2 g protein, 2g net carbs

Beef Broth

Beef broth is easy to make, and really good for you! The addition of coconut oil adds a ton of flavour, while also increasing your fat levels

Serving: 1

Serving Size: 1 cup

Prep Time: 0 minutes

Cook Time: 15 minutes

Ingredients

1 cup beef stock

Salt and pepper to taste

1 tsp dried thyme (optional)

2 tbsp coconut oil

Instructions

In a medium sized pot, warm all ingredients over medium high heat. Bring to a boil, and then reduce to low and simmer for 10-12 minutes.

Nutrition: 273 calories, 28.6 g fat, 4.9 g protein, 0.9 g net carbs

Weekly Shopping List

*Note- It can be more economical to purchase meat items in bulk. Portioning out your meat items and freezing them will save time and money later.

*Most of the recipes in this meal plan call for cooked chicken breast and cooked bacon. This has been done as a way to save you time during the week. Plan a prep day each week, read over your meal plan and recipes, and cook your proteins as needed in advance.

For cooked bacon:

Preheat oven to 350F. Lay 1 lb bacon onto a baking sheet lined with parchment. Bake 20-25 minutes, until cooked through. Allow to cool, and portion as needed for the week.

For cooked chicken:

Preheat oven to 350F. Pat the chicken breast dry, and season as you like (recommended per breast- 1 tsp dried thyme, 1 tsp salt, 1 tsp pepper). Pour ¼ cup water into the bottom of a baking sheet, cover with parchment, and lay down the chicken breasts (the steam from the water helps the chicken stay moist). Bake 20-25 minutes until cooked through. Allow to cool, and portion as needed for the week.

Pantry Staples For the Month:

Spirulina- 1 oz

Coconut Milk- 10 cans

Pickles- 1 jar

Kalamata Olives- 8 oz

Almond Butter- 1 jar (about 8 oz)

Stevia (*may sub for Erythritol) - 1 package about 2.5 oz

Sesame Seeds - 4 oz

Almonds - 8 oz

Pecans- 6 oz

Shredded Unsweetened Coconut - 1 lb

Walnuts - 1 lb

Pumpkin Seeds - 1 lb

Flax Seeds - 1 lb
Coconut oil- 1 oz

Canned tomatoes- 4x 8 oz cans
Olive oil mayonnaise or avocado oil
mayonnaise - 1 container, about 1 L

Tahini Paste - 1 container, about 1 lb

Italian Herbs- 1 package, about 300g

Dried Thyme- 1 package, about 300g

Cayenne Powder- 1 package, about 300g

Curry Powder- 1 package, about 300g

Cumin- 1 package, about 300g

Ground Ginger- 1 package, about 300g

Sugar Free Sriracha Sauce- 1 bottle

Gluten Free Tamari - 1 bottle

Coffee- 1 lb

Matcha Powder- 300 g

Salt

Pepper

Tortillas- 36 (keep wrapped and sealed until ready to use)

Nori sheets- 1 package

Almond Milk- 4 L

Beef Stock- either 3L prepared, or bouillon cubes

Chicken Stock- either 3L prepared, or bouillon cubes

Shiratake Noodles- 6 packages (keep refrigerated)

Week 1 Shopping List

Seafood, Meat and Eggs:

Eggs- 1 dozen

Salmon- 12 oz (4x 3 oz fillets)

Chicken breast, boneless skinless- 6]oz

Smoked Salmon- 1 lb

Bacon- 1 lb

Tofu- 1 lb

Ham- 1 package (about 6 oz)

Prosciutto- 6 oz

Dairy Products:

Cheddar cheese- 1 lb

Butter- 1 lb

Heavy Cream- 1 L

Mozzarella- 3 oz

Parmesan Cheese- 4 oz

Produce:

6 Avocados

2 Limes

2 Lemons

1 Head of Romaine

1 Package Fresh Spinach

1 Package Fresh Basil

2 peppers

6 jalapenos

1 pint cherry tomatoes

1 cucumber

1 package carrots

1 head broccoli

1 package (8oz) bean sprouts

2 roma tomatoes

1 lb carrots

Celery- 1 head

Week 2 Shopping List

Meat and Eggs:

Salmon- 8oz

Cod- 8 oz

Chicken Breast- 16 oz

Ground beef- 1 lb

Tuna, canned- 1

Bacon- 1 lb

Eggs- 1 dozen

Dairy Products:

None

Produce:

4 Portobello Mushrooms

2 roma tomatoes

1 Pint Cherry Tomatoes

3 lemons

6 Avocados

1 lb Spinach

1 head Romaine Lettuce

1 lb bean sprouts

10 stalks asparagus

1 orange

1 lime

1 red onion

Week 3 Shopping List

Meat and Eggs:

Cod- 6 oz

Shrimp- 1 lb

Ground Pork- 12 oz

Ham- 4 oz

Bacon- 1 lb

Eggs- 1 dozen

Salmon- 8 oz

Chicken breasts- 24 oz

Ground Beef - 8 oz

Dairy Products:

Butter- 1 lb

goat cheese - 8 oz

Cheddar Cheese- 1 lb

Produce:

1 orange

7 Avocados

1 Lime

½ lb Spinach

1 Package Fresh Basil

1 Bunch Cilantro

1 bunch green onions

1 Head of Broccoli

1 Head of Cauliflower

Portobello mushrooms x4

1 head celery

1 bunch carrots

1 tomato

1 package cherry tomatoes

1 red onion

Week 4 Shopping List

Meat and Eggs:

Chicken Breast-1 lb

Proscuitto- 8 oz

Cod- 6 oz

Bacon 1 lb

Eggs- 1 dozen

Shrimp-8 oz

Ham- 8 oz

Salmon- 6 oz

Smoked Salmon- 1 lb

Dairy Products:

Goat Cheese- 8 oz

Heavy Cream- 8 oz

Butter 1 lb

Produce:

1 bunch Asparagus

6 Avocados

1 package spinach

3 Packages Fresh Basil

1 Head Cauliflower

1 Carrot

1 Red Bell Pepper

1 Cucumber

1 Tomato

1 pint cherry tomatoes

4 Onions

2 lemons

1 lime

1 orange

CHAPTER 6
Questions You Will Ask

In this chapter, we will cover some commonly asked questions that pertain to the keto diet. This book is about helping you better understand your keto journey and getting the right information. Hopefully, your most burning questions will be answered in this chapter.

Is it OK to be in ketosis on a long-term basis?

In short, yes! As we talked about in other chapters, we are all born in a state of ketosis and it is not harmful at all. Naturally, as you stay true to the keto diet, your body will use up all its ketone stores and will begin to burn fat for fuel. This is called "fat adaptation". This is the ultimate goal of the kept diet and means that your body is now soley using fat as a source of fuel. You may even notice that your ketone monitors aren't registering ketones, anymore. Don't freak out! Over time, this is what is supposed to happen.

Is it OK to cycle in and out of ketosis?

Depending on your lifestyle, cycling in and out of ketosis is fine, especially if you are a major athlete or body builder. These folks are the only folks who actually need some glycogen before working out or competing. The quick release of sugar goes directly to their muscles and helps them to recover.

Some people find that carb-cycling helps them keep their body from becoming used to the keto diet and helps with weight loss stalls. You'll have to play around with what works best for you.

Can I be a vegetarian and eat a keto diet?

Honestly? Being a vegetarian or a vegan is pretty hard to accomplish while on a ketogenic diet. Many staple foods, like butter, cheese, and meat, are part of the diet. Since the keto diet requires you to cut out starching vegetables and almost all fruits, a vegetarian would be left with barely any food choices at the end of the day. I don't recommend vegetarians follow a keto diet for nutritional purposes.

How long before I see improved health and weight loss?

There is no cookie cutter answer for this question. Everyone is different, and our bodies adapt to new things at their own paces. You must factor in how much weight you need to lose and the severity of the health problems you are having. Some folks see results very quickly while others have to wait a little while as their body adjusts to the new way of eating.

Will I experience kidney stones on the keto WOE?

If you have suffered from kidney stones in the past the likelihood of them returning is probable. However, removing sugar from your diet and watching your mineral and protein intake can help decrease this risk. People who have never had kidney stones rarely develop them from the keto diet.
Why am I losing muscle on keto?

There will always be a degree of muscle loss on any weight loss diet. However, you can minimize this effect by eating adequate amounts of protein. Exercising most days of the week will also be beneficial to keeping your muscle alive and well.

TIPS AND STRATEGIES TO SUSTAINING YOUR KETO LIFESTYLE

Now that you are on the road to better health and weight loss through the ketogenic diet it is time to talk about how to sustain your newfound lifestyle.

Here are a few tips on how you can be successful and sustain all the progress you've made through keto:

1. Sometimes, ketogenic eating can be expensive. Just know that you don't need all the fancy products that you see being touted on keto blogs. So, you can't afford almond meal and MCT oil? No worries! Purchase the keto-friendly foods that you can afford. You can also purchase many keto foods in bulk and freeze, vacuum seal, or can them as this will save you a lot of money.
2. Always keep keto-safe foods within reach. When you are hungry and/or craving you want to have chopped up veggies, sliced cheese, or nuts at your disposal. If you don't have keto-foods ready to go you are more susceptible to reaching for a candy bar.
3. Meal prepping is essential to ketogenic success. Choose one day out of the week and make your meal plans and prep your food for the next 7 days. Sure, it may be labor intensive and time-consuming at first but you'll relish the ease of having your meals already prepped and ready over the course of the next week.
4. Would your family be open to keto? It is so much easier to prepare one type of food instead of two. See if you can't get them onboard the keto train. In fact, keto food tastes so good, my family doesn't even know when they are eating it. I have always made keto suppers for the family and myself. Unlike low-calorie diets, high-fat food is delicious. It's hard to believe that it is actually "diet food".
5. You do not need to exercise in order to be successful on the keto diet. However, it does help things move along a little quicker and it is good for you. Start out small with doing simple walking a few days a week. Gradually, you can move towards a more intense workout routine if you so desire.
6. Lastly, get yourself more keto recipe and research books. You want to keep your meals rotating so you don't get bored. Boredom leads to failure. Explore keto blogs, YouTube channels, and Facebook pages. Look up Dr. Eric Berg and Dr. Jason Fung who are known in the keto community for their expertise on the diet.

CONCLUSION

What Keto Has Meant for Me

Life changer. That is what keto has meant for me. I was tired of feeling sluggish, gaining weight, and having constant bloat around my middle. It hurt me every time I'd wander into a department store and try on clothes only to be disappointed by what I saw staring back at me in the dressing room mirror. Many times, I'd leave the clothes in a crumpled-up ball on the floor and walk out.
Before keto, I had no idea what metabolic syndrome was and that I was being affected by it. Nixing sugar from my diet totally helped repair this ailment. Today, I feel stronger, lighter, and far more fit than I ever have before.

I can run around the yard with my kids, go on hikes, and wake up rested all due to my ketogenic lifestyle. The days of being overweight, exhausted, and feeling frumpy are well behind me.

They can be for you, too.

This book is intended to help folks who are just starting out on the ketogenic diet. It is a guide to helping them meet their health and weight loss goals. It by no means replaces the expertise of your health care professional.

If you are already on a ketogenic diet this book will help you get more out of the lifestyle. Basically, it will help you cross over into more information and a better understanding of why you are choosing the keto WOE.

If you are a fast-paced person with a busy lifestyle, this book is for you as it provides you with a comprehensive quick recipe meal plan. More traditional? No problem. I have a meal plan for you, too.

Lastly, and most importantly, this book has been designed to help people sustain their keto lifestyle for the long haul. It is so important that you remember how you got sick and overweight in the first place and what keto did to change all of that.

Resources

1. https://www.ncbi.nlm.nih.gov/pubmed/17332207
2. https://www.ncbi.nlm.nih.gov/pmc/articles/PMC2633336/
3. https://www.ncbi.nlm.nih.gov/pubmed/11581442
4. https://www.ncbi.nlm.nih.gov/pmc/articles/PMC1819381/
5. https://www.ncbi.nlm.nih.gov/pmc/articles/PMC2367001/
6. https://www.ncbi.nlm.nih.gov/pubmed/14525681
7. https://www.ncbi.nlm.nih.gov/pubmed/6865776
8. https://www.ncbi.nlm.nih.gov/pubmed/14769489
9. https://www.ncbi.nlm.nih.gov/pubmed/14527626
10. https://www.ncbi.nlm.nih.gov/pmc/articles/PMC2633336/
11. https://www.ncbi.nlm.nih.gov/pmc/articles/PMC5329646/
12. https://www.ncbi.nlm.nih.gov/pmc/articles/PMC3826507/
13. https://www.journals.elsevier.com/diabetes-and-metabolic-syndrome-clinical-research-and-reviews
14. https://www.nap.edu/read/10490/chapter/8#275
15. https://www.healthline.com/nutrition/low-carb-ketogenic-diet-brain#section3
16. https://www.ncbi.nlm.nih.gov/pubmed/19332337
17. https://www.ncbi.nlm.nih.gov/pmc/articles/PMC3157418/
18. https://www.ncbi.nlm.nih.gov/pmc/articles/PMC4124736/
19. https://www.ruled.me/the-ketogenic-diet-and-cholesterol/
20. https://www.ruled.me/can-low-carb-diet-lower-blood-pressure/
21. https://www.ruled.me/keto-best-fatty-liver-diet/
22. https://www.ruled.me/3-reasons-keto-better-for-brain/
23. https://www.healthline.com/health/ketosis-vs-ketoacidosis#diagnosis
24. https://ketogasm.com/what-are-macros/
25. https://www.ncbi.nlm.nih.gov/pmc/articles/PMC3257631/

The Complete Beginners Guide To Intermittent Fasting For Weight Loss

Cure The Weight Problem And Reverse Chronic Diseases

Jason Legg

The Complete Guide
To Intermittent Fasting For Weight Loss

Introduction

Psst! Yes you!

Reckon you must be searching for ways to achieve weight loss and somehow you chanced upon this here. First I would like to say a warm welcome to this domain of intermittent fasting and I am absolutely stoked to know that you will be getting loads of value as well as actionable tips with which you can kick start and achieve significant progress on the weight loss journey.

I am by no means the final authority on intermittent fasting, and I would like to say the reason why I felt compelled to share what I know on this subject is because intermittent fasting literally saved my life.

Yes. You can call it a repayment of karmic debt or whatever you would like to term it as because this book as a labor of love is the end result of detailing what I know on intermittent fasting.

To cut the long story short, intermittent fasting was kind of forced upon me when I was diagnosed with all sorts of diseases and syndromes. All at the same time. Metabolic syndrome made its debut in my life, though that wasn't a real surprise considering my bulging waist line. Diabetes paid its call about a month later, and to top everything off, a minor cardiac arrest was the absolute crowning moment in those dark ages. The doctor's advice was to stick to meds and never miss a day. I was of course given the standard prescription for diet, meaning low fat , low calories in order to control weight gain.

It didn't work, and I panicked.

I started to toss aside the usual blind faith that I had in modern medical science and ventured into the world of natural weight loss for solutions to my problems. This and that diet came up, and believe it or not, I once drank olive oil for a straight five days. That was nasty. Eventually and fortuitously, I got hold of the concept of intermittent fasting when one of my neighbors sort of just casually dropped the subject when we were having our little chats. Little did I know it would consume me and I would be blessed once again with great health and a body that did not rely on external medication for proper function.

Intermittent fasting is a subject that has received plenty of widespread attention of late. People who have taken on fasting have managed to achieve some fantastic results in regards to both their health and weight. The phenomena of intermittent fasting is in no way a fad. Fasting has been practiced for centuries now and is considered by many ancient tribes as a means of survival, sacrifice, healing power, and spiritual cleansing. Intermittent fasting is in no way a new eating plan for you to try out for the next few weeks. Intermittent fasting is a way of life.

This book explores the many topics that surround intermittent fasting, such as the various methods of intermittent fasting and the multitude of benefits that have been discovered through numerous studies and research. There are also some useful tips on how to conduct your fast as well as the kind of food you can prepare and eat while taking part in intermittent fasting. The people who practice intermittent fasting today benefit in regards to weight loss and fitness. Studies have also found significant progress in regards to promoting other useful health factors such as inflammation, brain-cell creation, increased energy levels, and mental state. Intermittent fasting also encourages the natural fat-burning state of ketosis, which helps those who fast with shedding belly fat.

Apart from the various health benefits associated with intermittent fasting, you also want to give fasting a try because of a whole host of other reasons. One is the convenience of not having to eat as many meals as you would typically. Intermittent fasting allows you to skip meals, meaning that you will be able to save on the time and cost of preparing meals. Apart from the time and cost savings, you will also be eating much less than you would typically yet not experiencing those darn hunger pangs. This will allow you to automatically control your calorie intake just by following a simple eating timetable promoted by intermittent fasting.

This book goes into specific detail in regards to all of these benefits and how you can implement intermittent fasting to enjoy these benefits. It will help you to drastically improve your life in a healthy way. Intermittent fasting is a superb lifestyle choice and is indeed the way to go.

See you in the fasting nirvana! And oh, please enjoy the weight loss, improved health and better all-around lifestyle while you are in it!

Chapter 1: What is Intermittent Fasting

How Our Modern Diet is a Problem

It is estimated that more than one-third of adults in the United States are obese. This equates to over 78 million people who suffer from obesity. Obesity may be taken lightly by most people, but being obese can increase a person's risk towards certain medical conditions such as diabetes and heart disease. The chances of having a stroke rise in obese individuals. Another alarming statistic regarding obesity is that it is one of the leading causes of preventable death in America.

If you look back at the last few decades, it is possible to find a relationship between the rise in obesity and the way our diets have changed. Not only are we eating mostly processed food, often deep-fried, but we are also consuming larger amounts of food than we used to. The total caloric intake among individuals has gone up by 400 calories per day. The convenience and availability of cheap junk food has made it easily accessible for everyone to consume. However, the disadvantages of this modern diet are overlooked by most people.

The food we eat today is drastically different from the food that was consumed over 40 years ago. Most of the food then was fresh, some of it actually grown at home. Even though there were plenty of diners and fast food outlets back then, people still preferred eating good fresh food at home. In contrast, most of today's food is in some way processed, including the food that you choose to cook at home.

The type of food that we consume today is filled with additives, trans fats, colorings, and other various chemicals and ingredients that were not evident in food just a few decades ago. One of the most significant increases in our modern-day diet is the consumption of sugar. People in America consume 22 teaspoons of sugar on average per day. That makes up for 25 percent of a person's daily caloric intake. If you compare these statistics with past figures, then today's sugar intake has risen 20 percent since the seventies.

People today are obviously not consuming 22 teaspoons of actual sugar. The sugar that we end up consuming is usually found in juices, desserts, and sauces. This processed fructose is also evident in foods that are advertised as being healthy meals. Because of this, many parents will inadvertently give their kids food that's high in sugar.

Another significant contributor towards sugar consumption is soda and fruit juice drinks. Beverages like soda have large amounts of sugar in them and are usually considered as one of the worse sugar sources. Many people who know this tend to skip to a so-called healthier alternative by ordering juice instead of soda. The truth is, juice contains a very similar amount of sugar when compared to soda. And, you guessed it, soda and juice intake has also increased dramatically since the 1970s.

Soda drinks increased in popularity at a rapid rate over the last few decades, peaking around the year 2002. Interest in sodas has dipped ever so slightly since then. However, fruit juice has seen a decent increase in popularity since the late nineties and continues to grow in popularity as compared to the decrease in the popularity of sodas. People seem to be under the general impression that juice is much better for you than soda, but this is false.

If you ever thought of striking out that one thing from the modern diet in order to be healthier, then reducing sugar is the key.

The Food We Consume Today

The type of fats that we consume has also changed over the years. The primary consensus regarding animal fats and other saturated fats is that they can be dangerous for you because they are, most likely, a cause of heart disease. However, vegetable oils, such as corn oil and canola oil, that are processed are so dangerous that recent studies have shown that these daily cooking oils are liable to cause hormonal imbalances and metabolic changes in a person's body.

Repeated use of these oils has also contributed to the current obesity problem. The same can be said for trans fats, which are found in probably every single tasty treat or food in our modern diet. Studies have shown that trans fats, a form of polyunsaturated fats, increase bad LDL cholesterol while not increasing the good HDL cholesterol. Studies show that our use of vegetable oil has significantly increased since the 1960s.

There are also current studies that are focused on the relationship between trans fats and insulin resistance, which drives type 2 diabetes. The sad truth is that, today, many people have replaced heart-healthy butter with margarine that is filled with trans fats.

Some of the types of food that are known to include trans fats are:

- Chocolate
- Margarine
- Ice cream
- Burgers
- Cookies
- Cakes

- Cereals
- Bread
- French fries
- Pizza
- Fried chicken
- Pastries

Even though the consumption of trans fats has been regulated in recent years, we still consume way too much. The consumption of fast foods in the United States has consistently increased at a dramatic rate since the late sixties. A big reason for this is that our go-to food today is processed fast food. We like the convenience of foods that are cooked fast and available to eat on-the-go. No need to prepare a decent breakfast at home when you can fetch a burger at the drive-thru and eat in the car on the way to work. This way, you can get in an extra half hour of work at the office.

This is the perfect solution for productive people. Unfortunately, such food is loaded with trans fats. Even just grabbing snacks from a gas station takes its toll on us. We do this to avoid our hunger during our trip from work to home, instead of just waiting to get home and eat something healthy. These unnecessary processed foods are part of the cause of our terrible modern diet.

The modern diet is the primary reason behind obesity and people becoming sicker than before. More and more people are beginning to adopt the modern diet by abandoning traditional foods in favor of processed food. These processed foods are high in sugar, vegetable oil, and refined flour. On the other hand, eggs are considered to be one of the more nutritious foods out there. Yet our consumption of eggs has also gradually decreased.

Eggs are high in cholesterol, but they do not increase the bad cholesterol in the blood. Nevertheless, people still feel that eggs can cause a negative impact on your cholesterol. Because of this, people began to consume fewer eggs over the course of the years. New studies and diets are more accepting of eggs today and actually promote the consumption of eggs.

The History of Intermittent Fasting

It's clear that intermittent fasting has become something of a popular star today. Apart from the excellent weight-loss results, one of the primary reasons for fasting is the health benefits that one can enjoy. These are some of the elements that have caused intermittent fasting to receive plenty of attention and interest. When people look up intermittent fasting, one of the first things that these people research is the actual origin of intermittent fasting.

Yes, you probably have only recently heard of intermittent fasting, but the truth is, it has been around since ancient times. Back in the time when our ancestors were hunter-gatherers, people used to fast for long periods in between meals. They did this because food back then was not as readily available as it is today.

People used to hunt for food for days until a kill was made. The food that people gathered or claimed during a hunt was then shared over a period of a few days between everyone in the tribe. It was common for people not to find anything for an entire day when out hunting. These people would have to make do with the situation for that day and hope that the next day would be a much more productive day for hunting. If they could not find anything to hunt, then they would search for nuts and fruits that could help sustain them through their tiring hunting sessions.

Our ancestors may have been forced to fast because of their situation in regards to food, but, through fasting, they were able to cope with not having food readily available. Most of the time, these people managed perfectly fine with their fast, as their bodies had adapted to their eating pattern. Their eating pattern assisted in increasing fat oxidation while reducing body weight and accelerating fat loss.

These are some of the benefits that arise from intermittent fasting. Our ancestors didn't fast mostly because of these benefits, but merely as a way of survival. If fasting can be seen as a primary means of survival, then that alone will tell you how beneficial it can be. Another important part about fasting is feasting. What you eat when you do eventually eat is vital in determining the effectiveness of your fast.

Our ancestors made sure not to overdo it when it was time to eat. They ate rationally, to have enough food to go around, as well as to preserve food for more extended periods. They ate just enough food for them to get by. Only two meals a day was more than sufficient for them to remain nourished and healthy. This meant that these people ate enough food to enable their bodies to store the right amount of fat which would be used as a source of energy in the days to come.

This way of eating may seem irregular in today's age, but it was how we used to eat and how our body was designed to consume food. It is considered one of the best ways to help our body maintain itself, which is key to our health and wellbeing. Eating only when needed is the way to go.

Overeating is considered wrong and unnatural. Consuming large amounts of food forces excess fat on the body which leads to an unhealthy lifestyle. Being overweight and unhealthy can also cause a person to develop various diseases. It is known that our ancestors were much stronger than us. Most people back then had stronger bones than even our modern Olympic athletes. Our ancestors achieved their great physical conditions while fasting for long periods of time.

Other ancient civilizations, such as the Ancient Greeks and Egyptians, practiced eating patterns similar to that of intermittent fasting. They endured voluntary starvation with the hopes of allowing their bodies to recover from illness. They also understood the benefits behind fasting and undertook regular fasts so that they could enjoy those benefits.

Ancient Greeks and Egyptians also used intermittent fasting as a means of strengthening the body. These civilizations understood that when a person practices intermittent fasting, he or she becomes more alert and focused. This is due to a fasting person's body being able to release an increased amount of norepinephrine, a chemical that functions in the brain as a hormone and neurotransmitter.

Fasting in the Middle Ages

Intermittent fasting continued to be a part of many civilizations for years. It even managed to spread to other parts of the world. Intermittent fasting became popular during the Middle Ages as people took part in fasts for various reasons, primarily to reap the benefits associated with fasting. The Eastern Orthodox and Roman Catholic churches at the time had a significant influence on the diets of people from the Middle Ages.

The church prohibited meat and other animal products on a few different occasions throughout the year. An example of a specific event when meat was forbidden was during Lent, a period preceding Easter. Lent was also an occasion in which people were required to fast for 40 days. This is symbolic of how Christ fasted for 40 days while in the desert. Apart from Lent, most churches also advised that people should alternate between fasting and feasting.

One of the most popular times to fast was on Fridays. Most of the Christian churches saw fasting as a means of degrading the body while refreshing the soul. Fasting also served as a reminder of the humanity of Christ. Being able to fast meant that you and your body underwent abstinence and self-restraint.

Fasting in Religions

Throughout history, different religions have also practiced intermittent fasting. These religions have been fasting for centuries now. In Judaism, there are several days in the year that are reserved towards fasting. Yom Kippur, the Day of Atonement, is the most well-known full fast as it is a fast that is mentioned in the Torah. The purpose of the fast is to "afflict your soul." This can be seen as a form of repentance. The actual duration of the fast is 25 hours and it begins on the evening before Yom Kippur and after nightfall on the day of Yom Kippur.

Strict rules apply to the fast on Yom Kippur. There is no food at all allowed, not even water. Only the elderly, ill, and pregnant woman are exempt from the fast. Apart from Yom Kippur, there are more holidays and events spread out over the year that are associated with fasting. People are also allowed to engage in a private fast if they so wish, as long as they practice the fast within the set of rules.

In Islam, Muslims also practice fasting during the month of Ramadan. They begin their fast early in the morning, just before sunrise, (or before their morning prayer) and they end their fast in the evening, during sunset. All Muslims must take part in this compulsory fast daily for the 30-day duration of Ramadan until the day of Eid al-Fitr. The entire day of fasting prohibits all kinds of food and drink. Muslims cannot eat anything, nor can they even drink water.

There are various reasons behind fasting in the month of Ramadan. Ramadan is seen as a holy month in which the devil ceases to exist. It is a month in which Muslims are encouraged to practice as many good deeds as possible. One such good deed is the act of performing the Taraweeh prayer in the evening. Fasting is another good deed and is considered a form of abstinence and sacrifice. It is also seen as a means to cleanse the body of any external devices and toxins. Fasting and praying during Ramadan are how Muslims cleanse their bodies and their souls.

The Science of Intermittent Fasting

It makes sense for us to take part in intermittent fasting as our ancestors did for centuries. Some of the reasons why they took part in fasts were for survival and health benefits. Our hunter- gatherer ancestors also took part in intermittent fasting so that they could cope with periods of famine. There is a common argument that it certainly makes evolutionary sense if we, too, undertake similar fasts, as our bodies are designed to cope with such eating habits.

At the moment, there is a large body of research to support the health benefits of intermittent fasting, which is good for both your mind and body. However, the majority of the research has been conducted on animals and not on humans. This is why people are calling for more research and monitoring of individuals that are currently undergoing intermittent fasting. The research that is presently available shows that fasting assists in improving biomarkers of disease, preserves learning and memory functions, and reduces oxidative stress.

These findings are according to Mark Mattson, who is a senior investigator for the National Institute of Aging, a division of the US National Institutes of Health. Mattson conducted studies centered around the health benefits of intermittent fasting on the cardiovascular system and brain within rodents. In his studies, Mattson developed several theories about why fasting provides physiological benefits.

One interesting theory is that, during the fasting period, our cells are under mild stress. Because of this, our cells then respond by adapting to that stress. Our cells accomplish this by enhancing their ability to cope with stress and possibly enhancing themselves in order to resist disease more effectively. The stress that our cells may undergo during fasting does sound negative, but this type of stress can be comparable to the stress that our body undergoes during intense workout sessions in the gym or other vigorous exercise.

These sorts of high-intensity workouts place high levels of stress on your muscles and cardiovascular system. If you spend the right amount of time allowing your body to recover afterward, then your body will become stronger over time. Mattson says that there is a similarity between how our cells respond to the stress of exercise and how our cells respond to intermittent fasting.

Mattson has contributed to a specific study in which overweight adults with moderate asthma consumed only 20 percent of their daily caloric intake on alternate days. This meant that the subjects would perform a fast on one day, then eat normally the next day, then fast again the day after, and so on. The findings were that those who adhered to the diet managed to lose nine percent of their initial body weight over the course of eight weeks. Mattson also found a decrease in stress and inflammation, with an improvement of asthma-related symptoms and overall health.

In other studies, Mattson also explored the effects of intermittent fasting and energy restriction on weight loss and other biomarkers among young overweight woman. These biomarkers included conditions such as diabetes, breast cancer, and cardiovascular disease. The findings were that intermittent restriction was as effective as a continuous dietary restriction to improve weight loss. The results were just as positive towards insulin sensitivity and other health biomarkers.

Ketosis

Mattson also undertook studies of how fasting is related to neurons. He found that if you don't eat for 10 to 16 hours, then your body will begin to use its fat stores for energy. When this happens, then the fatty acids known as ketones get released into the bloodstream. This process has been shown to protect memory and functionality as well as to slow down disease processes in the brain.

Continuously fasting while on a low-carb diet allows your body to enter the state of ketosis. Ketosis occurs when your body switches over from its primary energy source, glucose, to another source of energy, known as ketones. As mentioned earlier, ketones are produced from the fat stores in our body. When our body runs out of glucose (or blood sugar), which mostly comes from the carbohydrates that we eat, then it will rely on ketones for energy.

The consensus is that when a person's body is in ketosis, then he or she will have to burn fat faster to consistently generate the ketones required for energy. If you wish to achieve a state of ketosis, then you will have to force your body not to produce any more glucose. A way of doing this is just to cut out carbs. Low-carb diets, such as the ketogenic diet, promote the state of ketosis by cutting daily carb intake to only five percent, overall, and increasing fat intake to 75 percent.

The keto diet makes it possible to have few to no carbs daily with increased consumption of fats. This means that your body will not have any more carbs to turn into glucose for energy. Instead, your body will rely on the fats you consume. This way, your body will remain in the fat-burning state of ketosis. Another way of achieving ketosis is through intermittent fasting.

Fasting for long periods of time means that your body will run out of its default source of energy, which is glucose. This means that while you are fasting, it will be possible for your body to transition to burning excess fat for fuel. Many people who practice the ketogenic diet on a daily basis also undergo intermittent fasting. The reason for this is that both promote the fat-burning state of ketosis very well.

It is important to remember that your body does not simply switch over into ketosis after just a single day of fasting. The process is long and can take up to seven days. In that time you will have had to watch the amount of carbs you ate which turn into glucose, while consuming the correct amount of fats that will be converted to ketones, to sustain yourself. Taking in large amounts of protein, instead of fats, will not work as our bodies will also convert excess protein into glucose.

Why You Want to Fast

The most common reason why a person wants to fast is to lose weight. If you do have issues with weight or you want to shape up a bit to fit into that gorgeous dress, then successfully implementing intermittent fasting into your life can be a way to achieve all of this. However, weight loss isn't the only reason you should be fasting. There are many other health reasons why you should fast. These are possibly some of the benefits that our ancestors enjoyed when they went on their periodic fasts.

Another excellent reason for why you should fast is that intermittent fasting is a natural calorie restriction method. You will notice that your caloric intake will automatically go down when you begin fasting, as long as you don't overdo your meals during your eating window. Let's take a more in-depth look at the benefits behind intermittent fasting.

The Benefits of Fasting

In recent times, people have begun to realize that there are plenty of benefits that one can enjoy while taking part in intermittent fasting. Some of the benefits include general food and caloric restrictions that can help promote weight loss as well as creating opportunities to skip meals. Not having to cook individual meals on a daily basis can directly equate to less effort in preparing meals as well as time and money savings.

If you plan to skip breakfast entirely on a daily basis, then you can save up on the expenses related to your first meal of the morning. It also means that you no longer need to wake up earlier to prepare your breakfast in the mornings before you rush off to work. You can now allocate your time in the morning for other activities. Apart from time and money savings, there are a few other benefits that you can enjoy while taking up intermittent fasting.

Weight Loss

Most people who take up intermittent fasting today are doing so to lose weight. If done correctly, intermittent fasting will allow you to eat fewer meals per day. This will drop your overall caloric intake. Apart from this, intermittent fasting enhances hormone function and facilitates weight loss. This is achieved through higher growth-hormone levels, lower insulin levels, and increased amounts of norepinephrine. These are the defining factors that assist the body in breaking down body fat to use it for energy.

Because of this, short-term fasting will increase your metabolic rate by up to 14 percent. That means that you will be able to burn even more calories on a daily basis. So if you are someone that pays careful attention to calories, then intermittent fasting has you covered on both sides. This is because intermittent fasting will force you to consume fewer calories while increasing your metabolic rate, helping you to burn those calories faster.

Research has shown that intermittent fasting over a period of three to 24 weeks causes people to lose between three to eight percent of their weight. People also managed to lose between four to seven percent of their waist circumference, meaning that they managed to lose plenty of belly fat. This is a massive benefit as belly fat is considered to be harmful fat in the abdominal cavity that can cause diseases. Studies have also shown that intermittent fasting will not cause you to lose as much muscle mass as a continuous caloric restriction.

Fitness

There are plenty of people who avoid intermittent fasting as they feel it will cause their fitness levels to deteriorate. This isn't necessarily the case for those people who do take part in intermittent fasting, as studies have shown that fasting does not negatively impact those who perform regular physical activities, especially if you cut down on your carbs as you fast and are in a ketosis state. Studies have shown that physical training while fasting can lead to higher metabolic adaptations.

Higher metabolic adaptations mean that your performance can increase in the long run. Taking part in physical training while fasting can also improve your body's response to post-workout meals. Consuming your pre-workout meal during your feasting periods will cause your body to absorb the nutrients even faster. This can lead to improved results. If you consume the proper nutrients, train the right way, and stick to regular fasts, then it is still possible to expect good muscle gains.

Reduces Inflammation

Excessive inflammation in our bodies can lead to many other chronic diseases such as dementia, Alzheimer's disease, diabetes, and more. Inflammation takes place in our bodies when white blood cells, and all of the other substances that they produce, begin to protect us from harmful bacteria and viruses. This sort of inflammation is necessary to dismiss any harmful bacteria. However, diseases, such as arthritis, trigger the very same inflammatory response even when there is no threat. These autoimmune diseases force the body's immune system to cause damage to its tissues as if it were trying to protect the body from a virus.

Intermittent fasting promotes autophagy, a process in which the body destroys its old or damaged cells. Killing off old cells may sound like a terrible notion. However, it can be seen as a way of removing old and unwanted dirt from your body. It's a simple method for the body to clean and repair itself. Old and damaged cells can create inflammation. Because intermittent fasting stimulates autophagy, then it is possible to reduce inflammation in your body while fasting.

When a person is fasting, their body ends up using all of its blood sugar stores because there is not food entering the body. Their body will then have to turn to fat for fuel. When this happens, the fat stores in the body get broken down further into ketones. Some ketones, such as hydroxybutyrate, block part of the immune system that is responsible for the regulation of inflammatory disorders such as arthritis and Alzheimer's.

When a person's body becomes insulin resistant, insulin and glucose build up in the blood, which then goes on to create inflammation. Fasting is known to assist in resolving insulin resistance. When a person is taking part in intermittent fasting, they are allowing their body to have a break from digesting foods. Because there is no food being consumed, the body will end up using all of its sugar stores, causing insulin levels to drop. Such a process can allow the body to re-sensitize itself again to insulin.

Burns Fat for Fuel

Studies have shown that fat is a cleaner and better source of energy than carbohydrates. Fat is known to produce more energy per gram than carbs do. This is probably why people on low-carb diets can control their hunger. Fats are also known to produce less free radicals during the energy-burning process. These free radicals are one of the causes of inflammation.

Free radicals are a form of waste that gets produced when your mitochondria (the body's battery cells) use carbs or fats to burn energy. Free radicals are also known to cause oxidative stress in the body. They are thought to be a cause of many other chronic diseases such as neurodegenerative diseases. Intermittent fasting also allows your brain to use ketones which are derived from fat, rather than sugar. Ketones are known to be a cleaner and more efficient fuel for your brain.

Brain-Cell Creation

Dr. Mark Mattson has found in his studies that fasting can increase the rates of neurogenesis in the brain. Neurogenesis is the development and growth of new brain cells and nerve tissues. This means that fasting can indeed assist you in creating more brain cells which will, therefore, improve your brain power. People who have higher rates of neurogenesis are known to have increased brain performance, focus, mood, and memory. Some studies show that intermittent fasting stimulated the production of new brain cells.

Increased Energy Levels

Fasting boosts neurogenesis as well as mitochondrial biogenesis. As mentioned earlier, neurogenesis is associated with the growth and development of new brain cells and nerve tissues. Mitochondrial biogenesis has to do with the creation of new mitochondria, which are known as the body's batteries for its cells. Each cell in your body has hundreds of mitochondria that power the cells to do their job.

Mitochondria in the brain are known to assist your brain in having more brain power. Fasting promotes brain power, which means that people who fast won't feel lazy and tired in the long run. Instead, they will be energetic and focused.

Mental State

Our brains are massive consumers of energy. Fats that are processed into ketones are considered to be the best energy-efficient fuel to run your brain and your body effectively. This means that your brain can continuously run on fuel that is derived from the fat that is stored in your body. It is even possible to use the fat that you consume as fuel. Using a preferred and effective energy source to power your brain can leave you feeling more focused and energetic.

When some people are under stress, they tend to turn to carbs as a way of seeking some form of release. Eating sweet or starchy food that contains carbs will allow the brain to make new serotonin. Serotonin makes us feel calmer, which in turn makes us feel as if we can cope. When fasting, your body will rely mostly on your fat stores for energy, meaning that you won't feel the need to snack on carbs to cope with mental fatigue or stress.

Muscle During Intermittent Fasting

There have been recent studies focused on the effects of intermittent fasting on males. One particular study was centered around the impact that 16-hour intermittent fasting had on men who were lifting weights in the gym. The study found that their muscle mass remained very much the same while their fat mass decreased significantly. The best results were achieved within the group that fasted for 16 hours as opposed to the group that fasted for just 12 hours.

People who are physically active and spend plenty of time in the gym are reluctant to take on intermittent fasting, as they feel that going on for long periods of time without food will, in fact, cause them to lose muscle mass. This is apparently not true, as per various recent studies. One particular study surprisingly showed that, when combining resistance training with 20 hours of fasting, the results were an actual increase in muscle mass, strength, and even endurance.

The subjects in that study only consumed about 650 calories per day. Some studies have also shown that untrained and overweight individuals benefit from intermittent fasting when comparing their muscle and weight-loss statistics to other individuals who just cut down their caloric intake. Undergoing extended periods of fasting has been proven to be more reliable than eating anytime while restricting calories.

The Benefits of Ketosis

Diets such as the keto diet were developed in the past as a way to treat people with neurological diseases such as epilepsy. Such a diet was meant for people who had difficulties controlling their epilepsy. The purpose of this was to promote the state of ketosis within those people who had epilepsy. Studies have shown that ketones aid in reducing the frequency of a person's epileptic seizures.

Similar studies have also shown that more than half of the people who are suffering from epilepsy managed to lessen the frequency of seizures by around half while on a diet that promotes ketosis. These exceptional results continued even after the subjects were taken off their diet.

There have been more studies that highlight the benefits associated with ketosis. Ketosis works well with controlling symptoms related to heart disease. Some of these symptoms are body fat, cholesterol levels, and blood sugar. At the present moment, people who are currently suffering from cancer and slow tumor growth are being advised to consider the ketogenic diet. The diet itself is not a means of curing the disease, but it serves as a means of making use of the advantages that are associated with ketosis.

Those who have studied ketosis have so far given a positive response to the advantages that are associated with it. Not only has there been a positive response concerning neurological studies, but there have been studies on the effects of ketosis on other health conditions, most of which have seen some positive results as well. Various researchers and medical practitioners are currently researching ketosis and its effects on the following medical conditions:

- Heart disease
- Parkinson's disease
- Epilepsy
- Polycystic ovary syndrome
- Acne
- Brain injuries
- Alzheimer's disease

This type of research has raised questions regarding intermittent fasting and ketosis and their application throughout history and various cultures. Many cultures and civilizations used to undergo intermittent fasts when they were ill or injured. People used fasting as a means of treating illness. The science and research was not as advanced as now, but the people back then already knew of the significant benefits of intermittent fasting and ketosis.

Chapter 2: Meet The Family

There are a few different approaches that one can take when practicing intermittent fasting. Taking on intermittent fasting does not mean that you are fully restricted to just a single method of fasting. In fact, you can select a method that best suits you and your lifestyle. All of the different intermittent-fasting methods are regarded as being useful by those people who have implemented them into their lives.

It is advised that you test out as many different methods as you can when you begin your intermittent-fasting journey. Some methods may not seem enticing to you on paper, but when put into practice, they may be the most suitable method. Not everyone experiences intermittent fasting the same way. This is due to certain lifestyle choices. Physically active people may not adapt to a specific fasting method in the exact same way that other non-active people do.

When it comes down to food, anything goes during your eating window. Most methods of intermittent fasting are more focused on the timing of your meals instead of the actual meals themselves. However, it is advisable to eat normally during your eating window. If you overdo it during these times, then you will have simply made up for the time that you did not eat. This will render the fast useless, especially if you really went all out and consumed more food than you would typically have consumed without fasting.

Intermittent fasting is not considered to be a dry fast. This means that you are allowed to drink water or coffee while you are fasting. During a dry fast, you are strictly prohibited from eating or drinking anything, including water. This isn't the case with intermittent fasting. There are people that actually drink low-calorie supplements while they are fasting.

If you do plan to take your diet and intermittent fasting seriously, then it is also advisable to stick to a low-carb diet. This way, you will not allow carbs to re-enter your body during times when you are feasting. That way your body will continue to remain in a state of ketosis, even while you are eating. Diets such as the ketogenic diet promote ketosis. This is because these diets are high fat, low carb-diets that focus on maintaining a fat-burning state within your body.

The 16/8 Method

This method will require you to fast every day, for around 16 hours. If you manage to accomplish this, then you will have restricted yourself to eating for only eight hours in the day. You will still be able to fit in about two to three meals within this eight-hour window. The easiest way to accomplish this method is to skip breakfast while refraining from eating anything after dinner.

No breakfast and no food after dinner roughly translates to having your first meal of the day at noon, with your last meal of the day at 8 p.m., just after supper. If you prefer to have your supper earlier, at around 6 p.m., then you can treat that supper as your last meal of the day. You can then have an early night and begin your day with your first meal at 10 a.m. It's best to adjust your eating times according to your lifestyle.

It's best to schedule your fasting times around the time you sleep. You naturally do not consume food while you are asleep. So the time that you sleep can be considered as part of your fasting time. If your sleep goal is eight hours per day, then perhaps schedule your fast to begin four hours before you sleep and to end four hours after you have woken up.

The 16/8 Method was initially made famous by fitness expert Martin Berkhan. The term that is currently associated with this fasting method is the Leangains protocol. This is the name that people from the world of fitness and nutrition use when discussing the 16/8 method of intermittent fasting. An example of an eating plan for this fast is as follows:

- 12 p.m. – Breakfast

- 4 p.m. – Second Meal

- 8 p.m. – Last Meal

Those who workout professionally or casually with weights can adjust meals according to their preference, as long as they are eating only within the available window. If you workout at around noon, then you can just have a pre-workout meal before you workout. Your biggest meal of the day can be after your workout, around 1 p.m.

Try not to feel discouraged about losing muscle mass when you do go for more extended periods without food. As mentioned before, studies have shown that intermittent fasting does not contribute to the loss of muscle mass. If you are someone who goes to bed early, then adjust the times of your eating window from 10 a.m. to 6 p.m. Once you have become comfortable with this eating plan, you can then adjust it further to shorten your eating window from eight hours to, say, seven hours.

The opposite applies in the case when you feel that eight hours may seem too much for you to adapt to right away. You can bump your eating window to nine hours. The purpose of doing this shouldn't be to consume more food, but rather because you wish to adapt your new intermittent- fasting method to your lifestyle gradually. An example would be those who are only allowed to eat at 10 a.m. at their workplace, and just get to have supper at 7 p.m.

If your lifestyle only permits you to eat at the above-mentioned times, leaving your eating window at nine hours, you can adjust to having your first meal at 1 p.m., but this may leave you feeling way too hungry in the morning. This can be discouraging for you, especially if you are busy at work with an empty stomach. It is okay to start off the 16/8 method of intermittent fasting with a nine-hour eating window. As the weeks go by, you may begin to enjoy the fast to a point where you will start trying to adjust your lifestyle and eating pattern to an eating window that's around eight hours or less.

Some people have their first meal early in the morning, at 6 a.m., which is around the time they wake up. These people stop all forms of eating at around 2 p.m. This fits in well with the 16/8 method of intermittent fasting as they are fasting for the full 16 hours, from 2 p.m. in the afternoon till 6 a.m. the next day. There is absolutely nothing wrong with this method of fasting. However, it can be challenging to keep up with social commitments that require you to have dinner with friends or family. Cutting off eating at 2 p.m. means no afternoon snacks or dinner.

Most people still feel more comfortable with merely avoiding to eat in the mornings. Not only is it more convenient, but it allows you the opportunity to have a good meal in the evening with your family. Also, eating in the afternoon and evening is a great way to relax from a hard day of work. Using up your eight-hour eating window in the morning means that you will not be able to eat in the evening and may possibly miss out on lunch as well. Not being able to enjoy supper and lunch with friends and family may discourage you from fasting.

The recommended fasting window for women is around 14 to 15 hours. This is about the estimated time that woman should fast to achieve the best results. When it comes to achieving the best results from the 16/8 fast, everyone should try and stick to a healthy diet and not overdo it when eating during the eight-hour eating window. Consuming large amounts of carbs or junk food during your eating window can make it difficult for you to fast the next day. Large amounts of carbs can leave you feeling hungry during periods when you are not eating.

It's best to practice a low-carb diet that can assist you in remaining full and satisfied during and after your eating window. Taking in too many carbs can also deprive your body of staying in a fat- burning ketosis state. The 16/8 method of fasting is also one of the most popular methods of intermittent fasts because it is the most natural kind of fasting method out there. Because the 16/8 intermittent-fasting method feels so natural, it has become one of the most straightforward and natural methods to adopt as it requires you to practice the fast daily, making it easier to adopt the new eating habit. It is perfect for beginners who wish to start their journey into intermittent fasting.

The 5:2 Diet

The 5:2 intermittent fast requires you to eat normally for five days of the week and to regulate your caloric intake for two days. The estimated caloric intake for the two days should be around 500 to 600 calories per day. Men on this fast can consume about 600 calories on each of the fasting days and women should stick to 500 calories. Probably the best way to achieve this is to have two light meals of around 250 to 300 calories on the days you choose to fast.

The 5:2 diet has become one of the more popular methods of intermittent fasting of late. This is because the fast allows you some flexibility. You will only be required to dedicate two days a week towards fasting. This makes it easier for people to schedule their lives accordingly. An example would be not to commit to lunch meetings with friends on the days that you are fasting. It is also just two days in the week in which you will have to say no to a person who is offering you something to eat.

Saying no to someone who is offering you food seems like an incredibly trivial problem. However, it can become a nuisance after a while as you have to always explain yourself to people by telling them why you are fasting. There's no issue when it comes to talking about intermittent fasting. But it can be distracting when someone new is trying to understand your eating habits while you are at work. If you chose to fast daily with the 16/8 method, chances are someone at work is going to ask "why you are not eating" in the mornings.

Monday and Thursday are the most common days to take part in the 5:2 intermittent-fasting method. There is no restriction as to when you should fast. However, these days are generally the ideal days for most people to fast. The most important rule regarding the days that you fast is that there must be at least one day in between the two fasting days. So you can select Monday and Wednesday as your two days to fast as long as you keep your caloric restrictions to a minimum on those two days.

As with most fasts, for the fasts to be effective, it is best to maintain moderate consumption of food during the periods when you are not fasting. If your first meal after your fast is a large, carb-heavy and unhealthy meal, then you will be rendering the fast t useless. Don't overcompensate during times when you do eat. Try to eat as you would normally eat when practicing a healthy and balanced diet.

There haven't been too many studies focused on the benefits of the 5:2 method. Yet, people, in general, feel that this method is a much better and natural choice over other kinds of calorie- restriction diets. One of the big reasons for this is that the 5:2 method is easier to implement in any individual's lifestyle. Intermittent fasting, in general, has its benefits even when practiced twice a week.

A 24-Hour Fast – Eat-Stop-Eat

The Eat-Stop-Eat method of intermittent fasting is just a single 24-hour fast that takes place at least once a week, as long as it is in between regular eating days. Going without food for an entire day is in no way an easy feat, but it is achievable. Some people actually practice this fast twice a week. To these people, it is almost like the 5:2 method of intermittent fasting, except for the fact that, instead of restricting calories, they don't eat anything at all.

The Eat-Stop-Eat method of intermittent fasting was made famous by fitness expert Brad Pilon. Taking part in a 24-hour fast usually means fasting from dinner on one day right up to dinner the next day. If you eat your dinner at 7 p.m., then that will be the time you begin your fast. As with the other fasts, no eating is allowed, except for water and coffee, right up until dinner the next evening. So you begin fasting after dinner at 7 p.m. and end your fast with dinner the next day, at 7 p.m.

You can adjust the times according to your lifestyle or schedule. Examples would be to fast from breakfast to breakfast or from lunch to lunch. However, it is important to adhere to a full 24- hour day of fasting. It is absolutely crucial that you make sure you have a normal, healthy supper the evening that you break your fast. It is easy to get tempted into preparing large meals while you are fasting. Your hunger can easily trick you into craving more food than you actually require.

It is important not to overcompensate when eating after you have performed your 24-hour fast. If you do eat much more than you usually would, then the fast will not have been a successful one. Try to stick to regular healthy eating habits and do your best to regulate your appetite. The Eat-Stop-Eat method of intermittent fasting is considered to be a popular method of fasting for many people. However, this method has its flaws.

With the Eat-Stop-Eat method, you are required to go without food for an entire day, which can prove to be difficult for most people. And because this fast only needs to be done once a week, it will take much longer for someone to adapt to this method. If you do wish to start off with this method, due to convenience, and you are having difficulties enduring a full-day fast, then you can begin with 16-hour fasts. Fast from dinner up until lunch the next day, then gradually increase your fasting window until you are ready to go a full day.

Alternate-Day Fasting

The alternate-day fasting method requires you to fast every other day. One day to eat, one day to fast, then the next day is to eat, and so on. The alternate-day fasting method is seen as a more advanced method of intermittent fasting. That is why it certainly isn't recommended for beginners. It's best for beginners to start off their intermittent fasting journey by merely fasting for small periods of time before they feel they are ready to take on more advanced methods such as this one.

During alternate-day fasting, you must fast an entire 24-hour day on the day of your fast. No food permitted, except for water and coffee. The alternate-day method is similar to the Eat-Stop-Eat method, in which you practice a full 24-hour fast. The big difference is that instead of just undergoing a single day of fasting per week, you have three to four full fasting days a week. This method may seem extreme, but it is achievable. There are variations of this method that allow you to consume about 500 calories during the days when you fast.

As with all of the other methods of intermittent fasting, it is imperative that you eat a normal, healthy diet on the days that you are not fasting. Overcompensating during these days will cause your body to make up for the days that it did not consume any food. This will be a massive waste on your part and will not make your fast effective enough to help you lose weight quickly.

The Warrior Diet

The Warrior Diet requires you to fast each and every day. However, you are allowed one large meal at the end of the day. This means no food the entire day, just water and coffee as usual, but a big meal at the end of the day to break your fast. There are other versions of the Warrior Diet that allow room for small portions of raw fruit and vegetables during the day while you are fasting. During the evening, you are allowed a single large meal within a four-hour eating window.

The Warrior Diet was one of the first methods of intermittent fasting to be popularized in recent times. Ori Hofmekler famously used this method of intermittent fasting. The type of food that is recommended for this diet is closely associated with the Paleo Diet. The food consumed is mostly unprocessed, with some fruits allowed.

Spontaneous Meal-Skipping

Spontaneous meal-skipping allows you the opportunity to take part in unplanned or unscheduled fasting periods in your life. The purpose of this is to unofficially fast by skipping meals in the hopes of enjoying some of the benefits associated with intermittent fasting. It is as simple as skipping meals from time to time. Some examples would be to skip breakfast and hold out until lunch, or to have a decent-sized breakfast and then fast until dinner.

If you do decide to skip out on lunch, only to eat dinner later on, then it is important to remember, once again, not to overdo it at dinnertime. Eating more than usual, due to your hunger, will add unnecessary calories to your daily intake. This is not what you want, especially if you have held out on calories during lunchtime.

P.S

If you have found any one thing of value or something which you have benefited from in this book so far, could I please seek your help here to leave a review over in Amazon

It would be super helpful to let more folk know about what was the one thing that you learnt or benefited from

Thank You Very Much !

How to Start Fasting

Apart from the various methods of intermittent fasting available, there are also different types of fasts available. The kind of fast you choose should be based on whatever it is you are trying to achieve as well as how you wish to approach your fast. Here are a few common types of fasts that are practiced today.

Water Fasting

This fast allows you only to consume water while you are fasting. If you take on the 5:2 method of fasting, then you can restrict yourself to just drinking water on the two days of the week when you fast. Some people include coffee as well, which is acceptable. Being able to drink water during the day may not seem like fasting to some people, but having water can help with bad breath and can keep you hydrated.

Juice Fasting

This fast allows you to consume either vegetable or fruit juice. Also known as juice cleansing, it's a diet that requires you to abstain from solid food consumption. Most people use juice fasting as a means of detoxification, which can be seen as an alternative medicine treatment. This method has seen plenty of criticism, as people usually go for days, and sometimes weeks, without food. Some people perform a juice fast as a way to detox for seven days.

This isn't the way to go as it can be potentially dangerous to your health by causing muscle loss, with the possibility of regaining even more fat once the detox has ended. There is also a significant amount of sugar in fruit juices. If you blend fruits yourself, there still will be plenty of sugar in the juice that you blend. If you plan to fast to lose weight, it's best to keep away from juices and stick to a healthy low-carb diet.

Partial Fasting

Partial fasting offers some benefits similar to intermittent fasting. However, the effects of the fast and detox will be slower than normal intermittent fasting. Partial fasting is also known as selective fasting, a cleansing diet, and a modified diet, to name a few. This type of fast is similar to spontaneous fasting in which people set fasting goals that they need to stick to.

Calorie Restriction

Calorie restriction is a common way for people to regulate their eating habits to lose weight. Intermittent fasting can be seen as a form of calorie restriction as your eating window is now much smaller than it used to be, restricting the amount of food that you will consume.

To get started with fasting, it's best that you experiment with the various methods and types of fasting available. The easiest method is the spontaneous meal-skipping method, and one of the most difficult methods is the alternate-day fast. Spontaneous meal-skipping can be a great way for you to get used to skipping meals such as lunch or supper. This way, you will gradually begin to get a sense of what it feels like to fast.

In some cases, while practicing spontaneous meal-skipping correctly and frequently, you may actually begin to reap some of the benefits of intermittent fasting, such as adequate calorie restriction, which in turn assists you in losing weight. Once you begin to start gaining confidence in not eating for long durations of time, you can then take on intermittent fasting for longer durations on a daily basis.

Abstaining from food can be difficult to achieve. The reason for this is that we are so accustomed to eating whenever we want. A person who fasts has a different mindset altogether. There is no temptation for food, just a focus on getting through the fast. The added benefits of intermittent fasting should replace the temptation for food. Instead of thinking about your next meal, think about how your fast is going to benefit you by helping you to lose weight.

Once you are used to fasting and have developed a good fasting mindset, then you can start taking on more advanced intermittent-fasting methods such as the 16/8 method or the 5:2 method. The 16/8 method is easy to implement into anyone's lifestyle. This method requires you to skip one meal only (such as breakfast). In doing so, you will drop your eating window to just eight hours.

The truth behind a smaller eating window is that you have to cut out some food from your daily intake, the most apparent food being junk food. If you are a person who snacks throughout the night, you will automatically have to ditch your midnight snacks to fast effectively. If you plan on keeping your junk food snacks, then they will have to replace real food. The last thing that you want is to be eating only junk food in place of any real food.

If a straight 16-hour daily fast is difficult at first for you, then perhaps try to fast for 12 to 13 hours per day. You could begin your fast at 6 p.m. and end your fast at 6 a.m. You will be asleep for most of the time, which will make your fast much easier to handle. If you are someone that likes to snack after six, you will have to try and cut out the snacks altogether or reserve a portion of your snacks for during the day.

Once you feel you have found a good routine, especially in regards to eating at night, you can then extend your fast a little further by only eating in the morning at 7 a.m., instead of 6 a.m. This will give you an extra hour of fasting. You can then push yourself further, right up to 10 a.m., to enjoy a full 16-hour fast. The 16/8 intermittent fast method is perfect for those who are trying to establish a good routine because this method requires you to fast daily. Implementing a daily fast will help you to develop a good habit towards fasting quickly.

The same cannot be entirely said about the 5:2 fast. It may be a bit more difficult to form a routine around this fast as you are only required to fast twice a week. On the other five days, your daily lifestyle and routine are the same. So, on these days, there's no proper detachment from your old lifestyle, with no sign of your new fasting lifestyle that is only reserved for other days. It's not that the 5:2 method is unachievable; it will just take a bit longer for most people. It's best to work your way to this more advanced method by trying out the 16/8 method, as mentioned above.

The alternate-day fast is meant for the seasoned pros who have gotten the act of intermittent fasting down to a science (just a figure of speech here). This method requires a full-day fast every other day. Yes, it is recommended for pros only, but you can still work your way up to this point and take on this fasting method once you are ready. Many average people take part in consecutive fasts because of their religion or culture. It is possible that you can achieve the alternate-day fasting method.

As with the rest of the methods, take your time and gradually work your way into the alternate- day fasting method. Fast for half days on your fast days, then implement heavy calorie restrictions, of around 500 calories, once you are ready. It is critical always to remember to eat normally and conservatively when you are not fasting and not to overdo it in a way that will overcompensate for the time you spent not eating.

It is also important to remember that you should see a doctor first before getting into fasting if you suffer from any medical condition. If you are a woman and you find yourself undergoing uncomfortable symptoms as a result of fasting, then it is best that you stop fasting and consult your GP. Women are advised to fast for shorter durations at first, for their bodies to appropriately adapt to fasting.

Fasting for General Health

Intermittent fasting, or any form of fasting, has been shown to have a host of different health benefits ranging from better brain function to general weight loss. Studies have found that fasting may assist in improving blood sugar control. This is something that can prove to be useful for those people who are at risk for diabetes. One study, in particular, required ten people with type 2 diabetes to take on short-term intermittent fasting. The fasting managed to decrease the participant's blood sugar levels.

Another study that was based on alternate-day fasting found that this method of fasting was just as effective at limiting calorie intake as it was at reducing insulin resistance. If you manage to decrease the insulin resistance in your body, then you will increase your body's sensitivity to insulin. This will allow your body to transport glucose from your bloodstream to your cells more efficiently.

Fasting has the potential for lowering blood sugar in most people. This can be seen as a great way to keep blood sugar steady, while preventing any spikes in blood sugar levels. It is important to remember that blood sugar level results can differ among individuals, especially between men and women. The results that one person may experience can be entirely different from a woman who might experience adverse effects on her blood sugar levels while fasting.

Intermittent fasting has the potential to enhance heart health. Fasting can have positive effects on a person's blood pressure, cholesterol levels, and triglycerides. One of the easiest and most recommended ways to reduce your risk of heart disease is to change up your current diet and lifestyle for a healthier diet. Research has shown that fasting on a regular basis can be beneficial, especially when it comes to heart health.

Studies have found that fasting can naturally increase human growth hormone (HGH) levels. HGH is a protein type that is related to many aspects regarding your health. Some of the aspects include metabolism, weight loss, growth, and muscle strength. One study, in particular, tested 11 healthy adults who had just fasted for 24 hours. The results showed that these adults were left with significantly increased levels of HGH.

Research (mostly limited to animals) shows that intermittent fasting can assist by boosting brain function (or brain health) and can even go as far as preventing neurodegenerative disorders. One study, in particular, showed that mice who practiced intermittent fasting for 11 months had improved brain structure and brain function. Another study based on animals showed that intermittent fasting can protect brain health. The same study also showed that fasting assists in increasing the generation of nerve cells which are used to help enhance cognitive function.

Others studies that were conducted on animals suggest that intermittent fasting can protect and even improve health conditions such as Alzheimer's disease or Parkinson's. Intermittent fasting is well known for being able to relieve inflammation. Because of this, fasting may also aid in preventing neurodegenerative disorders. Most of the studies that are undertaken towards animals have brought positive results in regards to intermittent fasting. However, there is still a need for studies to accurately analyze the effects that fasting can have on a human's brain.

More animal-based studies have yielded positive results in regards to extended lifespan as a result of fasting. A study has shown that rats that fasted every other day delayed their rate of aging. These rats managed to live 83 percent longer than other rats that did not fast. There have been other similar reports from animal studies that found that fasting can be effective in increasing longevity, as well as survival rates.

Speed Up Metabolism

A recent study found that people who successfully practice the 5:2 method of intermittent fasting manage to lower their risk of heart disease as well as attain a faster metabolism when compared to other groups that used older calorie-counting methods of restricting food consumption. These people didn't change their diets substantially by cutting down on carbs. They simply made sure that they performed their two fasts weekly.

On a weekly basis, after fasting for two days, you will have consumed fewer calories in that week as compared to not having fasted at all. However, this is only accomplished if you perform the fasts correctly and don't overeat on the non-fast days. It is advisable to have around 500 calories on the days that you fast. This should be sufficient to keep you going for the rest of the day.

Fasting for Weight Loss

Intermittent fasting can be seen as an effective way to reduce calories, which in turn can assist you in losing weight. Fasting on a regular basis will ensure that you consume fewer calories overall. If you successfully skip meals while maintaining normal eating patterns while you are not fasting, then your calorie intake should be well regulated. If you overcompensate by overeating during times when you are not fasting, then you may still be consuming the same amount of calories that you would have before fasting.

A 2014 study found that intermittent fasting can, in fact, lead to significant weight loss. The study states that intermittent fasting managed to help people reduce body weight by three to eight percent over a period of three to 24 weeks. A more in-depth look into the weight-loss figures showed that people who performed regular intermittent fasting lost about 0.25 kg/0.55 pounds per week. People who took part in alternate-day fasting actually lost 0.75 kg/1.65 pounds per week. People also managed to lose belly fat. The loss totaled between four to seven percent of a person's waist circumference.

Intermittent fasting methods are natural ways of sticking to healthy diets on a regular basis. People who fast on a daily basis using the 16/8 method of intermittent fasting usually drop their total meals per day from three-plus to just two. This can be one meal in the morning and one in the evening. Some people eat snacks in between, but because the eating window isn't that long, there isn't a reason to snack that hard, especially if you take on a healthy, filling diet. Intermittent fasting is more of a lifestyle choice, which makes it easy for people to stick to a new dieting lifestyle for a longer time.

Fasting for Muscle Gain

Most studies on intermittent fasting have been done in regards to weight loss. If a person takes part in intermittent fasting without exercising, then weight loss will be a combination of both fat mass and lean mass. Lean mass includes everything, including muscle (excluding fat). This sort of lean-mass loss isn't only evident in intermittent fasting, but with other traditional diets as well. However, there have been a few studies that have shown that intermittent fasting does cause small amounts (around one kg/two pounds) of lean mass to be lost through consistently fasting for several months.

To confuse matters even further, other studies related to lean-mass loss have shown no loss when performing intermittent fasting. There are some researchers that believe that intermittent fasting is actually more effective at maintaining lean mass during weight loss when compared to non-fasting, calorie-restriction diets. However, as mentioned earlier, the research in this regard is still in its infancy, and more research is needed to prove this. In general, it is believed that intermittent fasting will not cause you to lose more muscle than any other diet will.

There is next to no research that promotes muscle gain when taking part in intermittent fasting. Probably one of the main reasons for this is that most studies focus more on the weight-loss aspect instead of muscle gain. That being said, there was one study that focused on intermittent fasting and weight training. Eighteen young men, who had never previously taken part in weight training, performed an eight-week weight training program.

The men in the study followed either a normal diet or a time-restricted diet, similar to intermittent fasting. The time-restricted diet required them to consume all their food within a daily four-hour window. At the end of the study, the group that practiced time-restricted eating had managed to maintain their lean body mass while increasing its strength. On the other hand, the group that ate a normal diet managed to gain lean mass (2.3 kg/five pounds) while also increasing its strength.

These results show that time-sensitive restrictive diets, similar to intermittent fasting, aren't necessarily the best in regards to muscle gain. One of the possible reasons for these results is that time-restricted eating means that the men were, in fact, consuming less protein than is needed for muscle gain. Another reason why the men with the restricted eating pattern were not able to gain muscle mass is that you need to consume more calories than you can burn, especially protein, to build muscle mass.

Intermittent fasting makes it difficult for you to consume the required amount of calories needed to build muscle, especially if your feasting window is very short and you consume low- carb meals that fill you up. This means that you will have to make a much larger effort to consume enough protein when you are eating less than usual. All being said, it doesn't necessarily mean that it is impossible to grow muscle mass while fasting. There still has to be a specific study aimed towards proving this first, before we know the actual results of muscle growth.

There has been research centered around weight training and how it can help prevent muscle loss when you are losing weight. There are a few studies that have shown muscle loss prevention in men who took part in intermittent fasting. An eight-week study, geared towards finding out the outcomes of intermittent fasting while weight training three days per week, split 34 men into two groups. The first group consumed calories only within an eight-hour window, while the other group was on a normal diet.

Both groups were allocated the same amount of calories and protein for daily consumption. The only real difference was the men with a shorter eating window. The study found that neither group lost strength or lean mass. The group that was on a time-restricted diet did, however, lose fat (1.6 kg/3.5 pounds). The group on the normal diet did not see any change. This study proves that weight training for three days per week actually helps to maintain muscle during fat loss as a result of intermittent fasting.

Another study was done on people who took part in alternate-day fasting while spending between 25 to 40 minutes on an exercise bike or elliptical trainer at least three times per week. These people maintained lean mass during weight loss. In general, if you wish to maintain muscle mass while fasting regularly, then it is advisable to perform regular exercise.

A popular question in regards to intermittent fasting and exercise is, should you exercise while fasting? Many debates have come as a result of this pressing question. Some people state that it is better to exercise while fasting, as your body isn't being bogged down by any sort of food or drink. Others argue that they need to eat something small, to have some kind of energy before they train.

One study placed 20 women on treadmills over a four-week period. Some of these women were fasting while exercising, while the other women performed non-fasted exercises. The participants in this study exercised for three days per week at one hour per session. The study found that both groups lost the same amount of weight and fat, with neither group having a change in lean mass. According to these results, it doesn't seem to matter if you exercise while you are fasting or not.

Nevertheless, people, in general, feel that training while fasting can impair your exercise performance, especially if you are a professional athlete. This is probably one of the reasons why most of the studies on intermittent fasting and weight training have not required subjects to exercise while they are fasting. If you do wish to train while fasting, you should be fine as long as you break your fast shortly afterward.

Fasting for Women

Intermittent fasting may affect women and men differently. There is evidence out there that states that intermittent fasting may not be as beneficial for some women as it is for men. One study found that blood sugar control worsens in women after three weeks of intermittent fasting. Such results were not the case in men. There has also been some talk centered around women who experience changes to their menstrual cycles once they begin intermittent fasting.

It is said that most of these sorts of shifts occur due to the extreme sensitivity of female bodies to calorie restriction. Fasting for long periods of time brings down a woman's calorie intake which affects their hypothalamus, a part of the brain. Such an event can disrupt the secretion of hormones, such as the gonadotropin-releasing hormone. This hormone also assists in releasing other hormones, such as the luteinizing hormone and the stimulating follicle hormone.

When these hormones are compromised in any such way, it makes it difficult for them to communicate with a woman's ovaries, which then results in irregular periods, poor bone health, infertility, and other related health conditions. At this moment there aren't any human-based studies available to prove that intermittent fasting can, without a doubt, cause adverse effects on women.

There have only been tests performed on lab animals, which have shown that alternate-day fasting for three to six months caused a reduction in ovary size as well as irregular reproductive cycles in female rats. It's best that woman take a more conservative, mild, and modified approach to intermittent fasting. Begin your intermittent fasting journey with shorter fasting windows and gradually extend your fasting times as your body similarly adapts to intermittent fasting.

Intermittent Fasting Benefits for Woman

Heart disease is among the leading causes of death worldwide. Some of the leading factors surrounding the development of heart disease are high blood pressure, cholesterol, and high triglyceride concentrations. One study found that women and men who took part in intermittent fasting managed to lower their blood pressure by six percent after eight weeks. The study also showed that intermittent fasting also reduced LDL cholesterol (by 25 percent) and triglycerides (by 32 percent).

It is important to note that no specific test or evidence fully links intermittent fasting with improved LDL cholesterol and triglyceride levels. There was a study that found no significant improvement in LDL cholesterol and triglycerides in women and men who undertook a 40-day intermittent fast during the month of Ramadan. People in general have reported improved heart health once they have begun fasting. However, there is no official evidence backed research or study out there that signifies the results that intermittent fasting has on a persons heart health. Official high-standard studies, with more capable testing methods, are needed to fully determine the effects of intermittent fasting on heart health.

It is possible that intermittent fasting can also effectively help manage the risk of diabetes. It is similar to how calorie consumption can help reduce some diabetic risk factors. A study that consisted of more than 100 overweight women found that intermittent fasting, over a period of six months, helped the women reduce insulin levels by 29 percent. The women also experienced a 19 percent reduction in insulin resistance, but their blood sugar levels remained the same.

Intermittent fasting may have its benefits, but it may not be as beneficial for women as it is for men. Another study found that blood sugar actually worsened for women after 22 days of intermittent fasting. This was through the alternate-day method of intermittent fasting. Despite this, it is still believed that the reduction in insulin resistance and insulin itself can still reduce the risk of diabetes, especially for individuals with pre-diabetes.

In regards to weight loss, there still aren't any effective weight-loss studies available that are specifically focused on women who perform intermittent fasts. Various studies and reports highlight the weight-loss experienced by adults in general over both short and long periods of time. The average weight loss of overweight adults after a year of intermittent fasting is seven kg (15 lbs). Short-term losses in body weight were around three to eight percent.

Best Methods of Intermittent Fasting for Women

As mentioned earlier, intermittent fasting for women is not a simple transition into a new style of eating. It is advised that women start fasting for smaller periods of time to allow their bodies time to adjust to their new eating habit. Women can also consume small amounts of calories on fast days, if they wish, before taking the leap into a full fast.

The different methods of intermittent fasting were discussed already, but there are a few adjusted methods that apply mainly to women.

Crescendo Method

Fast for 12 to 16 hours on either two or three days in a week. Any day is fine, as long as fasting days are not consecutive. An example would be to fast on Monday, Wednesday, and Friday. The best way to achieve a day's fast is not to eat anything in the evening and to skip your breakfast. If you have a late breakfast at 10 a.m., after your last meal at 6 p.m. the day before, then you can easily achieve 16 hours.

Eat-Stop-Eat – The 24-Hour Protocol

This is a full fast, at least once a week. It is also permissible to fast twice a week, if need be. Some people do push harder by fasting three times a week. This is not advised for women. The maximum number of days per week for women should be two days. It isn't necessary for women to fast the full 24-hour day. Just as with the crescendo method, women can start off with a 14- to 16-hour fast once a week.

However, fasting just once a week, for 14 hours, may be too less for you to adjust accordingly. The break from one fasting session to the next will be an entire week. This is far too long of a break for a person to settle into a decent rhythm. Try to advance to a larger fasting window as quickly as you can, or try out two days a week of fasting.

The 5:2 Diet

This is also called the "Fast Diet," which requires you to fast on two non-consecutive days. An example would be to fast on a Monday and Thursday. The fasts that you perform on these days allow you to consume around 500 calories. This can be one 500-calorie meal during each of your fasting days, or you could opt for two small 250-calorie meals. You are then allowed to eat normally, as you would on the other five non-fasting days.

Alternate-Day Fasting – Modified

Alternate-day fasting requires you to eat on one day, fast the next day, then eat again on the following day, and so on. You are required to fast for an entire day on your alternate-fast days and to eat normally on feast days. This is an excessive and advanced method and isn't usually advised for beginners or women in general. However, you can modify this fast to include about 500 calories on the days that you fast.

500 calories is about 25 percent of your normal daily intake and can either be had in one meal or split into two meals. This means that you will eat normally on one day, then restrict your intake to 500 calories the next day.

The 16/8 Method

The 16/8 method, also known as the Leangains method, consists of daily fasting for about 16 hours. This brings down your eating window to about eight hours. This is known as one of the easiest methods to adjust to as you fast daily, so implementing the fast in your daily life will be easy. Women are advised to begin this method on a shorter fasting window of 14 hours, to adjust to this method correctly.

If you choose to fast moderately by completing modified versions of intermittent fasts, then you should more or less be safe from any uncomfortable physical symptoms. There have been studies that have reported some side effects that groups of women have experienced while practicing intermittent fasting. Some of these side effects include mood swings, headaches, lack of concentration, and hunger on fasting days.

Apart from the studies, there have been complaints from women online who reported that their menstrual cycle stopped while they were on an intermittent fast. If you have moved from a moderate level to a more intense level of intermittent fasting and are beginning to experience uncomfortable symptoms, then you should move back to your moderate routine. Most of the symptoms can be overlooked, but if they get so bad that they actually make it difficult for you to work or carry out daily duties, then start toning it back a bit.

If you are someone who has a medical condition, then it is best to consult with a doctor first, before trying out intermittent fasting. Women who have had a history of eating disorders should consider this as well. Others that should receive a medical consultation before taking on intermittent fasting are:

- Women who are pregnant and breastfeeding

- Women who are trying to conceive

- Women who are underweight

- Women who have nutritional deficiencies

- Women who have diabetes

- Women who have low blood sugar levels

There hasn't been any serious medical condition that has come about as a result of intermittent fasting. Women should be safe, for the most part, when practicing intermittent fasting, especially if done moderately. If you do experience dramatic changes, such as loss of your menstrual cycle, then you should stop as soon as possible.

A Step-By-Step Guide to Intermittent Fasting

Step #1 – Consult a Doctor Before Starting an Intermittent Fast

It's best to seek out proper medical advice from your doctor before embarking on any diet. Intermittent fasting may have many health benefits, but it doesn't mean that you should overlook your own personal doctor's advice. It is possible that a doctor may advise against fasting if you have some form of the pre-existing medical condition.

Intermittent fasting can have a dramatic effect on your metabolism. Intermittent fasting can also affect a woman differently when compared to the effects it has on men. People who already have type 1 diabetes may not be able to handle long hours of fasting as they will have difficulty maintaining healthy insulin levels because they are not consuming food regularly enough to get their insulin going at a balanced rate.

Step #2 – Choose the Intermittent Fasting Method That Best Suits You

It's best to go with an intermittent-fasting method that will be easy to adopt and will suit your lifestyle. The 16/8 method, as well as the 5:2 method, are among the easiest to adopt and are considered beginner fasting methods. If you are looking for a lifestyle change, then the 16/8 is the way to go as it will require you to fast every day. This means that fasting will be a part of your daily life as you will need to implement it into your daily schedule and routines.

If you are not such an intense person but want to get into the world of intermittent fasting, then the 5:2 method is perfect, as it will require you to revisit your new fasting lifestyle for only two days in the week. Keeping up a weekly routine can definitely work, which is why the 5:2 method is an effective way of losing weight. You never know, you may enjoy this method so much that you might even begin to fast more on a regular basis.

The best method for absolute beginners who simply want a taste of intermittent fasting is the spontaneous meal-skipping method. This method gives you the flexibility to fast when you want. We are conditioned to make sure that we eat every single meal that is available to us. The spontaneous meal-skipping method allows us to skip meals from time to time, to get a taste of what fasting is with the hopes of also reaping some of the benefits.

Whatever method you choose, if you are inexperienced in fasting, it is advisable that you begin fasting for shorter periods than the methods require you to. Instead of fasting for 16 hours, try eight hours, and instead of going for a full day, do half-day fasts. Ease your way into fasting first, before you c begin to take on much more intense fasting sessions. Also make sure you drink enough water during your initial fasting sessions so that you remain hydrated throughout your fast.

Step #3 – Fast When You Are Asleep

One of the main reasons why the 16/8 method of intermittent fasting is so effective is that most of the time spent fasting is during the time you are asleep. When you sleep, your body obviously does not consume any food or unwanted calories. It also gives you the opportunity to fast for a short period while you are awake.

There are plenty of people that fast from sunrise to sunset. This means that these people have to wake up extra early to eat, then eat again in the evening. This sort of a routine actually breaks up your fasting times into shorter times, meaning that you are only allowing your body less time to burn fat. Try to fast for periods before and after you sleep. This way you can take advantage of your sleeping time without food.

Step #4 – Keep Track of Your Calories

Most diets require you to keep a close eye on your calorie intake. Intermittent fasting will automatically decrease your calorie intake as long as you usually eat during your eating window. However, it is easy to fall off the wagon when it is time to break your fast, especially if you are taking part in long, extended fasting periods. Counting your calories means that you will be aware of those moments when you unwillingly overeat.

If you are someone who always has, in some way or another, practiced healthy eating after doing some research, then you will already have an idea of the number of calories that are in your meals. If you are new to counting calories, then one of the quickest ways to get into counting calories is by using an app similar to MyFitnessPal or Lifesum. These are great apps that allow you to simply input the food that you are eating into the app.

The app will then calculate the calories for you. Some apps will even break down your daily calorie intake into macronutrients such as fat, protein, and carbs. This is ideal if you want to be on top of the exact nutrients that your body is receiving. However, you must be cautious as your exact calorie readings are usually just an estimate and should be seen as a guide. Calories differ due to the different brands of foods, and it is possible that you or the app could have made a calculation or input error.

Step #5 – Exercise

Exercise is recommended for all types of diets and weight-loss programs. Not only does working out help boost your weight-loss efforts, but it also promotes good health and longevity. This is why it is undoubtedly a great idea to exercise or to continue exercising while you begin your intermittent-fasting journey.

If you are a bit skeptical towards working out while you are fasting, then schedule your gym visits for a time that is within your eating window. An example would be to fast from 6 p.m. till 10 a.m. the next day (16-hour fast). You can then schedule your gym session for either 4 p.m. or 5 p.m., after work. This way you can have a few light snacks in the afternoon, before your gym session.

These snacks can help you to maintain good levels of energy before you get to the gym. Your last meal of the day can be right after you train, which will be ideal. You can also schedule your gym session for midday, when your energy levels are relatively high. Your meal at 10 a.m. should be sufficient to take you through to your workout. You can then snack on something afterward, like a post-workout protein snack.

There may come a time when you will want to workout in the morning while you are fasting. You can certainly do that, as long as it is not a high-intensity workout. A light run or cardio should be okay.

Chapter 3: Essentials of Eating

Scheduling Meals

When you begin your intermittent-fasting journey, you will be able to feel fuller for much longer. This will allow you the opportunity to keep your meals very simple. You can adjust your meals according to the intermittent-fasting method that you may choose. If you are planning on fasting for less than half a day, then you will be able to eat every meal of the day, including some additional snacks. An example would be to have an eating window from 8 a.m. to 6 p.m.

Once you have begun to ease into your fast, which mostly takes place in the evening, you can then slowly begin to extend your fasting hours. This is how most people who start with intermittent fasting begin to progress through to more advanced and longer fasts. Instead of fasting through the night and ending your fast at 8 a.m., try to push a little further, till about 10 a.m. This will give you a full 16-hour fast. Once you have mastered these times, you can then boost the time to 12 p.m.

If you only begin eating at 12 p.m. and stop eating at 6 p.m., then you will have narrowed your eating window to a mere six hours. This means that you will have to miss out on breakfast. If you are not a breakfast person, then this may be great news. However, there are plenty of people that insist that breakfast is their most important and favorite meal of the day. You can still eat the same meal at either 10 a.m. or 12 p.m., but you will have to skip out on lunch because you will already be full from your breakfast.

Not having lunch is not as difficult as you may think, as you will have had a late breakfast. After a few weeks of fasting this way, you will actually be fine with not having lunch because you will be feeling full, and waiting till dinner to eat won't be so bad. You can instead have an early dinner and begin your next fast. This will bring you to just two meals a day, which is perfect for those who wish to take part in intermittent fasting.

There's no problem with having snacks such as nuts and seeds in between your two meals for the day. You can even have another meal, if you like. However, it is best to limit your food and calorie intake during these times. You will naturally feel full during the midpoint of your eating window. As you progress on your intermittent-fasting journey, you will notice, as the weeks pass, that your entire mentality towards eating and food will change. You will begin to find a new love for food and will respect, conserve, and enjoy food in a whole new way.

The 5:2 method of fasting is another popular intermittent-fasting method. This is a suitable method for most people, as you only have to fast twice a week, meaning that there won't be much change to your current eating habits and routine. Just a whole-day sacrifice, twice a week. For the other five days, you will need to eat clean, meaning that you must try not to consume too much junk food on these days. It's best to stick to a healthy low-carb diet on these days.

On the days that you do fast, restrict yourself to 500 calories. If you are just starting this method of intermittent fasting, then it is advisable to consume 700 calories each day, until you are confident that you can go lower. Five-hundred calories is the sweet spot, as you can overcompensate at times because of calculation errors. One meal in the evening is fine, or you can break up the 500 calories into two small meals.

Popular advanced variations of the 5:2 plan don't allow you to eat anything during the two nonconsecutive days of the week. If you choose Monday and Thursday as your two fasting days, then you will be prohibited from eating anything on these two days. No food at all from the time you wake up till you go to bed, then clean eating for the rest of the five days. This may sound excessive, but it is entirely achievable, especially if you keep up with water consumption.

For those who are really into intermittent fasting and have mastered many methods of fasting, there is an advanced every-other-day plan which allows you eat on one day then do a full complete fast the next day, with no food at all, and to eat normally the following day. This is an excessive method of intermittent fasting, as you will have full days without food every alternate day. Those who have undertaken this method of fasting say this method produced excellent results.

When it is time to eat, you should try and stick to healthy fats, clean meat, and vegetables, with some fruit. On your full-fasting days, it's just water. With the option for black tea or coffee. You can also sip on some herbal tea if you like, as long as there is no sugar or milk. As mentioned earlier, mindset plays a huge role when fasting. As you advance into fasting and start getting better at it, fasting an entire day can become second-nature for you.

Use an app such as MyFitnessPal or Lifesum to track your meals. These apps give you proper breakdowns of your meals in regards to calories, fat, carbs, and protein. The Fitbit app also has an excellent food-tracking feature. Once you have come to understand how much calories are in the food that you are eating, you will then be able to simply pick out the right food to eat at the right times.

Intermittent Fasting and the Ketogenic Diet

The state at which your body switches over from its primary energy source in glucose (derived from carbs) to an alternate energy source in ketones (derived from fats) is known as ketosis. Once you have achieved a state of ketosis, your body will then rely on fats for energy. This means that you will turn your body into a fat-burning machine. To achieve this, you will have to cut out the carbs that are usually used to fuel your body.

There are two ways in which you can heavily restrict your carb intake. One way is to fast regularly, and the other way is to take on a low-carb diet such as the ketogenic diet. The ketogenic diet (keto diet) is an extremely low-carb, medium- to low-protein, high-fat diet. Practicing this diet in tandem with intermittent fasting means that you can allow your body's glucose reserve to deplete fully. In doing so, your body will then begin to start converting fat into ketones for energy.

Relying only on intermittent fasting to achieve a fat-burning state of ketosis isn't so simple. Your body needs time to switch over into ketosis, which is usually about two to seven days. Fasting regularly, while consuming plenty of carbs during your eating window, won't allow you to remain in a ketosis state. You will have to adjust your diet accordingly to remove unwanted carbs. The keto diet is the way to go if you wish to achieve this.

What is the Keto Diet?

The keto diet, short for the ketogenic diet, is a low-carb, high-fat diet. The purpose of this diet is to restrict carbs to a bare minimum to promote ketosis, a fat-burning state that uses ketones derived from fat, either from your body's fat stores or from the food you eat. This is why the keto diet consists of up to 75 percent of fat consumption. The calorie breakdown looks something like this:

- 60 - 75% fat

- 15 - 30% protein

- 5 - 10% carbs

The keto diet does allow for protein, but at a controlled and reduced amount. Consuming too much protein can cause the excess protein that you consume to be converted into glucose. This can disturb the process of ketosis. The keto diet relies on the fats that you consume for energy. Your body will process these fats into ketones which can be used to fuel your body and brain. If you carefully follow the keto diet eating plan, then your body will transition over into ketosis, which usually takes about two to seven days.

How Does Ketosis Work?

As mentioned before, the physical state of ketosis usually arises when your body doesn't have any carbs to feed your cells to produce energy. As a solution for this, your body will begin to generate ketones, organic compounds that your body then uses in place of the missing carbs. So instead of your body shutting down due to a low carb/glucose energy source, it will, in a smart way, turn to fat/ketones. When this happens, your body will have to burn fat faster than usual so that it can consistently generate the appropriate amount of ketones.

Ketones can be seen as an alternative fuel for your body, which, on a regular basis, relies only on carbs which are broken down into blood sugar or glucose. When your body is in short supply of glucose, it will then look to an alternate energy source such as ketones. This is the main reason that the keto diet only allows for an extremely low amount of carbs so that you can force your body to begin working towards using its alternate energy source.

Your body and your brain rely on either glucose or ketones as an energy source and not simply carbs or fat itself. Whether it's carbs or fats, your body will break down whatever food you eat into molecules which can then be used as energy. So if you successfully practice the keto diet, you will be able to force your body to switch its fuel supply to run entirely on fat, which is further broken down into molecules known as ketones. The reason the switch over to a ketosis state takes a few days is that your body is busy finishing off its carb/glucose reserve.

When achieving a ketosis state, your body's insulin levels will be low. As a result, it will be easier than ever for your body to access the stored energy (fat stores) to burn them off. Achieving this is perfect for those who are looking to lose weight. Another benefit behind this is having a steady supply of energy, which can also assist you in regulating hunger.

Types of Keto Diets

There are a few different types of keto diets, each designed to suit people from all different kinds of backgrounds with different lifestyles. Because of this, it can be easy for you to transition into the keto diet.

Some versions of the keto diet actually allow you to consume carbs as well. These versions are great, especially if you are an athlete or bodybuilder. These modified and targeted diets are seen as advanced versions of the keto diet and are best suited for those professional athletes that may adopt them.

Standard Ketogenic Diet – SKD

This is the standard version of the keto diet that everyone knows about. This version consists of a very low carb intake, with moderate protein and high fat. Your calorie consumption should look like this: five percent carbs, 20 percent protein, 75 percent fat.

High-Protein Ketogenic Diet

The high-protein ketogenic diet is very similar to the standard ketogenic diet. In this diet, you just adjust your protein intake from 20 percent to 35 percent, while keeping your carb intake to a minimum. Your calorie consumption should look like this: five percent carbs, 35 percent protein, 60 percent fat.

Cyclical Ketogenic Diet – CKD

This diet allows for higher carb refeeds during some periods. Carb refeeds meaning meals that allow for a higher percentage of carbs (about 250 grams of carbs compared to the current diets 50 grams). The keto diet only allows for 5% of carbs. This means that your body will go for a long time without carbs. A short carb refeed can restore some balance to a diet based on prolonged carb restriction. An example of this would be to follow the keto diet correctly for five days of the week while consuming carbs for the remaining two days of the week.

Targeted Ketogenic Diet

This version of the keto diet allows you to consume carbs around the time when you perform your workouts or physical activities.

The most recommended diets from this list are the standard keto diet and the high-protein keto diet. Apart from all of the benefits of these two diets, they are, in fact, the most researched diets on the list, as the rest of the diets are advanced modified variants of the keto diet. There has not been that much research conducted on the cyclical and targeted keto diets.

Research has shown that the keto diet is much more effective in losing weight when compared to other low-fat diets. One of the reasons for this is that the keto diet is a high-fat intake diet. Consuming food that is high in fat will naturally leave you feeling less hungry later on. The same cannot be said for other calorie-restriction diets which, in most cases, leave people hungry as they continuously count calories. On a keto diet, it is still possible to lose weight even without restricting one's calorie intake.

One study, in particular, showed that people on the keto diet were able to lose more than two times the weight of those other people who were on a low-fat diet. The same study showed that the participants' HDL cholesterol and triglyceride levels also improved. The keto diet allows your body to remain in ketosis. This means that your body's increased levels of ketones will assist in lowering your blood sugar levels while improving insulin sensitivity. These beneficial factors of a keto diet are among the reasons behind the diet's ability to help people lose weight efficiently while living a healthy lifestyle.

Exercising While You Are Fasting

Those of us who love spending time in the gym also love spending equal amounts of time in the kitchen. Eating healthy meals all the time is more or less a part of living healthy and keeping healthy. Intermittent fasting isn't necessarily an end to any of these. You can still enjoy great food and exercise on a regular difference. The only major difference is that you will not be able to eat during specified eating windows.

So how does this affect your workout regime? Are you someone who has to have a pre-workout shot before you enter the gym? Do you need a blast of protein right after the gym? Can you still build muscle if you train while you fast?

When you are physically active, your body mainly uses glycogen, which is stored carbohydrates, as fuel for exercise. The only exception to this is when your glycogen reserves have been fully depleted. This is possible if you haven't eaten in a while. So, with the exception of not having any glycogen fuel, your body will seek out alternative energy sources in the form of fat. The *British Journal of Nutrition* posted a study which had men run before eating breakfast. These men managed to burn up 20 percent more fat than men who ate breakfast before they ran.

Your body also has the potential to break down protein when in short supply of glycogen. This means that intermittent fasting will cause you to lose fat as well as muscle when you workout and fast. If you decide to go out on a run while fasting, chances are your body will begin to burn protein. Working out while fasting can also possibly slow down your metabolism, which can have an effect on how you lose weight in the long run. When you workout, your body will require more calories. But if you are fasting, then your body will have to adapt to fewer calories, which means a slower metabolism.

It's important to be careful when looking up advice regarding physical training while fasting. There are mixed feelings towards this exact subject as there has not been any solid proof of the actual muscle gains or losses from working out while fasting. Similar studies were done in which men who trained while fasting didn't lose any muscle mass or lean mass. Instead, they maintained their lean mass and only lost body fat.

However, the problem with most of these studies is that these men usually eat right after working out. There still has to be a study that analyzes men who workout while they fast without them eating anything after the workout. There also has to be a study with the effects of pre-workout and post-workout supplements with men who workout while they are fasting.

Tips on Working Out While Fasting

Working out is definitely recommended for those who practice intermittent fasting as workouts can help boost weight loss. However, it's best to workout within an eating window, just to be safe. Some people may find cardio workouts great during periods while they are fasting. This is okay as long as you try to eat something shortly after you have trained.

So, no need to throw in the towel, keep going with your workouts. Working out regularly is just as important to your health as intermittent fasting is, both physically and mentally. Here are a few tips on planning your workouts in order to get the most out of them while fasting.

Tip #1 Cardio Intensity

It's best to keep your cardio intensity low if you are fasting while you workout. Keep track of your breathing as this can be a good clue on how far your body can go while fasting. It can be easy to get carried away and overdo your cardio effort levels as your body is light from no food, making it easier to accomplish your cardio routines. This is why you should pay attention to your breathing.

You should be okay if you plan on going for a small walk or jog while fasting or even a low-effort elliptical session. Stop exercising if you feel lightheaded or dizzy while you are working out. This could be your body warning you to stop. We like to push past these symptoms in order to gain the next level of fitness. Just don't overdo the intensity or duration of your workout if you feel this way while fasting.

Tip #2 Go High Intensity Once You Have Broken Your Fast

There certainly isn't anything wrong with light exercise while fasting, especially if you keep yourself well hydrated. However, you shouldn't try high-intensity workouts during your fasting window, as mentioned above. You can step things up when you are working out during your eating window. Some intermittent-fasting programs, such as the Leangains program, advise you to schedule meals around your workouts in order to maximize fat loss while still staying fueled up.

The closer you schedule moderate to intense workout sessions to your last meal, the better. This way, you will be able to have some leftover carbs, in the form of glycogen, to help fuel your workout. Consider snacking on some light carbs after an intense workout so that you can feed your glycogen-tapped muscles.

Tip #3 Eat High-Protein Meals

Regardless of whether you are fasting or not, you will need to consume decent amounts of protein if you wish to build muscle. As mentioned earlier, your body can drain its glucose, fat, and even protein reserves when you are fasting and working out. This is why it makes sense to stock up on protein, to compensate for any protein loss from fasting. You can also create some outstanding muscle mass while you are at it.

A pre-workout snack may just be a good idea, especially if you are fasting. Yes, you are not allowed to eat anything while you fast, but you are about to embark on a gym session while on an empty stomach. Check the ingredients of your pre-workout snack or drink before you have it. If it has carbs that are less than 50 calories, then you should be okay to consume such a supplement while you are fasting.

While you fast, it is okay to consume a total of 50 calories. However, this should only really be made up of beverages such as coffee or tea. You can substitute these with small amounts of supplements when you fast. Just don't overdo it and go above the 50-calorie mark. When in your eating window, try to consume between 20 to 30 grams of high-quality protein, especially after training.

If you want to take your workout to the next level, then try and schedule your workouts between the two meals within your eating window while ensuring you consume the right amount of protein in these meals.

Tip #4 Keep on Snacking

If you do schedule your workout during your eating window, then you can even schedule snacks about three to four hours before your workout. Intermittent fasting promotes small snacks between meals. Having a healthy, simple snack that has fast-acting carbs, with blood sugar stabilizing protein, a few hours before you workout can give you a good blast of energy once it is time to workout. No junk food though!

Try to complement your workout by chowing down on a post-workout snack that contains around 20 grams of protein as well as 20 grams of carbs. Such a snack promotes muscle growth and can assist your body in finding its glycogen stores. These simple snacks can help you to remain energized.

Types of Foods for Intermittent Fasting

It is always important to remember that, when changing your diet for a diet that you have never done before, it is best to consult with a GP or health professional first before you make your decision. This doesn't just apply to the type of food that you will eat while fasting, but to any lifestyle diet change. Your body has to adapt to the change in nutrients that it will be receiving and if you have a medical condition, then that adaptation may not be as simple as you may think.

That being said, when it comes to intermittent fasting, the restrictions that you will face are mostly placed on when to eat rather than on what you can eat. Intermittent fasting isn't, in fact, a diet, but more of a lifestyle choice that assists you in cutting down on your calorie intake by decreasing your daily eating window. This means that you can still eat whatever you want during those eating windows. However, the question is, should you eat whatever you want?

Consuming too many varieties of junk food during your eating window will boost your overall calorie intake. Having chocolate and ice cream in the afternoon, after a good period of fasting, does sound tempting, especially after a long hard day of fasting. However, you will be wasting your fasting efforts as the junk food you consume will compensate for the calories that you missed out on. Moreover, when you feel sated from the junk food, that means the opportunity to for the body to replenish its required minerals and vitamins from nutrient-dense natural foods will be gone. It's best to work towards maintaining a well-balanced and healthy diet while fasting.

A proper, healthy diet can help you to maintain energy levels throughout the day and is also key to losing weight. The focus should be on nutrient-dense food such as vegetables, fruits, nuts, beans, seeds, whole grains, beans, dairy, and lean proteins. If you are known for eating an unhealthy diet, then try to switch things up by looking for food that can assist with improved health such as food that is high in fiber, whole foods, and even unprocessed food. These kinds of foods are good for your health and also help you stay full after you eat. Here are a few examples of these healthy types of food.

Fish

Most dietary guidelines recommend that you consume at least eight ounces of fish per week. In doing so, you will be providing yourself with generous amounts of vitamin D as well as healthy fats and protein. Fish can also be considered good for your cognitive function and is labeled as brain food by many people.

Avocados

Avocados are considered to be among the highest calorie fruits. For that reason, avocados may not be a good choice for those trying to watch their weight, but the fruit does have a decent amount of monounsaturated fat. This is part of the reason why avocados are very satiating to eat. Adding half an avocado to your lunch can assist in keeping you feeling full for hours longer than other fruits or vegetables.

Potatoes

Not all white foods are as bad as you think. Just like avocados, potatoes are among the most satiating foods available. There are studies that prove that eating potatoes as part of a healthy diet can, in fact, aid with weight loss. One fact, in particular, is that when potatoes are cooked in healthy ways, they actually won't cause any harm to weight-loss plans. Some examples of healthy methods of cooking potatoes are baking them, boiling, steaming, and roasting. Potatoes are known to be complex carbohydrates and can aid in weight loss.

Eggs

Eggs are considered an excellent source of protein and are easy and quick to cook. One medium- to large-sized egg has about six grams of protein. Consuming protein is a great way to build muscle. One study, in particular, found that men who ate eggs for breakfast over a bagel were less hungry after breakfast. These men also ate less throughout the day. There are more current studies aimed towards the benefits of eating eggs and also toward debunking the idea that eggs are harmful because of cholesterol.

Whole Grains

Eating carbs while on a diet isn't always a bad thing, especially if you consume whole grains that are rich in fiber and protein. Eating just a little will go a long way in keeping you full. One study, in particular, found that eating whole grains instead of refined grains may actually assist in increasing your metabolism. Experiment with different types of whole grains such as bulgur, kamut, and amaranth.

Nuts

Nuts are known to have more calories than most snacks. However, nuts contain healthy fats that are good for your body. Studies show that polyunsaturated fat in walnuts can alter the physiological markers that are related to satiety and hunger. Nuts are also known to carry some key benefits like the ability to reduce metabolic syndrome risk factors such as cholesterol levels and high blood pressure.

Berries

All types of berries are known to contain crucial nutrients. Strawberries are an excellent source of immune-boosting vitamin C. Studies have shown that people who consume food that is rich in flavonoids, such as blueberries, have smaller increases in their BMI over a 14-year period than those who do not eat berries. The bottom line is that berries are good for you for many reasons such as being low in carbs yet high in fiber and antioxidants. Most berries have proven benefits towards heart health as well.

Beans and Legumes

It is known that food such as chickpeas, black beans, peas, and lentils can assist in decreasing body weight without calorie restriction. Beans and legumes may consist of carbs, but they are low-calorie carbs which won't hurt your eating plan. These are the sort of carbs that can assist in supplying you with energy, without all the excess calories.

Cruciferous Vegetables

Food such as broccoli, cauliflower, and Brussels sprouts are filled with fiber. These are also the kinds of foods that can help keep you regular by assisting in preventing constipation. Food with fiber can also make you feel full. This is especially useful if you intend to go without food for a while due to fasting.

Fluids Allowed When Fasting

Most people who take part in intermittent fasting consume water while they fast. Consuming water is prohibited when undergoing certain religious fasts. However, that isn't the case with intermittent fasting as it is advised that you stay hydrated with water while you fast, as long as it is only water that you consume while fasting, and not food. Not consuming water may cause you to become dehydrated which can result in headaches and general fatigue. You don't want to be experiencing this while you have not eaten.

If you are undertaking a 16-hour fast, then not drinking any water will not get you into any trouble as far as dehydration is concerned. The chances of you becoming dehydrated depend on many factors, such as the weather and your behavior, and whether you are active or not. If you have a decent amount of water during the evening before you start fasting, then you should be okay the next day.

Apart from water, the only other beverages that are acceptable are coffee or tea. Drinking these hot beverages is acceptable while fasting as they do not have that many calories in them and will not genuinely affect your weight-loss efforts. Unfortunately, you cannot add any other ingredients to your coffee or tea while you are fasting. This means no cream, sugar, or milk. These items contain added calories that you should stay away from when you are fasting. It is a massive no to other beverages such as soda and juices.

Chapter 4: Getting Around Speed Bumps

The Common Mistakes of Intermittent Fasting and How to Avoid Them

#1: Eating Junk Food

When you initially start fasting, you will most likely find yourself counting down the minutes until you're allowed to eat again. As a result, your mind will cause you to develop cravings for things that you like to eat because they taste good and will satisfy you, i.e., junk foods such as chocolate, potato chips, and fizzy drinks, to name a few. It's natural for your body to crave what it's being denied, but this is where an element of self-control is needed, as well as a basic understanding of the concept of intermittent fasting.

When you fast, your body becomes an efficient, self-cleaning machine. It breaks down not only fats but also its damaged components and converts them to energy. This process cleans and repairs the entire body, promoting it to work as efficiently as possible for optimum health. Hence, what you put into your body is of great importance.

To achieve the best results from intermittent fasting, you have to try and consume foods that are high in nutrients and low in fat and sugar. Nutrient-rich foods will provide your body with the nourishment it needs, especially in the fasted state, and also will keep you fuller for longer. Even though you are eating fewer meals a day, filling up those meals with junk food will only lead you towards more unhealthy food cravings. This is because junk food doesn't provide your body with the nourishment it needs and will cause you to feel hungry again more quickly. This can only lead you to cheat by breaking your fast.

What Steps Can You Take to Avoid Giving in to Junk Food Cravings?

The digital age is a complete blessing in this instance as there are quite a few calorie-counting apps now available to help you track your intake every time you eat a meal. These apps can be most useful by giving you an idea of how many calories you are consuming per meal item, so you will be able to make better choices when deciding what to eat, and how much to eat, i.e., portion size.

Another useful tip is meal prep. Preparing your meals ahead of time can save you the frustration that comes from fasting and being hungry, and thus can save you from giving in to your cravings. By having a meal ready, you don't have to go through that sometimes arduous and time-consuming process of cooking a meal after an extended period of fasting. This frustration can lead you to binge on junk food while you're cooking and this can lead you to go over your maximum calorie intake before you've ever eaten your meal.

Lastly, I would advise you to indulge your body and give in to those cravings, but only after you have eaten a proper, nutrient-rich meal. Your hunger will be sated, and therefore you will be less likely to overindulge.

Even though intermittent fasting works best because you eat less, it doesn't mean that you can eat what you want. Nutrient-rich all the way!

#2: Over-Restricting Calorie-Intake

A big concern when you are trying out the intermittent-fasting method is not eating enough food during the eating window. Sometimes people can go overboard and start over-restricting their calorie intake because they feel this will help them lose weight faster. This is completely untrue. When you don't consume enough calories per day, your body goes into emergency mode. So instead of using your body's fat stores to create energy, it stores the fat for use in the future and proceeds to feed on its own muscle mass. This will, in turn, cause your metabolism to slow down, which is the complete opposite of what you want.

A slower metabolism means you will lose weight at a very slow pace or sometimes not at all, and your fast will be for naught. Frequently, a slower metabolism can cause other adverse or undesirable effects on your body and will not be good for you in the long term. Signs include dry and cracked heels, hair loss, fat storage in places you've never noticed before, and sugar cravings, to name a few.

So the important thing to remember when trying out the intermittent-fasting method is to eat enough food during your eating window. You need to listen to your body and feed your metabolism to lose weight. The trick is to listen to your body and to feed it the right kind of foods that will promote an increased metabolic rate.

How Do I Make Sure I Am Eating Enough?

Once again, you can make use of those calorie-counting apps so that you can determine how much to eat for each meal, and make sure you're meeting your daily quota of calories, and therefore, energy.

Another idea is to consult a dietician. Although this might not be an option for those wishing to save money, it has the added benefit of professional advice based on you and your body specifically. A dietician will be able to tell you what foods will be good for you according to your blood type and body mass index, and will take into consideration any comorbidities you might suffer from.

If you're not one for gadgets and gizmos, scales and measuring cups, and you want to make intermittent fasting work for you in the simplest way possible, all you need are your hands. This guideline works as such:

- The size of your palm determines the size of your protein portion.

- The side of your fist determines your veggie portion.

- The size of your cupped hand determines your carb portion.

- The size of your thumb determines your fat portion.

If you're a man, it is recommended that you use two times the allotted portion size per protein, veggie, carb, and fat. If you're a woman, one portion size for each is recommended. Even though intermittent fasting works best because you eat less, it doesn't mean that you should eat as little as possible. Remember to listen to your body.

#3: Eating Too Much During the Eating Window

A common trap that many people fall into when they start the intermittent-fasting method is that they overeat when they break their fast. They may be eating all the right foods, rich in nutrients, but they are eating way too much. This can occur because we all have some kind of emotional attachment to food; for some of us, it may be a bit more pronounced than others.

We've all heard the adage that some people eat to live, while others live to eat. Some of us use food to deal with our emotions and how fulfilled we feel in our lives. For example, you'll find newly-wedded couples indulging in dinners of pasta and wine more than once a week because they're all happy and in love. And how many of us have taken to polishing off a whole tub of ice-cream after a bad breakup?

So because you're depriving your body of food, the very thing that sustains it, your emotional state can dip very low, and in an effort to uplift your spirits, you can go overboard and binge. The primary focus of the intermittent fast is to listen to your body. Your body is designed to tell you when to stop eating, and it does this by releasing hormones to make you feel full or sated.

How Can I Avoid Overeating?

The aforementioned method of using your hands to gauge appropriate portion sizes for each food type will work really well here. You can once again make use of the calorie-counting apps and dietician visits for professional guidelines.

Another thing you can do is prepare something you really like to eat for each meal, keeping in mind that it is not high in fat or sugar. This is to ensure that not only will you be eating the right kind of foods but that you will also enjoy your meal. Sating both your physical and emotional hunger will leave you feeling more fulfilled and less likely to develop cravings. Win-win!

#4: Not Drinking Enough Water

The intermittent-fasting regimen will cause a decrease in the amount of hydration you would normally get from eating fruits and vegetables. Therefore you should make an extra effort to drink more than the recommended daily eight glasses of water a day. If you don't, your body will go into a dehydrated state, in addition to already being in the fasted state. This can lead to headaches and unclear thinking, muscle cramps, constipation, kidney stones, and even cause an increase in hunger pangs and junk-food cravings. You will be able to survive with no water for 16 hours. However, it is not advised to do this that often. It's best to stay hydrated.

When your body is in the fasted state, it starts to break down damaged components and toxins, and water is essential for these processes to flush them out of your system. It is recommended to drink approximately 11 cups of water for women, and 16 cups of water for men each day. The Centers for Disease Control and Prevention recommend "letting your thirst be your guide" as a way to stay hydrated. Not only will drinking more water keep you hydrated, but it will keep you fuller for longer by helping to stave off those hunger pangs.

How Can I Include More Water Intake Daily?

You can try to drink a full glass of water before and after each time you eat a meal in your eating window. You can also stay hydrated by including more water-based soups or broths in your eating window. These are not only satisfying to the soul but are also good low-calorie options. While you are fasting, you can motivate yourself to drink more and more water when you would normally have a meal. You can use the clock to set targets for water consumption, or in between completing your daily tasks at work or home.

You can also stay hydrated by drinking tea or coffee, but to keep the calories down, these have to be black.

No milk, cream, or sugar! Artificial sweeteners can be used but in moderation. You can also try fruit-infused water to keep things exciting and satisfy your taste buds. Many people opt for strawberries or lemon, but tastes and combinations vary.

#5: Obsessing Over the Clock

In the beginning, the intermittent-fasting method may be harder for some and can lead to obsessing over the clock. The stress of this new change on your body, combined with the inevitable hunger, will leave you counting down the minutes and seconds until you can finally eat again.

How Do I Stop Obsessing?

If you want to stay true to your fast and have it work best for your body, it's important to occupy your mind by engaging fully in your work or daily tasks. You can even use the time to set new goals for yourself to accomplish each day to help divert your attention away from the hunger. You can try to fill up your time by doing things you find enjoyable such as reading or catching up on a TV show.

Any pleasurable activity that will keep you busy is recommended so that you will not be emotionally starved as you are physically starved. This will also associate the fasting with pleasurable activities, which helps with overall motivation. Take all this newfound time to accomplish something you've always wanted to do but have never done, or use the time to do things you usually don't have time for, like walking your dog or starting that organic garden you always wanted. Take the time to feed your soul!

Frequently Asked Questions

Which is the best type of intermittent fasting?

The best type of intermittent fasting that is agreed upon by the majority of the fitness and dietary worlds is the 16/8 Method or the Leangains Protocol.

Why?

- The main reason is that it is a type of fasting that you can implement every day, without any "cheat days," and it therefore has the greatest potential of becoming a permanent lifestyle.

- It allows your body to utilize your fat stores for energy consumption on a daily basis during the fasting hours when food is unavailable. This results in losing weight at a steady daily pace and therefore is a more sustainable form of weight loss.

- It is also easier to maintain because it incorporates your sleeping time into the 16-hour fast. This means that you will not be subjected to hunger pangs while you are asleep. And you can choose your eight-hour eating window to suit yourself. For example, if you are someone who needs to start the day with breakfast, you can set your eating window from 8 a.m. to 6 p.m. Or if you feel you can skip breakfast altogether, you can choose to eat between 11 a.m. and 7 p.m., giving you enough time to prepare dinner after getting home from work.

How can I prepare myself for intermittent fasting?

- Do your research properly. You're already off to a great start by reading this book but you can also find out more from people all over the web, which will give you a wider understanding of the concept as a whole.

- Consult your doctor on whether this option is suitable for you. Fasting and subsequent hunger pangs can cause a lot of stress and therefore may not be the best option for people already suffering from stress and anxiety disorders, especially those suffering from eating disorders. It can also be dangerous in type 1 diabetics, patients suffering from stomach and intestinal problems, and those with clinical myopathy (muscle- wasting disease).

- Pick an eating window that suits you best. As mentioned before, the eating window can be tailored to suit your specific lifestyle so try and choose one that will be easiest to maintain for you personally.

- Get into the habit of consuming more water. As mentioned previously, approximately 11 cups of water a day should suffice if you are a woman; and if you are a man, around 16 cups a day should do it.

- Make a list of things you can do to fill up the time and keep your mind busy while you are fasting. This can be a fun activity which will allow you to set goals you previously wouldn't have thought about.

- Take a picture of yourself before you start fasting so you can determine if this is working for you and to monitor your progress. This can also have the added benefit of keeping you motivated to stay on track.

How and what should I eat during the eating window?

The eating window is not meant for you to cram as much as you can during that time. And while it's important to eat the foods you love, you have to exercise caution and make sure you're not overindulging in things that are deemed unhealthy. Try to eat balanced meals that are rich in nutrients and which have components that you like in particular. Strive to incorporate lean proteins, fruits and vegetables, eggs and dairy, and healthy fats into your diet so that you have a variety of nutrients from different sources and a variety of meal options so things don't get boring.

For example, if your feeding window is from 10 a.m. to 6 p.m., you can use liquids like tea, coffee, or fruit-infused water to keep yourself full until 10 a.m. At that point, you can choose to have a proper breakfast and a lighter meal for lunch, or a small meal to keep you full until lunchtime so that your main meals are lunch and supper. Others choose to have a good meal for supper and resume drinking liquids after the feeding window closes, which in this case is at 6 p.m. You can choose what works for you.

What is a circadian rhythm and how does it relate to intermittent fasting?

A circadian rhythm can be defined as the physical, mental, and behavioral changes that occur in living beings over a daily cycle, i.e., a 24-hour period. They are built-in cycles that respond to an organism's exposure to external sources such as light and temperature. For example, we have a built-in circadian rhythm of sleeping patterns that respond to light in that we sleep at night and are awake during the day.

So, with regards to intermittent fasting, it is a frequently mentioned term because most research supports the use of our body's circadian rhythms, i.e., sleep-wake cycles when planning your fasting schedule. There also exists a circadian rhythm to hunger which can be tracked by the hunger hormone ghrelin. Research has shown that ghrelin is lowest in the mornings when you wake. So, contrary to popular belief, we are not the hungriest in the mornings and therefore do not need to start the day with a large breakfast. Ghrelin levels typically peak at around 1 to 2 p.m. and begin to dip again afterward towards the evening. This suggests that the day-and-night cycle also affects hunger, in that we are hungrier during daylight hours.

So by choosing to schedule your eating window with your body's circadian day-and-night cycle-related rhythms, the 10 a.m. to 6 p.m. feeding period can work best here where you focus on the main meal at around lunchtime and a smaller meal at dinnertime. The key to intermittent fasting has always been about listening to your body, and in this way, you are listening and responding to your ghrelin (hunger hormone) levels and are thus feeding your body accordingly.

Will intermittent fasting cause me to lose muscle mass?

In the fitness community, it's a common belief that intermittent fasting leads to muscle loss. When you lose weight by any method, it's important to remember that you lose both lean mass and fat mass. This is true for intermittent fasting as well as other diets. Studies have shown that you don't lose any more muscle mass when intermittent fasting as compared to being on any other weight-loss diets.

Is it true, however, that intermittent fasting may not be the best way to gain muscle mass if that is your primary goal. Because of the smaller amount of calories consumed with the intermittent- fasting regime, your body won't be getting enough calories, and in particular, protein to help you build muscle.

Can I workout when I am intermittent fasting?

Yes, you can do this. If you want to maintain your muscle mass as you lose weight, studies prove that weight-training is recommended to help you do this.

Should I workout when I am intermittent fasting?

Within the intermittent-fasting community, there is great debate about whether you should exercise when you are intermittent fasting if weight loss is your primary goal. Studies conducted to determine if weight loss is greater when exercising when fasting, as opposed to when not fasting, show that weight loss results are ultimately the same.

So it all boils down to what you prefer. Many people choose to workout because they enjoy it and because they want to maintain their body's muscle mass, as mentioned above. Others opt to not exercise in the fasted state because it can sometimes decrease levels of endurance and performance.

How can I include my working-out time when intermittent fasting?

The best way you can achieve this is actually to plan your meals around your workouts. So if you have chosen the 16/8 method, as recommended above, you should plan to exercise in the morning, before your eating window commences.

Cardio is best done on an empty stomach, so morning runs or spin classes are a great option. However, if you know that you will be working out the next day, it's advisable to make sure you have enough available energy to do so. You can do this by eating enough complex carbs for your last meal the day before. It's essential to plan ahead, to make sure that your body has enough nutrients and energy for the demands of the intensity of the workout.

With this in mind, it's also important to not pick a high-intensity workout for the morning because this is at the end of your fasting period, where energy stores are at a low. So if you are working out intensely, without the energy reserve to back it up, you may feel lightheaded and could actually pass out.

Cardio is not the greatest option when you have just eaten a meal because your muscles will demand most of your blood flow; blood flow that is needed for digesting and absorbing what you ate. As a result, you can end up feeling very bloated or nauseous, and may become sick.

So the key is to plan ahead: try to incorporate more complex carbs into your eating window when you know will be working out. For those days that you choose to take a rest, you can opt to fill your meals with more proteins, fats, and fruits and vegetables.

Is it safe to intermittent fast if I am pregnant?

There hasn't been enough research to determine if intermittent fasting is harmful when pregnant because it's unethical to put pregnant women on a diet (of any kind) for research purposes.

When you are pregnant, you certainly are eating for two, so naturally, your body's demand for nutritional value will be much greater. And it's important to meet those demands to ensure the healthy development of your baby. As a result, intermittent fasting should be avoided when pregnant.

Why do I get headaches when I intermittent fast?

When you first start intermittent fasting, your body can have some trouble adapting to this new schedule and lower calorie intake and therefore, many in the initial stages complain about headaches.

When you fast, your blood sugar levels take a dive and the first organ to feel this is the brain. The added elements of dehydration and increased stress hormones when you fast can also contribute to this. So try to drink as much water as you can by sticking to the aforementioned guideline of 11 cups for women and 16 cups for men per day. You can also try to incorporate liquids into your meal options like soups, and broths, to keep hydrated for longer. After a few days, the headaches will disappear.

I was told that intermittent fasting improves brain function, so why do I feel mentally sluggish?

In the initial stages of intermittent fasting, the brain has to adjust to all the changes mentioned above and therefore you may feel as though you are more sluggish in your thought processes. This will pass as the days go by and you will experience an increase in our brain function.

Is intermittent fasting a long-term solution for weight loss?

Yes, because it's not a diet in the typical sense of the word, but rather a lifestyle choice. And it has the whole host of added benefits mentioned previously that will make your lifestyle choice a healthier and more fulfilling one, leading you to feel better about yourself in all respects. Even if you do have a very unhealthy diet, intermittent fasting will still be able to automatically cut down on your overall calorie intake. However, this will only work if you don't overcompensate by eating larger meals when breaking your fast.

If you want to speed up the fat-burning and weight-loss process, then it is recommended that you eat a healthy low-carb diet in conjunction with fasting. This way, your body will remain in a fat-burning state for longer. Loading your body with carbs during your eating window will take your body a few steps backwards after you have endured a day fast.

Why should I intermittent fast if I don't need to lose weight?

Many choose to go the intermittent-fasting route as a lifestyle choice because of its added benefits. There are plenty of people who are reasonably slim and fit, yet they still choose to fast because they want to experience the healthy lifestyle choice that is associated with intermittent fasting. Here are some of the reasons why you should fast, regardless of you wanting to lose weight or not.

- Not only does it just improve brain function and mental sharpness but it also helps to prevent neurodegenerative diseases such as Alzheimer's and Parkinson's disease.

- It can naturally lower "bad" LDL cholesterol.

- It enables you to control your blood sugar levels better and can thus reduce the risk of you developing diabetes. It also helps diabetic patients by naturally decreasing insulin resistance.

- It can improve your body's ability to metabolize toxins.

- It reduces the body's oxidative stress levels. Oxidative stress is widely thought to increase the risk of heart disease and cancer, as well as diabetes.

- It can also reduce inflammation in the body, which is a key element in the development of many diseases.

- It has great potential to reduce the risk of chronic diseases and thus the potential to increase your overall lifespan.

- It automatically reduces your food and calorie intake, meaning less meals to prepare. If you begin preparing less food on a daily basis, you will begin to benefit from all that time saved from having to cook the meals that you will be skipping. You will also manage to save money this way. Every meal that you skip on a daily basis will add up as a monetary saving. Just imagine the cash you can potentially save over weeks and months.

- Studies have shown that fasting increases a person's brain function, which in turn increases their awareness and alertness. Fasting on a daily basis can certainly help you to be more energetic and sharper at work.

Chapter 5: Intermittent Fasting Hacks and Tips

If you have taken part in regular intermittent fasts, then you may have hopefully noticed some form of weight loss as a result of the fast. This is actually quite a delicate phase of your new intermittent-fasting lifestyle because you can either get too excited by your weight loss and fall back into unhealthy eating, or you can get a good taste for your new weight-loss venture and look forward to taking things to the next level.

The results that you may have achieved thus far may seem great, but it is possible to still build upon those results without even spending that much more time in the gym or kitchen. You already have that intermittent-fasting mentality. Now it's time to improve upon that with some extra intermittent-fasting hacks and tips that will help you to take your new weight-loss regime to the next level.

Tip #1 Break Your Fast the Right Way

When you break your fast at the beginning of your eating window, you should stick to foods that will not cause your blood sugar to spike. The same goes for your insulin levels, which aren't something that remain consistent when you eat food. Intermittent fasting has been proven to assist in lowering insulin levels. Seeing that insulin is considered a fat-storage hormone, your body will, in fact, stop burning fat when your insulin levels become elevated.

It can become impossible to burn fat if there are large amounts of insulin present in your body. One of the main reasons for fasting is that it can help to burn fat because, as mentioned, fasting reduces insulin levels. However, if you complete a near-perfect fast that helped you achieve great insulin levels, only to eat the wrong food when breaking your fast, then you will cause your insulin levels and blood sugar to spike. When this happens, your body will actually begin to store fat instead of burning it.

If you want to keep the fat-burning process going, then it's best to stick to wholesome single- ingredient types of food when you break your fast. Most of these foods are positioned away from the other processed foods that you will find in a grocery store. Carbs are among the foods that have the most significant impact on your body's insulin levels. Some dairy products will also have a sizeable impact on your insulin, with protein having a moderate impact. Fat has the smallest effect on your insulin.

You can maintain decent insulin levels when breaking your fast if you do not overindulge in dairy or carbohydrates. A good hack for this is to consume as many vegetables as you can at breakfast so they will fill your stomach up while removing your hunger. After this, you can then move on to your protein and fat sources. If you still do feel hungry, then you can have some dairy or more fat. By doing this, you will be able to limit your insulin spikes during your eating window.

It's easy to get carried away and overdo it when you break your fast as you will have been thinking about eating food for a while. Try your best to limit yourself when you do eventually eat. If you find this difficult to do, then stick to the type of food as listed above.

Tip #2 Fast for Longer Periods

Because your fasting efforts will assist you in lowering your insulin levels, this will cause your body to burn fat for energy, meaning that that longer you fast, the more fat you can consume. When you feel you have mastered short-term intermittent-fasting protocols, you can then work your way up to extended fasting hours which can last you between 24 and 48 hours.

The 16/8 method requires you to fast for 16 hours a day. If you feel that 16 hours has become too easy for you and you are seeking out a real challenge, then ramp things up to 20 hours per day. There are people that swear by a 20-hour daily fast. They manage to accomplish this daily feat by shortening their eating window to just four hours. You can still spread out a couple of small meals in this short timeframe.

Once you have proven yourself with the four-hour eating window, you can then upgrade to OMAD status, which is One Meal A Day or what we mentioned as the Warrior Diet in an earlier section. This means that you will be fasting a full 24 hours, with just a single meal for the entire day. It doesn't end here. If you truly want to become an intermittent-fasting master, then you can push your fasting window up from 36 hours to 48 hours.

As with all of the fasting methods, the 36- to 48-hour fast may seem difficult and downright impossible to take on, but if you work your way to it and are ready for the challenge, then it can actually be easier than it looks. The more you get used to long periods of fasting, the more your fast will, in fact, blunt your hunger in such a way that it will actually feel like an appetite suppressant. Fasting for long periods of time like this will mean that your calorie consumption for the week will go down to a minimum. As mentioned earlier, long fasting hours mean longer fat- burning hours as well.

Tip #3 Fasting Workouts

Fasted workouts have not received much praise due to some findings from studies which claim that working out while you are fasting does not burn more calories than regular training during your eating window or within non-fasting individuals. One of the reasons for this is that most of these results have been flawed due to the fact most of the participants in those studies were given a meal-replacement shake right after their workout, which would have boosted their insulin levels.

There aren't that many studies focused on participants that continue to fast after training. Whatever the case may be, working out during or after your fast will help accelerate your fat burning as long as you keep to a good low-carb diet. Exercise can increase your appetite. Try your best to keep that appetite in check as you fast and train in the gym.

Tip #4 Strength Training

One of the fastest ways to completely deplete your glycogen stores in your body is to challenge your body by lifting heavy weights. Intense workouts with heavy weights will help bring your muscles close to failure. This sounds terrible, but your cells can rebuild to be much stronger afterward. This sort of training, combined with fasting, can assist in using up your current glycogen stores, as fasting is another excellent way of using up these glycogen stores.

By using up your glycogen fat stores, your body will then switch over to fat stores, which will trigger a fat-burning reaction. It's possible that weight training can also help you build more muscle, which will allow you to store more glycogen in your muscle cells instead of fat cells. If you are someone who is physically active, but you don't lift weights, it is advised that you do so. Try to start off small and slowly progress to heavier weights over time.

Tip #5 Avoid Artificial Drinks

Stay clear from energy drinks, soda, diet soda, juices, and other flavored beverages, even the ones that claim to be low in sugar as these drinks still contain plenty of artificial sweeteners that are not good for your health. Some of the negative ingredients in these drinks include Splenda, which can stimulate your appetite. It's best not to have any drinks with sugar, such as fruit juice, especially when you are fasting.

The best and safest plan is to drink plenty of water to keep yourself well hydrated. The great news about intermittent fasting is that it allows you to drink water as you fast, unlike other traditional and religious fasts. Intermittent fasting also allows you to have black coffee and tea, as well as herbal tea as long as there is no sugar or milk. Swap sugary sodas and juices for these alternatives that you can enjoy during and after fasting periods.

Tip #6 Keep Busy During Fasting Hours

This is a tip that is so close to the truth, to be genuinely successful when fasting: you should keep yourself busy during fasting windows. Keeping yourself busy with work or your favorite pastime or activity may keep your mind off food. Anything, for that matter, that can distract you from thinking of food is best. In doing so, you will allow yourself the opportunity to adapt to fasting as well as help yourself develop that intermittent-fasting mentality that can help drive you to fast for more extended periods.

If you choose to start your fast in the evening, then you will spend most of your fasting window, if not a significant portion of it, asleep. This is why plenty of people begin their fasting window in the evening. Having your first meal between 10 a.m. and 12 p.m. may seem like a long stretch, especially if you are idle and have nothing better to do. Try and fill up your morning with some productive work to keep yourself busy before you break your fast. Those last few hours can become a handful while you patiently await your meal.

Tip #7 Sleep and Stress

Sleep is essential whether you take on intermittent fasting or not. It is crucial to our well-being and health as sleep assists us in repairing our bodies as well as helping us to lose weight. Your body will burn plenty of calories while you sleep, which will, in turn, assist in boosting your metabolism. Your body will undergo plenty of changes due to the fat burning that it will undergo from fasting. Rest up to ensure your body remains in good health.

One of the biggest triggers for overeating is stress. Many people stress-eat on a regular basis. And the food that people go for during stressful times is either unhealthy or full of carbs. The carbohydrates themselves won't help relieve the stress, but they help us endure stress because consuming carbs allows the brain to produce new serotonin. Serotonin actually makes us feel calmer; as a result, it makes us believe that we can cope. Avoid the trap and develop a healthy mindset that will allow you to control your stress while you are fasting and feasting.

Tip #8 Intermittent Fasting on a Ketogenic Diet

Most people who take on intermittent fasting usually practice balanced and flexible diets which have room for plenty of kinds of food. However, most diets focus on protein and have considerable amounts of carbs in them. Fasting will help you burn fat, while carbs will slow down this process. This means that you will be in and out of a fat-burning state. The keto diet promotes the fat-burning state of ketosis. Taking on the keto diet while fasting can help ensure that you remain in a constant fat-burning state.

If you want to begin the keto diet, then you will have to make sure that you consume the recommended macronutrients (minimal carbs with maximum fat). This can be seen as an effective way of feeding your body more fat for energy as your body is currently burning out all the fat. The "keto fast" has become a well-known dietary combination practiced by many people who are seeking outstanding results.

Tip #9 Don't Tell Anyone Who is Not Supportive

It's natural to seek out approval and support from your fellow peers. It is probably just as natural for your fellow peers to reject your ideas and your actions. It happens all too often: you start out a new venture in life and can't wait to tell everyone. Then the first person you speak to shoots down your new venture. This unneeded criticism is most likely not true, but you begin to feel discouraged.

Making changes in life is difficult. Starting out a new eating plan, like intermittent fasting, is a whole new lifestyle change that will leave you feeling awesome once you are fully into it. However, the hardest part, as with most things, is getting started. Gathering the willpower needed to start something new isn't easy as there is still so much doubt in your head. Now imagine a stranger, or even worse, a close friend shoots down your idea. It can leave you feeling depressed, which can cause you to abandon your new intermittent-fasting plan.

The thing is, those who do practice intermittent fasting love to share about it. So it can be difficult to contain yourself at times. But it is best to continue your fast on your own, without too many people knowing. At first. You should obviously tell your partner that you are taking part in intermittent fasting. Don't force your partner to join, though. This is your journey to fulfill.

Practice fasting during periods when you don't really have to socialize with people, like late at night and early in the morning. Reserve your eating window for times when you and your friends and family will most likely eat together. An example would be lunch and supper. This way, you won't have to explain intermittent fasting to people at a dinner table. You will risk the entire group going into a debate as to why should you or should not be fasting in the first place.

Try to find a good rhythm with your fasting and try and achieve excellent results first, before you begin to tell people. This way you will feel more comfortable when speaking to people who may wish to shoot down the idea or just debate with you. Who knows, the results that you achieve may be so great that people might start approaching you to ask you what your secret is.

Using Hand-to-Portion Food

Calorie counting has become the standard method of measuring our food consumption while offsetting it with the calories that we burn in a day. People say that the best way to lose weight is to count calories. To most, it's as simple as calories in vs. calories out. If you restrict your calorie intake to less than what you burn, then you will eventually lose weight. If you consume more calories than you can burn, then you will gain weight. However, when it comes to weight loss, it isn't that simple, and the same goes for counting calories.

When it comes to counting calories, you need to figure out how many calories are in the food you eat. This means you have to conduct plenty of research while taking down notes and figures related to the calories that you are eating. You will then have to add your figures up to make up your daily intake. There are quicker methods available, such as food-tracking apps like MyFitnessPal and Lifesum. However, even these apps don't know the exact calories in your food for sure.

The reason that these apps could give out wrong figures is that it is possible that the app and the research behind the figures are miscalculated, or you could have made an error while inputting the figures into the app. Research has shown that calorie databases can be out by 25 percent because of incorrect labeling, food quality, and other lab-related errors. There can even be significant variances among the different brands of foods. It's also easy to forget to write down some small snacks or sweets that you may have consumed on the fly.

There has been some praise recently given to new calorie and food measurement systems that depart from the normal calorie counting. One, in particular, does not consist of using measuring cups or scales, nor does it require smartphone apps or calculators. All you need is your hands. How it works is your palm determines for protein portions; your fist determines your vegetable portions; your cupped hand determines your carb portions; and your thumb determines your fat portions.

To determine your protein intake, you will need to use a palm-sized serving. This can be protein-dense food such as meat, fish, eggs, beans, or dairy. It is recommended that men have two palm-sized portions for each meal. One palm-sized portion of meat is recommended for women for each meal. It's important to remember that a palm-sized portion is the same thickness and diameter as your palm.

When it comes to your vegetable intake, it is recommended that men consume two fist-sized portions of vegetables with each meal. This applies to veggies such as spinach, broccoli, or carrots. For women, one fist-sized portion of veggies is recommended. The portion of vegetables must equal the same thickness and diameter as your fist.

You will use your cupped hands to determine the number of carbs you wish to consume. This is meant for carbohydrate-dense food such as starches, grains, fruits, etc. Two cupped hands are recommended for men while one cupped hand is recommended for women for most meals. With fat intake, its thumb-sized portions of fat-dense food such as butter, oil, nuts, and seeds. Two thumb-sized portions are perfect for men while one thumb-sized portion is right for women.

In general, the bigger you are, the bigger your hand is, the more you will need to consume. So not everyone will consume similar amounts as food. Your hand is your own personal measuring device for the food you wish to consume. Some people may confess to having large hands that are not proportionate to their body size. However, our hand size does somewhat correlate pretty closely with our general body size. This includes our muscle and bones.

Time- and Money-Saving Meal Prep

Making your meals from scratch at home takes up plenty of time and may not be as economical as you initially thought it would be. For this reason, most people would rather just eat out as it is convenient and, in some cases, cheaper. The problem with this is that you can quickly get caught up purchasing the wrong type of food, like high carb, unhealthy junk food. You also run the risk of upsizing your portions and overeating. Try reassessing your home cooking to prepare meals on the cheap quick and easy. Here are some tips below.

Tip #1 Keep Cooked Meat on Hand

Try cooking a whole bunch of meat or chicken in one go and then freezing it for later use. An example would be to prepare all of the chicken you just purchased from the grocery store as soon as you get home. You can then place your cooked chicken into small meal-sized portions (hand-measured, as explained above) into separate bags or freezer boxes. This way, you can merely defrost your meat the next time you wish to eat.

When you are eventually ready to eat, you can just remove a single meal-sized portion of the meat from your freezer, defrost, then heat up. You can cook your sides as you wait for your meat to defrost. This way you do not eat excessively, as you have already determined your portions. You will then only eat the portion that you defrost because you are obviously restricted here due to your earlier portion allocation. This way you will not over eat, or even waste food like before when you were not freezing your cooked meat. You would not waste as well if you did. It is a win-win situation.

Tip #2 One-Pot Meals

There will be times when you are not prepared to take on one of those quick-reheat dishes as you may have just run out of pre-cooked meat. An excellent quick and cheap solution for this scenario is to create a one-pot meals. Get together a whole lot of ingredients, throw them into a pot, and cook. There are plenty of great one-pot recipes out there that can even be made using a crock-pot. Having the ability to just throw everything together into a single dish, and you're done, means that meal prep will be kept as easy as possible and, in most cases, cheap.

Tip #3 Stock Up on the Essentials

It is absolutely crucial that you keep stock of your essential ingredients and food items at all times. If you find yourself missing a few simple ingredients, you may feel discouraged towards preparing your home-cooked meal. This might just be the thing to force you to go and eat take out again. The more you rely on cooking at home, the more you will be able to figure out the exact ingredients you need at all times.

You will even be able to pick up on which ingredients are running low so that you can make a grocery run and stock up. If you want to take things further, you can shop when your essential items are on sale. You can pick up your mayo and mustard in bulk when the prices are at rock bottom. This way you can ensure that you are fully stocked up on your essential items while saving on costs in the long run.

Tip #4 Cook in Double Batches

A great way to stretch your food a bit further is to cook in double batches. This means that instead of cooking just a single meal for yourself, you cook a larger portion that is twice as much. This way you can eat one portion that very evening and have the second portion later in the week. This works great if you cook yourself a lasagna. Baking a lasagna in the oven is no quick and easy feat. You can, however, bake once and eat twice.

This way you will get the most out of one cooking session. You can also freeze the remaining portions for use at a much later stage. This way you can even increase the portion size further and cook more than double. The excess food that you will not be able to be eating that evening can just go straight into the freezer.

Nutrient-Dense Food Swaps

There are many different types of food swap and substitution scenarios that can help you boost health while preventing disease. An example is bacon, which can itself be a meal. Bacon can also be a condiment, side dish, and even a dessert. Here are a few examples of fascinating swaps that you can implement into your daily diet and meal-prep routines.

Cauliflower Rice

Riced vegetables are becoming more popular. Not only do these vegetable-based rices allow us to easily consume the right amount of veggies, but they also serve as a great way to reduce our carb intake. Selecting rice cauliflower instead of rice in your food bowls can save you around 200 calories and carbs. It will also, in turn, increase the nutrient density of your meal.

Bean Chips

Bean-based chips are a new game changer in the munchies department that replaces the old- time favorite potato chips and pretzels. Bean-based chips also give you a significant boost in whole-food ingredients such as whole beans. Black bean chips have five grams of protein with only 85 mg of sodium and only ten digestible carbs. Try to stick to baked versions which go well with guacamole or even hummus.

Bean-Based Pasta

Bean-based pasta options are now becoming more available in the pasta aisles all around the world. In the past, the primary option was the healthy 100 percent whole-wheat version of pasta. Now, the nutritional figures totally favor the bean option.

Not only are they gluten-free, but bean-based pastas also contain about 20 grams more protein and eight grams more fiber. Bean pasta is also bound to fill you up faster than other traditional whole-wheat options. It is also a superb source of plant-based protein.

Ground Turkey or Tofu

Swapping ground beef for ground poultry means less saturated fat. This is good news for those who wish to keep their waistline intact. A recent study conducted in 2017 showed that too many unsaturated fats in a diet can possibly cause fat gain to your gut. Chicken breast and turkey meat are among the choices with the least amount of saturated fat.

Roasted Chickpeas

Eating plenty of salads can be seen as an excellent way to consume some low-calorie nutrients. However, even the best of salads can be flawed because of the inclusion of refined grains such as croutons. Swap out your croutons for delicious roasted chickpeas instead. You can either make them yourself or buy them. Including chickpeas in your salad can add fiber to your meal which can, in turn, assist in increasing your satiety while delivering healthy fats that can help metabolize your fat-soluble vitamins.

Sweet Potato Toast

Sweet potatoes are filled with antioxidants such as vitamin A and C, fiber, and potassium. Having this vegetable instead of bread can help you to reduce the grains in your diet while helping you to lose weight. Try it out for yourself by cutting a raw sweet potato into thin slices. You can do this by keeping the fiber-rich skin on. Toast until brown and then top as you would normally top a piece of toast. Some examples of toppings are avocado, eggs, cheese, etc.

Specific 5:2 Minimal Calorie Day Food Choices

With the 5:2 method of intermittent fasting, you will be required to fast for two nonconsecutive days in a week, while eating normally for the five remaining days. Most people try not to eat anything these days. However, you are allowed to consume around 500 calories each day. Five-hundred calories does not seem like much, and is perhaps less than a single meal for some people, but if planned correctly, you can manage a few small meals into the allotted 500 calories.

An example would be to have a small breakfast under 100 calories, lunch that is under 200 calories, and dinner which is between 200 to 300 calories. An example of a breakfast below 100 calories includes eating raisins, Greek yogurt, and almonds, which totals around 94 calories. Or you can opt for a spinach omelet that comes in at 94 calories as well.

Crushed new potatoes and shoots is a great lunch option that totals 170 calories. Or you could opt for a chicken miso soup which is a mere 12 calories. For dinner, you can have a simple vegetable chow mein (170 calories) or a Moroccan root tagine with couscous (238 calories). Small fruit snacks such as tangerines are great for in-between snacks to keep you going.

Conclusion

Thank you for absorbing the information found here. Hopefully, you were able to find all of the relevant information that you were looking for right here in these pages. This book has covered as much information as possible in regards to intermittent fasting. Information provided included the benefits of intermittent fasting and the science behind intermittent fasting.

The topic of intermittent fasting is very in depth as it covers various methods and ways in which you can begin your fasting journey as well as methods that are best suited for the more advanced. If you haven't started fasting yet, then try and make today your first day. Go ahead and abstain from food now, even if it is for just half a day. Do it regularly, and you will for sure reap the benefits.

Once your mindset has shifted to a more poised and balanced fasting mindset, then you will be able to handle long hours without food like a champ. If you are someone who doesn't care much for eating healthy, you can still fast. Because you have now become aware of your eating habits, you will automatically become aware of your eating. Hence, you might even adjust your food selection so that you can eat healthier.

The first few months might be a little difficult for you if you have never fasted before. Try easing into your fasts, as the book has suggested. Once you have progressed to someone who can fast for most of the day, try your utmost best to keep up with intermittent fasting. You will notice some real changes to your body and to your energy levels if you consistently fast for six months or more. Start fasting now and stick to it if you want to get the most out of intermittent fasting.

Good luck, and all the best on your intermittent-fasting journey.

P.S

If you have found any one thing of value or something which you have benefited from in this book, could I please seek your help once again to leave a review over in Amazon

It would be super helpful to let more folk know about what was the one thing that you learnt or benefited from

Thank You Very Much !

CPSIA information can be obtained
at www.ICGtesting.com
Printed in the USA
LVHW060110201020
669244LV00011B/526